William J. Hozack

Martin Krismer

Michael Nogler

Peter M. Bonutti

Franz Rachbauer

Jonathan L. Schaffer

William J. Donnelly

Minimally Invasive Total Joint Arthroplasty

William J. Hozack (Editor)

Martin Krismer (Editor)

Michael Nogler (Editor)

Peter M. Bonutti (Editor)

Franz Rachbauer (Editor)

Jonathan L. Schaffer (Editor)

William J. Donnelly (Editor)

Minimally Invasive Total Joint Arthroplasty

With 352 Figures and 12 Tables

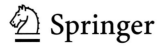 Springer

William J. Hozack, M.D.
Professor of Orthopedic Surgery
Rothman Institute Orthopedics
Jefferson Medical School
925 Chestnut Street
Philadelphia, PA 19107, USA

Martin Krismer, M.D.
Full Professor
Medical University Innsbruck,
Department for Orthopaedics
Anichstrasse 35, A-6020 Innsbruck, Austria

Michael Nogler, M.D., M.A., M.A.S., M.Sc.
Associate Professor
Medical University Innsbruck,
Department for Orthopaedics
Anichstrasse 35, A-6020 Innsbruck, Austria

Peter M. Bonutti, MD, FACS
Bonutti Clinic
1303 West Evergreen Avenue
Effingham, Illinois 62401
Associate Clinical Professor
Department of Orthopaedic Surgery
University of Arkansas

Franz Rachbauer, M.D., M.A.S., M.Sc.,
Associate Professor
Medical University Innsbruck,
Department for Orthopaedics
Anichstrasse 35, A-6020 Innsbruck, Austria

Jonathan L. Schaffer, M.D., MBA
Managing Director, e-Cleveland Clinic
Information Technology Division
The Cleveland Clinic
9500 Euclid Avenue, Desk A-41
Cleveland, Ohio 44195, USA

William J. Donnelly, Dr.
Orthopedic Surgeon
Brisbane Orthopaedic Specialist Services
Level 7, Suite 1, Holy Spirit Hospital
Wickham Terrace, Brisbane, QLD 4000 Australia

ISBN 3-540-21007-5
Springer Medizin Verlag Heidelberg

We thank FAKTUM. Der Mediendienst, Germany for providing us with some of the figures.

Cataloging-in-Publication Data applied for
A catalog record for this book is available from the Library of Congress.

Bibliographic information published by Die Deutsche Bibliothek
Die Deutsche Bibliothek lists this publication in the Deutsche Nationalbibliografie;
detailed bibliographic data is available in the Internet at <http://dnb.ddb.de>.

Springer Medizin Verlag.
A member of Springer Science+Business Media
springer.de

© Springer Medizin Verlag Heidelberg 2004
Printed in Germany

SPIN 10987728
Cover Design: design & production GmbH, 69121 Heidelberg, Germany
Typesetting: TypoStudio Tobias Schaedla, 69120 Heidelberg, Germany

Printed on acid free paper 18/5141 – 5 4 3 2 1 0

Contents

Contents

List of First Authors

Arnold, William
Department of Orthopedic Surgery
Thomas Jefferson University and
Rothman Institute Orthopedics
Philadelphia, PA
USA

Austin, Matthew
Department of Orthopedic Surgery
Thomas Jefferson University and
Rothman Institute Orthopedics
Philadelphia, PA
USA

Baerga-Varela, Luis
Sports, Spine and Orthopedic
Rehabilitation
Kessler Institute for
Rehabilitation
West Orange, New Jersey 07052
USA

Bargar, William
Sutter General Hospital
1020 29th Street Suite 450
Sacramento, CA 95816
USA

Berger, Richard
3660 N Lake Shore Dr #4301
Chicago IL 60613
USA

Bonutti, Peter M.
Bonutti Clinic
1303 West Evergreen Ave.
Effingham, IL 62401
USA

Buehler, Knute C.
Orthopedic and Neurosurgery
Center of the Cascades
2600 Neff Road
Bend, Oregon 97701
USA

Callaghan, John J.
Department of Orthopaedic Surgery
200 Hawkins Drive
Iowa City, IA 52242
USA

Chauhan, S.K.
Department of Orthopaedics
Brighton and Sussex University
Hospitals
Eastern Road, Brighton
BN2 5BE
United Kingdom

Cossey, A.J.
Lower Limb Arthroplasty
Sportsmed SA
32 Payneham Road
Stepney SA 5069, Adelaide
Australia

D'Antonio, James A.
613 Davis Lane
Sewickley, Pa. 15143
USA

Donnelly, Bill
Brisbane Orthopaedic Specialist
Services
Arnold-Janssen Centre
Holy Spirit Hospital
259 Wickham Terrace
Brisbane QLD 4000
Australia

Dorr, Lawrence D.
The Arthritis Institute
501 E. Hardy Street
Inglewood, CA 90301
USA

Dreinhöfer, Karsten E.
Department of Orthopaedic Surgery
Rehabilitationskrankenhaus Ulm
University of Ulm
Germany

Dunbar, Michael J.
Clinical Research Scholar
Dalhousie University
Suite 4822 New Halifax Infirmary
Hospital
QE II Health Sciences Centre
1796 Summer Street
Halifax, Nova Scotia B3H 3A7
Canada

Frueh, Walter
Rothman Institute
925 Chestnut Street
Philadelphia, PA 19107
USA

Heynen, Garry F.
Level 3 Ascot Hospital
90 Greenlane Road East
Remuera, Auckland
New Zealand

Jaramaz, Branislav
Institute for Computer Assisted
Orthopaedic Surgery (ICAOS)
The Western Pennsylvania Hospital
4815 Liberty Avenue
Mellon Pavilion, Suite 242
Pittsburgh, PA 15224
USA

Keggi, Kristaps
Orthopaedic Surgery, pc
1201 West Main Street
Waterbury, CT 06708
USA

Kessler, Oliver
Stryker SA
Scientific & Clinical Affairs
Florastr. 13
8800 Thalwil
Switzerland

Klein, Gregg R.
Department of Orthopedic Surgery
Thomas Jefferson University and
Rothman Institute Orthopedics
Philadelphia, PA
USA

Krebs, Viktor E.
Adult Reconstruction Section
Department of Orthopaedic Surgery
The Cleveland Clinic
9500 Euclid Avenue, Desk A-41
Cleveland, Ohio 44195
USA

Krismer, M.
Department of Orthopaedic Surgery
University of Innsbruck
Anichstraße 35
6020 Innsbruck
Austria

Langlotz, F.
M. E. Müller Research Center for
Orthopaedic Surgery
Institute for Surgical Technology and
Biomechanics
University of Bern
Switzerland

Lieberman, Jay R.
Department of Orthopaedic Surgery
David Geffen School of Medicine at
UCLA
12-138 Center for Health Sciences
Los Angeles, CA 90095
USA

Lucas, D.
Department of Orthopaedics
Brighton and Sussex University
Hospitals
Eastern Road, Brighton
BN2 5BE
United Kingdom

Mahoney, Ormonde
Athens Orthopedic Clinic
125 King Avenue
Athens, Georgia 30606
USA

McAllister, Craig M.
Evergreen Orthopedic Center
12911 120th Ave NE #H210
Kirkland, WA 98034
USA

Moctezuma de la Barrera, José Luis
Vordere Poche 11
79104 Freiburg
Germany

Mont, Michael
Sinai Hospital of Baltimore
2401 West Belvedere Avenue
Baltimore, MD 21215
USA

Murphy, Steve
Center for Computer Assisted and
Reconstructive Surgery
New England Baptist Hospital
125 Parker Hill Avenue
Boston, MA 02120
USA

Nessler, Joseph P.
1131 Mill Creek Circle
Saint Cloud, 56303
Minnesota
USA

Nogler, Michael
Department of Orthopaedic Surgery
University of Innsbruck
Anichstraße 35
6020 Innsbruck
Austria

Rachbauer, Franz
Department of Orthopaedic Surgery
University of Innsbruck
Anichstraße 35
6020 Innsbruck
Austria

Ranawat, C.S.
Dept. of Orthopedic Surgery
Lenox Hill Hospital
130 East 77 Street 11th Fl
New York, NY 10021
USA

Repicci, John A.
Joint Reconstruction Orthopedics
4510 Main St
Buffalo, New York 14226
USA

Rosenberg, Aaron G.
Rush Medical College
1725 W Harrison #1063
Chicago, Illinois 60612
USA

Schaffer, Jonathan L.
e-Cleveland Clinic
Information Technology Division
The Cleveland Clinic
9500 Euclid Avenue, Desk A-41
Cleveland, Ohio 44195
USA

Sledge, John
Sports Medicine North Orthopaedic
Surgery, Inc.
471 Broadway, Route 1 North
Lynnfield, MA 01940
USA

Timperley, A.J.
Princess Elizabeth Orth. Cent.
Barrack Road
Exeter, Devon EX2 5DW
United Kingdom

Tria, Alfred J.
210 Brooks Bend
Princeton, NJ 08540
USA

Turnbull, Allen
11/468 The Kingsway Miranda
2228 Sydney
Australia

Walker, Peter S.
VA Medical Center
Annex Building 2, Room 206A
423 East 23rd Street
New York, NY 10022
USA

Wixson, Richard L.
Northwestern Center for Orthopedics
676 North St. Clair Street, Suite 450
Chicago, IL 60611
USA

Wolf, Alon
Institute for Computer Assisted
Orthopaedic Surgery (ICAOS)
The Western Pennsylvania Hospital
Mellon Pavilion, Suite 242
4815 Liberty Avenue
Pittsburgh, PA 15224
USA

Introduction

Minimally Invasive Total Hip and Knee Replacement

Change is inevitable, but progress does not necessarily follow. We are currently witnessing two dramatic changes within the world of total hip and knee replacement. Minimally invasive surgical techniques have been popularized in the media and on the web and the effect has been to focus an increased interest in the preservation and handling of the soft tissues during hip and knee replacement. Computer-assisted hip and knee replacement surgery has developed to the point where it can be seamlessly integrated into the operating room. Together these two changes – minimally invasive surgery and computer-assisted surgery – create an optimism that an evolution is underway towards a better and more functional total hip and total knee replacement operation. This book was assembled in an attempt to address this optimism.

What is minimally invasive surgery of the hip and knee? As the reader peruses the chapters of this book, he will begin to understand that the concept of minimally invasive surgery is fluid and constantly changing. Most people agree that minimally invasive surgery should lessen the impact of the operation on the patients' quality of life and disruption of daily routine. How each individual surgeon chooses to achieve this goal varies quite considerably. Surgeons focus their efforts in various directions in order to minimize soft tissue and muscle trauma, skin incision length, and capsular disruption while trying to maintain the ultimate goal of a well-aligned, well fixed hip or knee replacement. This book was organized not only to give the reader an overview of current attitudes and approaches to minimally invasive surgery, but also to provide a discussion of the true value of these new approaches.

The first section of this book was designed to answer the question as to whether minimally invasive approaches to hip and knee replacement were needed. The next several sections detail specific minimally invasive approaches to the hip and knee and also present a corporate perspective on minimally invasive surgery. Neither specific surgical technique nor corporate philoso-

phy is highlighted, but rather a compilation of expertise has been assembled for the reader to evaluate. Within the text of this book, many issues will be presented, some of which are incision length, single versus multiple incision, muscle sparing versus muscle splitting, in situ bone cuts versus dislocation of the joint, and intra-medullary versus extra-medullary instrumentation. As long as the judgement of time has not provided a single best solution the issue, there is a place for a variety of techniques, approaches, and opinions. Therefore, the editors invited those experts to contribute whose names are already associated with minimally invasive total joint surgery, and who are well known for their high level of competence in the field. Although the role of navigation in minimally invasive arthroplasty is not well defined, there is a strong belief that the combination of minimally invasive surgery and computer-assisted surgery together may be the future, combining the principles of high precision surgery with the advantages of soft tissue and muscle sparing surgical approaches. The diminished visualization in less invasive surgery may be compensated by the advantages and enhanced visualization provided by navigation. The final sections of the book provide perspectives on whether minimally invasive surgery is a winning concept and whether new instruments and new prosthetic designs are required. The ethics surrounding this phenomenon of minimally invasive surgery, and the issues of marketing and how such a new concept should be introduced to the orthopedic and lay population are discussed. Finally, the issue of teaching minimally invasive and computer-assisted surgery is explored.

The primary purpose of this book was to assemble a comprehensive collection of current knowledge on minimally invasive arthroplasty technique. As are the editors, the authors comprise a global group of experts on minimally invasive and computer-assisted surgery of the hip and knee from North America, Europe and Australasia. Our goal was to include all important trends. We leave the task of formulating the individual approach to each reader. As long as the scientific evidence regarding definitive outcomes is lacking, and as long as some of these techniques are still in the early phases of development, this book will claim only that it is a repository of information on minimally invasive surgery available to assist reconstructive surgeons in their decision-making for individual patients. This book has been assembled under a very tight time schedule in an attempt to present opinions, techniques, and results that are as current and up to date as possible. For this the editors are grateful to the authors who accepted this additional workload and completed this work in a timely fashion.

Total hip and total knee arthroplasty will continue to evolve in directions previously thought not possible. The integration of computers into the operating room, the use of minimally invasive techniques, specific instruments and future developments in implant design will all change as part of this natural evolutionary process. It is important in this time of significant change that we maintain sight of the ultimate goal – that of safely improving patient's quality of life with a procedure that already has well published excellent results. The potential advances offered by minimally invasive surgery must be evaluated in a responsible manner, with appropriately designed and performed studies and peer reviewed publications as the foundation stones upon which are built the next generation of total hip and knee replacements.

March, 2004

W. J. Hozack, M. Krismer,
M. Nogler, P. M. Bonutti,
F. Rachbauer, J. L. Schaffer,
W. J. Donnelly

Part I   Is There a Need for Minimally Invasive Approaches in Total Joint Arthroplasty?

Rehabilitation after Minimally Invasive Surgery

L. Baerga-Varela, G.A. Malanga

Introduction

Total joint replacement surgery has given many patients relief from joint pain as well as great improvement in their level of function. It has become one of the most successful and frequently performed orthopedic surgeries. Over the past few decades, it has evolved greatly due to improvements in materials, prosthetic joint designs and surgical techniques. A recent trend towards minimally invasive arthroscopic, laparoscopic and angioplastic surgeries has triggered an interest in the development of minimally invasive total joint replacement surgical techniques. These surgical techniques are designed to allow a total joint replacement of the hip or knee through a smaller incision with potentially less tissue damage. Proponents of minimally invasive surgery believe that these new techniques hold the promise of decreased tissue damage, blood loss and post-operative pain, as well as faster post-operative recovery, shortened length of stay and improved cosmetic results due to a smaller scar. Skeptics of these new techniques worry about the addition of new risks to an already very successful surgery, poor visualization during the procedure, increased difficulty of the technique and a possible increase in operative time [1]. This chapter will discuss the effects minimally invasive total joint replacement surgery may have in the rehabilitation process and outcomes of patients undergoing total joint replacement surgery.

Developments in Total Joint Replacement

At the beginning of the 19th century, several surgical treatments of the painful hip were attempted, such as osteotomies and implantation of interpositioning materials, including soft tissue, wood and gold foil. The first

attempt at a total hip replacement was performed by Wiles in 1938. Charnley introduced the use of a metal femoral head and a high-density polyethylene, reporting a 96% success rate at 10-year follow-up in 1973 [2]. Currently, total joint replacement surgery through the standard posterolateral, lateral and anterior approaches is extremely successful.

Total hip arthroplasties have increased from 80 000 yearly procedures in 1976, to 125 000 in 1993 and approximately 250 000 currently [2, 3]. These numbers are expected to increase considerably as the "baby-boomer" generation reaches the age of peak incidence of debilitating osteoarthritis. Individuals in this very physically active generation will also have very high expectations of their functional status after total joint replacement. Many of them will not be satisfied with short-distance ambulation and transfers, but instead will expect the ability to participate in more challenging physical and athletic activities. The challenge for prosthetic designers, orthopedic surgeons and rehabilitation specialists will consist of helping this generation achieve its goals.

Not only have total joint replacement surgical techniques, prosthetic designs and materials improved greatly over the past few decades, but the rehabilitation process has changed considerably as well. There has been a trend to initiate therapy and improve pain control, strength and ROM earlier in the rehabilitation process. The introduction of cemented prostheses allowed earlier weight-bearin g, sometimes as soon as the first or second post-operative day. A report from the Hospital for Special Surgery from 1990 to 2000 showed a trend to earlier achievement of functional milestones after total hip arthroplasty. In 1990, total-hip-arthroplasty patients were able to achieve unassisted transfers, walker ambulation and stair climbing in a mean of 7.7 days. By the year 2000, these goals were achieved in a mean of only 4.4

days. The length of stay was also reduced from a mean of 9.7 days in 1990 to 5.3 days in 2000 [4]. Advocates of minimally invasive joint replacement surgery purport that these less invasive surgical techniques will further shorten the time to achieve functional goals and length of stay.

Principles of Joint Replacement

The current principles of joint replacement consist of early pain control, mobilization, range of motion and functional training, including independent transfers, ambulation with gait aids, stair climbing and activities of daily living. Pain control is crucial not only for patient comfort, but also to ensure better participation and gains during therapy. Early mobilization and institution of range of motion exercises post-operatively are also essential. Range of motion is usually started immediately post-operatively and ambulation commences approximately 1 to 2 days post-operatively. Precautions must be maintained during the rehabilitation process, especially in hip arthroplasties to avoid dislocations due to capsular weakness from the necessary surgical disruption of the capsule. After posterior approaches, care must be taken to avoid hip hyperflexion or internal rotation and after lateral approaches hip adduction and internal rotation must be avoided.

One of the main goals of minimally invasive joint replacement surgery is to decrease the amount of surgical trauma and tissue damage. Many different techniques and approaches have been described for both the hip and knee. During standard posterior approach to the hip, a long incision is made, the gluteus maximus is split along its fibers and the external rotators of the hip are detached from their femoral insertion [5]. Although many different minimally invasive posterior approaches have been described, the dissection of the gluteus maximus is much smaller and not always are all the external rotators of the hip detached. The size of the incision is dependent mainly on the size of the acetabulum to be inserted through the incision [1, 6]. In the standard anterior approach the iliac origin of the tensor fascia lata and both heads of the rectus femoris, the direct and the reflected head, are detached from their origins [5]. Several different minimally invasive anterior approaches, involving one, two or three incisions, have been described. These approaches utilize the planes between the tensor fascia lata and the sartorious or between the tensor fascia lata and the rectus femoris, thus decreasing

tissue damage [1, 7]. Once again, the size of the incision is determined by the space necessary to safely insert the acetabular component. During total knee arthroplasty, minimally invasive techniques strive to maintain the integrity of the extensor mechanism and the suprapatellar pouch, which are many times violated in the standard approach [8]. Preserving muscle integrity will be very important to the patient who hopes to continue to participate in high demand activities. By eliminating the need to recover the function of these muscles, the patient can more quickly progress to higher level rehabilitation, such as proprioceptive and pylometric training, with the goal of maintaining high-level function while muscularly controlling joint forces and potentially protecting these prosthesis from early wear and failure.

Pain Management

Minimizing tissue damage from surgical trauma has the potential effect of reducing post-operative pain which is also a major goal of the minimally invasive surgical procedures, A decrease in pain levels can be expected with smaller skin-and soft-tissue incisions. A reduction in pain can positively affect rehabilitation at many different levels. Firstly, by reducing the amount of pain, the patient may be able to better participate in therapy, ensuring a decrease in missed sessions secondary to pain, as well better performance and attention during each session. By reducing the amount of medication necessary to control pain, the known side effects of pain medications, such as decreased alertness, sleepiness, nausea and constipation, among others, can be minimized. All these side effects can have a negative impact on the participation and gains during the rehabilitation of post-joint arthroplasty patients. Another deleterious effect of pain on the rehabilitation process is weakness of the muscles surrounding the affected joint secondary to pain inhibition. The weakness caused by pain inhibition not only affects functional gains due to weakness during functional activities, but also causes muscle imbalances across the joint. These muscle imbalances and weakness can result in altered biomechanics which can result in antalgic gait patterns. For example, pain inhibition of the quadriceps (especially the vastus medialis) results in a quadriceps avoidance gait. This again results in altered biomechanics and neuromuscular engrams which can be difficult to retrain or eliminate, even after the pain has disappeared.

Currently, to our knowledge, there are no published studies that compare the level of pain between a standard and a minimally invasive joint-replacement surgery as one of the measured outcomes. Nevertheless, many surgeons anecdotally report decreased pain levels with minimally invasive techniques [1, 3]. Although a reduction in pain is expected with the decrease of tissue trauma achieved with these procedures, further prospective randomized studies with pain levels as a major outcome measure will be helpful to further elucidate this issue.

Joint Stability

Another advantage of preservation of muscle tissue integrity during joint arthroplasty is to reduce the amount of mechanical derangement of the main joint movers and stabilizers. This should result in better preservation of strength, and biomechanical stability around the joint. By maintaining closer to normal biomechanics and joint stability, quicker achievement of functional milestones can be expected. During hip replacements, the capsular incision still has to be large enough to accept the acetabular component, and thus there is still a risk of dislocation through the capsular violation. For this reason, the usual precautions still must be maintained. Nevertheless, improved biomechanical stability due to better preserved stabilizing musculature may reduce the inherent risk of dislocation. On the other hand, component malposition has been correlated with an increased risk of dislocation. Skeptics of the minimally invasive techniques worry about the increased difficulty in prosthetic positioning, the inability to eliminate osseous impingement and osteophytes and the inability to thoroughly assess stability due to decreased joint exposure. All these difficulties may result in component malposition, prosthetic joint instability or increased risk of dislocation [1]. However, Kennon et al. reported 28 dislocations in 2132 patients (1%) during the first 6 months after total hip replacements done through a minimally invasive anterior approach which is no greater than the normally quoted 1–2% for the standard approaches [7].

Mobilization

As discussed earlier, over the past decade, the number of days to achieve functional outcomes and to discharge has decreased significantly. Physical and occupational therapy are started earlier and more aggressively. Discharges as early as 3 days post-operatively are not uncommon. Minimally invasive total joint replacements are expected to reduce the amount of time needed to achieve functional milestones and thus reduce the length of stay. By decreasing tissue damage, post-operative pain and post-operative weakness, this type of procedure promises a quicker rehabilitation process. Some advocates of minimally invasive surgery believe that patients may leave the hospital within 24 hours of the operation. Berger implemented an accelerated rehabilitation protocol for his patients after a minimally invasive two-incision approach. Patients were allowed to leave the same day or the day after surgery as long as they met the discharge criteria. The criteria required the patient to transfer in and out of bed from a standing position, transfer from a sitting to standing position, walk a minimum of 100 feet and ascend and descend a full flight of stairs. Out of 88 patients, 100% were discharged to home during the first 23 hours. Eighty-five percent were discharged the day of the surgery and 15% were discharged the next day [3]. The benefits of early discharge to home are obvious in terms of both cost effectiveness and patient satisfaction. This type of accelerated rehabilitation with early discharge to home requires attention to the patient's home situation and well-coordinated services, especially in the older, single and medically complicated patient.

The early mobilization that may be achieved by minimally invasive procedures may also have a positive impact in other areas of rehabilitation. By facilitating early ambulation, common complications of inactivity such as muscle atrophy, neuromuscular and cardiovascular deconditioning, constipation, ileus, pneumonia, decubitus ulcers and deep venous thrombosis may be avoided.

Complications

Deep venous thrombosis is a relatively common complication of total joint replacements with a prevalence quoted between 5% and 60%. This is felt to be secondary to local trauma of the vascular endothelium during surgery, potential hypercoagulable states after tissue trauma and venous stasis secondary to inactivity. Kennon et al. report a 0.8% incidence of clinically relevant thromboembolic disease in their series of 2132 minimally invasive total hip-arthroplasty surgeries through an anterior approach.

All their patients were prophylaxed with a 65 mg daily dose of aspirin. They believe that their low number of thromboembolic events are due to short operative times, avoidance of femoral vein retraction and improved limb positioning, achieved with their anterior approach [7]. It should be noted that in this series only clinically relevant thromoembolic events were reported, thus, non-clinically relevant deep venous thrombosis were not looked for or reported. Even though, early mobilization is not enough to prevent deep venous thrombosis by itself, in combination with the usual prophylaxis, it may help reduce the incidence of this common complication.

Conclusions

Total joint replacement surgeries have evolved greatly over the past few decades, and minimally invasive techniques represent the newest development in this highly successful surgery. By reducing the initial trauma at the time of surgery, the benefits include: less tissue damage, reduced pain, faster rehabilitation with earlier accomplishment of functional outcomes, decreased length of stay and possibly reduced complications resulting from immobilization. An ever increasing, more active and demanding patient population will be seeking these very promising techniques for both short- and long-term effects on function and quality of life.

References

1. Berry DJ, Berger RA, Callaghan JJ, Dorr LD, Duwelius PJ, Hartzband MA, Lieberman JR, Mears DC. Minimally invasive total hip arthroplasty. Development, early results, and a critical analysis. J Bone Joint Surg Am 2003; 85-A(11): 2235–2246
2. Zimmerman JR. Rehabilitation of total hip and total knee replacements. In: DeLisa JA (ed) Rehabilitation medicine: Principles and practice, 3rd edn. Philadelphia: Lippincott-Raven, 1998: 1677–1693
3. Berger RA. Total hip arthroplasty using the minimally invasive approach. Clin Orthop Rel Res 2003; 417: 232–241
4. Ganz SB, Wilson PD Jr, Cioppa-Mosca J, Peterson MG. The day of discharge after total hip arthroplasty and the achievement of rehabilitation functional milestones: 11-year trends. J Arthroplasty 2003; 18(4): 453–457
5. Hoppenfeld S, deBoer P. The hip and acetabulum. In: Hoppenfeld S, deBoer P (ed) Surgical exposures in orthopaedics: The anatomic approach. 2nd edn. J.B. Lippincott, Philadelphia. 1994: 323–399
6. Goldstein WM, Branson JJ, Berland KA, Gordon AC. Minimal incision total hip arthroplasty. J Bone Joint Surg 2003; 85 [Suppl 4]: 33–38
7. Kennon RE, Keggi JM, Wetmore RS, Zatorski LE, Huo MH, Keggi KJ. Total hip arthroplasty through a minimally invasive anterior surgical approach. J Bone Joint Surg Am. 2003; 85-A [Suppl 4]: 39–48
8. Tria AJ Jr, Coon TM. Minimal incision total knee arthroplasty: early experience. Clin Orthop. 2003; 416: 185–190

Treatment and Rehabilitation Concepts – USA

W. Arnold, W.J. Hozack

Introduction

A key goal of minimally invasive arthroplasty surgery is the concept that operative changes should translate into an overall improvement in the postoperative course of patients. That is, less surgical dissection in the operating room should lead to less post-operative pain, shorter length of hospital stay, less need for in-patient rehabilitation and quicker return of functional status. These goals need to be achieved while maintaining, if not surpassing, the low complication rate of current hip and knee arthroplasty surgery. These goals are certainly attractive to the patient and the surgeon. Furthermore, they are also attractive to hospitals constantly under pressure to expedite care without sacrificing quality. While the concept of minimally invasive surgery emphasizes operative technique, it is truly a more inclusive concept that requires changes in anesthesia, pain management and physical therapy to achieve its full potential. It requires cooperation at several levels from the entire team of health professionals who will interact with the patient prior to, during and after the surgical procedure. Most of all, it requires a true commitment on the part of the patient to maximize results.

Patient Expectations

As with current arthroplasty surgery, a challenge of minimally invasive surgery involves properly managing patient expectations. Many patients come to the first physician–patient encounter with unrealistic goals, often fueled by Internet and mass media hyperbole. Therefore, proper patient education is essential. Pre-operative classes that strive to disseminate realistic goals while also placating unrealistic fears easily address this. The expected post-operative course can be explained to the patient in a detailed fashion. Additionally, patients can be screened pre-operatively to address post-operative disposition plans. This can be especially helpful for pre-screening potential sites for those patients who will likely require post-operative in-patient rehabilitation. The patient is also sent for a session of pre-operative physical therapy in which the post-operative rehabilitation exercises are explained. This all helps to involve patients in their post-operative care prior to surgery. These programs also help to create a mindset within patients that stresses their contribution to the overall success of the surgery. Such programs have proved helpful for our traditional arthroplasty patients. The programs are likely even more important with respect to minimally invasive surgery. While sparse, the available literature on minimally invasive arthroplasty certainly suggests that results are optimized in certain patient groups, specifically those with a body-mass index of less than 30. Therefore, it is important to temper the expectations of patients who may not fall within this group.

Anesthesia Techniques

The goal of anesthesia in hip- and knee-arthroplasty surgery is to provide adequate pain relief and muscle relaxation during the surgical procedure. Ideally, the type of anesthesia used should also minimize post-operative nausea and confusion, both of which delay rehabilitation efforts. Currently, regional anesthesia in the form of spinal anesthesia or selective nerve blocks (e.g., femoral nerve block, lumbar plexus block) comes closest to approaching these goals. Regional anesthesia also avoids the potential pitfalls of general anesthesia in a patient population that tends to be elderly with multiple medical co-morbidities. The exact type of regional anesthesia employed is generally dependent upon the expertise of the anesthesia staff involved. It has been our experience that spinal anesthesia works well for both hip- and knee-arthroplasty surgery. When used for hip-arthroplasty patients, spinal anesthesia has the potential to provide adequate analgesia for both the surgical procedure and often for the immediate post-operative period, especially when a longer acting agent is employed. When used for knee arthroplasty, the spinal anesthesia is complemented by the placement of an epidural catheter, since the post-operative pain experienced by knee-arthroplasty patients is usually more variable and often more substantial than that experienced by hip-arthroplasty patients. Patients are provided additional mild sedation during the surgical procedure as needed. It has been our experience that the muscle relaxation obtained using this anesthesia regimen is excellent and greatly facilitates the performance of the operative procedure. This is especially important for minimally invasive surgery as tissues that are not relaxed can further minimize an already small surgical workspace. Non-relaxed tissues also tend to require more vigorous retraction, thereby increasing the risk of subsequent damage to the tissue. This tends to negate the proposed benefit of minimally invasive surgery in terms of minimizing muscle damage.

Surgical Factors

The actual surgical approaches to the hip and the knee are described elsewhere in this volume. However, it is nonetheless relevant here to highlight specific surgical practices. With regard to hip arthroplasty, it has been our experience that a direct anterolateral approach provides an excellent surgical exposure. This is also true when this approach is used in a minimally invasive fashion. The importance of minimizing muscular trauma cannot be over-emphasized. Failure to do so results in greater post-operative pain, an increased risk of heterotopic ossification and an increased risk of a post-operative limp. Maintaining muscular integrity has always been a goal of arthroplasty surgery; however, it becomes one of the defining criteria in minimally invasive surgery. There is no point in attempting a minimally inva-

sive procedure if a patient's body habitus (e.g., obese patient, muscular patient) precludes doing such surgery at the risk of excessive tissue damage. The same argument may be made with regard to minimally invasive knee arthroplasty. Another surgical practice worth mentioning is that of minimizing eversion of the patella during knee arthroplasty. This decreases the amount of soft-tissue trauma done to the extensor mechanism during the surgery and thereby improves quadriceps function during post-operative rehabilitation.

Other treatment practices deserve special mentioning. At our institution we have long abandoned the use of surgical drains in knee arthroplasty. This has recently been reviewed by Esler et al. [2]), who found no efficacy for drain use in cemented knee arthroplasty. This recent study reaffirms the results of earlier studies in this regard [3, 4]. While this policy toward drain use may simply reflect surgeon preference with regard to traditional arthroplasty, it becomes important in a practical sense in minimally invasive arthroplasty as the use of drains may hinder aggressive physical therapy and early mobilization and discharge (sometimes within 24 h). Also the more limited dissection of minimally invasive surgery with its subsequent less blood loss would seem to further minimize any benefit a surgical drain might provide. Along this line of thought, we also no longer emphasize the use of autologous blood for minimally invasive arthroplasty. This is in agreement with a recent study by Billote et al. [5] who showed that pre-operative autologous blood donation provided no obvious benefit to non-anemic hip-arthroplasty patients. No longer requiring autologous blood donation and transfusion provides a monetary benefit while also decreasing the burden to patients in terms of their pre-operative preparation while avoiding transfusion risks.

Pain Management

The management of post-surgical pain in hip and knee arthroplasty is a key element in maximizing the benefits of minimally invasive surgery. It is obvious that early post-operative physical therapy as well as decreasing the length of post-operative hospitalization relies critically upon adequate post-operative analgesia. As mentioned previously, such analgesia must be obtained while minimizing post-operative confusion, hypotension and nausea. This often becomes a delicate balance. It has been our experience that intravenous narcotics often tip this balance towards undesirable side effects, especially in elderly patients. Therefore, strategies have been implemented to become less dependent upon intravenous narcotics for analgesia. Some of these are employed pre-operatively. We have adopted the policy that patients on a significant narcotic medication regimen, when they are first seen in the office, will not be offered surgery until this regimen is appropriately minimized with the assistance of a pain-management specialist. Otherwise, these patients frequently have unmanageable post-operative pain and cannot participate appropriately in their post-operative care. It is also essential for all patients in their pre-operative education to form realistic expectations with regard to post-operative pain management. Pre-operatively, starting medications such as Bextra or Vioxx the night before surgery appears to assist in minimizing post-operative pain and facilitating post-operative rehabilitation. In terms of the surgery itself, the benefit of longer acting agents, such as Duramorph in the spinal anesthetic, has previously been discussed.

Post-operatively, attempts have been made to rely more upon oral rather than intravenous narcotic medications for analgesia. Total knee arthroplasty patients are started on valdecoxib (Vioxx), a cyclooxygenase-2 specific anti-inflammatory medication, post-operatively on the day of surgery. The benefit of valdecoxib in reducing the need for post-operative narcotic in total-knee-arthroplasty patients has been demonstrated in the literature [6]. A protocol employing oral controlled-release oxycodone (Oxycontin) has also been implemented for hip- and knee-arthroplasty patients. The use of oral controlled-release oxycodone has been demonstrated in the in-patient rehabilitation setting to improve pain relief, improve early functional range of motion and decrease the length of the in-patient stay in total knee arthroplasty patients [7]. These pain medications are supplemented on an as well needed basis with oral immediate-release oxycodone, hydrocodone, codeine or propoxyphene. The analgesia obtained in most cases is excellent with minimal side effects. While these strategies have improved the care for all of our arthroplasty patients, we have seen the greatest effect upon our hip-replacement patients where the use of this pain-management regimen has often decreased the hospital stay by one day. Additionally, the pain control obtained is often sufficient enough for these patients to excel in their physical therapy such that they are dis-

charged to home rather than to an in-patient-rehabilitation facility. This has been especially the case in patients treated with minimally invasive arthroplasty surgery.

Physical Therapy

While obviously emphasizing the importance of early patient mobilization, a further major purpose of immediate post-operative physical therapy is to help determine patient disposition. It is the patient's ability to adequately perform activities of daily living, along with appropriate support as needed, which determines whether a patient is discharged to home or to an in-patient-rehabilitation facility. The ultimate deciding factor in this regard is patient safety. Given the increasing pressure to decrease the length of hospital stays, this decision towards patient disposition needs to be made relatively quickly in the post-operative period. Therefore, the physical-therapy and occupational-therapy regimens used at our institution have been tailored to expedite this decision process. These regimens for both traditional arthroplasty and for minimally invasive arthroplasty are outlined in ❑ Tables 2.1 and 2.2. Emphasis is placed on attaining specific minimal goals in the hospital with the idea that more rigorous therapy will be accomplished in the ensuing weeks. While the early goals are somewhat minimal, the immediate post-operative regimen is nonetheless rigorous in the sense that no maximal goals are set and patients are encouraged to advance forward with their rehabilitation as quickly as they are able. Active patient participation is essential. As mentioned previously, adequate analgesia without accompanying undesirable medication side effects is of the utmost importance in this regard. Stated specifically, a patient who cannot adequately participate in the first two physical therapy sessions because of pain, nausea or hypotension will likely be slated towards a disposition of in-patient rehabilitation.

The need to expedite post-operative care for minimally invasive arthroplasty patients has led to a reconsideration of certain prior care protocols that were used for traditional arthroplasty patients. Some of them are worth mentioning although not all of these changes were made specifically for minimally invasive surgery. At our institution, primary arthroplasty patients may bear weight as tolerated. This greatly facilitates the post-operative physical therapy regimen for these patients. We

Table 2.1. Physical/occupational therapy intervention for traditional total hip/knee replacement

	POD 1	POD 2	POD 3
PT Evaluation	Note prior level of functional mobility Perform therapeutic exercise program Assess bed mobility, transfers, and ambulation Attempt short distance ambulation from bed to chair with standard walker Monitor vital signs pre-, during and post treatment Establish aftercare recommendation and indication for Inpatient Rehabilitation vs. Home PT services upon discharge from hospital	*AM*: Initiate treatment either bedside or in department gym based upon patient tolerance to being out of bed for at least one hour on POD 1 Perform full therapeutic exercise program Progress ambulation distance to patient tolerance with standard walker Monitor vital signs throughout treatment — Emphasize out of bed activity greater than 1 hour and progress patient's mobilization as appropriate	*AM*: Continued progression of mobilization in department gym with emphasis on simulation of patient's home environment Progression of stair training to include negotiation of a full flight of stairs. Perform car transfers Review of therapeutic exercise program Initiate discharge plan pending patient's level of independence with all of the above
		PM: Continued progression of ambulation distance in patient room (i.e. >20 feet) Consider use of crutches based on patient's gait pattern, balance, and comfort level Continued performance of full therapeutic exercise program	*PM*: (*if indicated*) Continued mobilization with emphasis on achieving patient independence throughout all aspects of functional mobility
OT Evaluation	N/A	Initiate evaluation either bedside or in department gym based upon prior patient tolerance to physical therapy Assess upper body strength for negotiation of ambulatory devices Begin to educate patient on possible effects of THA/TKA on function (i.e. dressing, bathing, household management) Assess functional transfers to and from bed, commode/toilet, and tub/shower stall depending on patient's home set-up Establish aftercare recommendation and indication for Inpatient Rehab vs. Home OT services upon discharge from hospital (confirmed with PT) Patient educated to and/or issued, depending on disposition plan, to lower extremity bathing and dressing adaptive equipment (long-handled reacher, long-handled shoe horn, long-handled sponge, leg lifter, and sock donner) Patient educated to and demonstrates use of durable medical equipment to enhance function during recovery (i.e. tub seat and raised commode) Monitor vital signs pre-, during, and post-treatment	Monitor progression of independence with functional transfers to and from bed, commode/toilet, and tub/shower stall depending on patient's home set-up Monitor progression of independence with lower extremity bathing and dressing via adaptive equipment Address patient and family concerns regarding rehabilitation placement and/or return to home Monitor vital signs throughout treatment Continued performance of functional tasks with emphasis on achieving independence throughout all aspects of daily living Initiate discharge plan pending patient's level of independence with all of the above

POD postoperative day, *PT* physical therapy, *OT* occupational therapy, *THA* total hip arthroplasty, *TKA* total knee arthroplasty

2

◼ **Table 2.2.** Physical/occupational intervention for minimally invasive total hip/knee replacement

		POD 1	POD 2
PT Evaluation		*AM:* Note prior level of functional mobility Perform therapeutic exercise program Assess bed mobility, transfers, and ambulation Monitor vital signs pre-, during, and post- treatment Attempt ambulation and progress distance to patient tolerance Consider use of crutches based on gait pattern, balance, and comfort level Establish aftercare recommendation and indication for Inpatient Rehab vs. Home PT services upon d/c from hospital Assess appropriateness for BID session based upon patient performance in AM in conjunction with determination of home discharge	*AM:* Initiate treatment either bedside or in department gym based on patient tolerance POD 1 ▬ Monitor vital signs throughout treatment ▬ Perform full therapeutic exercise program ▬ Progress ambulation with crutches to household distances (i.e.150 ft) ▬ Attempt stair training with progression to negotiation of a full flight if indicated ▬ Perform car transfer ▬ Consider use of a single point cane based on gait ▬ Consider use of a single point cane based on gait pattern, balance, coordination, and comfort level ▬ Initiate discharge plan pending independent performance of all of the above
		PM: (*if indicated*) Continued progression of ambulation to patient tolerance. Perform full therapeutic exercise program	*PM:* (*if indicated*) Continued mobilization with emphasis on achieving patient independence throughout all aspects of functional mobility
OT Evaluation		N/A	Initiate evaluation either bedside or in department gym based on patient's tolerance to physical therapy POD 1 Assess upper body strength for negotiation of ambulatory devices Begin to educate patient on possible effects of THA/TKA on function (i.e. dressing, bathing, household management) Assess functional transfers to and from bed, commode/toilet, and tub/shower stall depending on patient's home set-up Establish aftercare recommendation and indication for Inpatient Rehab vs. Home OT services upon discharge from hospital (confirmed with PT) Patient educated to and/or issued, depending on disposition plan, to lower extremity bathing and dressing adaptive equipment (long-handled reacher, long-handled shoe horn, long-handled sponge, leg lifter, and sock donner) Patient educated to and demonstrates use of durable medical equipment to enhance function during recovery (i.e. tub seat and raised commode) Address patient and family concerns regarding rehab placement and/or return to home Monitor vital signs pre-, during, and post treatment Initiate discharge plan pending patient's level of independence with all of the above

POD post-operative day, *PT* physical therapy, *OT* occupational therapy, *THA* total hip arthroplasty, *TKA* total knee arthroplasty

have also recently re-evaluated the need for post-operative hip precautions. We recently performed a randomized, prospective study involving 303 hip arthroplasties (265 patients) through an anterolateral approach [8]. Patients were randomized to a restricted group in which traditional hip precautions were employed or to an unrestricted group in which minimal hip precautions were employed. Only one early hip dislocation occurred, and this involved a patient from the restricted group. Consequently, we now employ the minimal hip precaution protocol for our hip-arthroplasty patients. The changes in the post-operative physical therapy regimen for minimally invasive surgery patients as compared with traditional arthroplasty patients are shown in ◻ Tables 2.1 and 2.2. Overall, while not all of these changes were made specifically for minimally invasive surgery, they certainly have coincided nicely with the introduction of minimally invasive surgery at our institution. Taken as a whole these changes have simplified the post-operative course of our patients, thereby minimizing the disruption of surgery to their lives.

Medical Issues and Patient Selection

There is little question that immediate post-operative progress in joint-arthroplasty patients is dependent upon pre-operative patient health. While perhaps not the main goal, it is nonetheless implied that one of the purposes of minimally invasive surgery is to decrease the post-operative hospital stay as well as the need for in-patient post-operative rehabilitation. The logic employed is quite straightforward: less surgical dissection leads to less post-operative morbidity. This translates into less need for post-operative in-patient rehabilitation. Berger recently reported the results for 100 cases in which minimally invasive hip arthroplasty was performed [1]. Seventy-five patients went home the day of surgery and none of the patients required in-patient rehabilitation. The average age of the patients was 55 years old and the average weight was 176 lbs. It cannot be overlooked that this does not represent the usual arthroplasty patient population. However, arguments over the potential benefit of minimally invasive surgery need not to be relegated to the question of whether patients can go home within 24 hours. The ability of a patient to go home within 24 hours of surgery probably has less to do with the actual surgery and more to do with post-operative pain management as

well as the patient's pre-operative medical condition. This honest appraisal cannot be overlooked when evaluating the results of minimally invasive surgery. Truthfully, most experienced surgeons can predict, to a relatively good degree, which of their patients will do well post-operatively in terms of going home after a short hospital stay. It makes little sense to preclude patients from the potential benefits of minimally invasive surgery simply because they do not fit a specific profile.

This highlights the importance of patient selection for surgery. It has been thoroughly explained up to this point that minimally invasive surgery embraces a concept of patient care that goes well beyond the operating room to involve aggressive post-operative pain management and physical therapy. A significant number of arthroplasty patients simply may not fit the patient profile appropriate for this aggressive treatment philosophy. The usual limiting factors in this regard are age and medical co-morbidities. Nonetheless, such patients may benefit from the minimally invasive surgery protocol insofar as it can be safely applied. It can be argued that this patient group has been somewhat ignored in the debate over minimally invasive surgery simply because the overall results in this group pale in comparison to those results obtained in a younger, more medically fit group. This is only expected at a time when the results of minimally invasive surgery are being tested against those of traditional arthroplasty. Nonetheless, the philosophy at our institution has been to offer minimally invasive surgery to all appropriate arthroplasty patients. Of course, the aggressiveness of the post-operative care protocols is tailored to the individual patient. While certain patients will never go home within 24 h of surgery and a number of them will still require in-patient rehabilitation, it still seems that such patients benefit from minimally invasive surgery. Therefore, within reason, perhaps the greatest impediment to minimally invasive surgery is more dependent upon a patient's body habitus than upon a patient's pre-operative medical condition. This of course assumes that the patient's pre-operative medical condition has been optimized prior to surgery. For those patients with considerable medical co-morbidities, it becomes important to minimize the actual surgical time. Therefore, for a given surgeon if the time to perform a minimally invasive arthroplasty surgery is significantly longer than that required for a traditional arthroplasty surgery, it may be a better service for higher risk patients to perform the latter.

While known medical co-morbidities can be addressed pre-operatively, perhaps the medical co-morbidity of greatest concern post-operatively to hip- and knee-arthroplasty patients is that of deep venous thrombosis with its subsequent risk of pulmonary embolism. A large number of anticoagulation protocols have been applied in treating arthroplasty patients. We currently employ an anticoagulation regimen in which warfarin is given as a loading dose (usually 5–10 mg) on the day of surgery and then is dosed according to a sliding scale based upon laboratory values of the prothrombin time International Normalized Ratio (INR) obtained from intermittent blood draws. Patients are currently anticoagulated for a total of 6 weeks post-operatively. This regimen has a long history of success at our institution. At the same time, it is recognized that other anticoagulation regimens may be used, usually based upon individual surgeon preference and experience. While the introduction of low molecular weight heparin for anticoagulation is attractive in some ways (fewer blood draws), it is less attractive in other respects (need for injection, potentially higher risk of post-operative bleeding). The use of aspirin as an anticoagulant is simple and also has its proponents [9]. While the specific anticoagulation protocols chosen by orthopedic surgeons will likely continue to vary, their use in patients treated with minimally invasive surgery may prompt a re-evaluation of these protocols, just as it has prompted a re-evaluation of previous physical therapy and pain-management protocols. Certainly, with the current emphasis on less invasive surgery and more rapid recovery, it is possible that the risk of thrombophlebitis will diminish and less aggressive regimens of anticoagulation, such as aspirin, will suffice. Ultimately, the anticoagulation protocols adopted may rely more upon expediting patient care and less upon traditional preferences so long as the efficacy and safety of the overall treatment remains paramount.

Discussion

The purpose of this chapter has been to highlight many of the non-surgical aspects required to maximize the benefits of minimally invasive arthroplasty surgery. Overall, the advent of minimally invasive surgery has challenged several of the treatment protocols previously employed for traditional hip and knee arthroplasty. These changes have essentially been made to better expedite patient recovery and minimize the overall disruption of surgery to patients' lives. All of this must be achieved while never compromising the current standard of patient safety.

Minimally invasive surgery represents only the latest in a number of innovations with regard to arthroplasty surgery. What is clear is that joint arthroplasty as a whole encompasses several treatment regimens. This has been the main emphasis of this chapter. It is also clear that advances in one component of joint arthroplasty can be stifled if other components of arthroplasty fail to advance. Specifically, the benefits of operative advances made in minimally invasive arthroplasty surgery simply cannot be realized if appropriate changes do not occur with regard to pain management, pre-operative preparation and physical therapy. Surgeons cannot simply concentrate only on the advancements made in the operating room. To do so compromises the full potential benefit that minimally invasive arthroplasty surgery can offer to patients. Simply stated, minimally invasive arthroplasty surgery must be more than just a small incision.

References

1. Berger RA (2003) Total hip arthroplasty using the minimally invasive two-incision approach. Clin Orthop 417: 232–241
2. Esler CN, Blakeway C, Fiddian NJ (2003) The use of a closed-suction drain in knee arthroplasty. A prospective, randomised study. J Bone Joint Surgery Br 85: 215–217
3. Beer KJ, Lombardi AV Jr, Mallory TH, Vaughn BK (1991) The efficacy of suction drains after routine total joint arthroplasty. J Bone Joint Surgery Am 73: 584–587
4. Adalberth G, Bystrom S, Kolstad K, Mallmin H, Milbrink J (1998) Postoperative drainage of knee arthroplasty is not necessary: a randomized study of 90 patients. Acta Orthopaedica Scandinavica 69: 475–478
5. Billote DB, Glisson SN, Green D, Wixson RL (2002) A prospective, randomized study of preoperative autologous donation for hip replacement surgery. J Bone Joint Surgery Am 84: 1299–1304
6. Reynolds LW, Hoo RK, Brill RJ, North J, Recker DP, Verburg KM (2003) The COX-2 specific inhibitor, valdecoxib, is an effective, opioid-sparing analgesic in patients undergoing total knee arthroplasty. J Pain Symptom Management 25: 133–141
7. Cheville A, Chen A, Oster G, McGarry L, Narcessian E (2001) A randomized trial of controlled-release oxycodone during inpatient rehabilitation following unilateral total knee arthroplasty. J Bone Joint Surg Am 83: 572–576
8. Peak EL, Parvizi J, Ciminiello M, Purtill JJ, Sharkey PF, Hozack WJ, Rothman RH. The role of patient restrictions in early dislocation following total hip arthroplasty: a randomized, prospective study (submitted for publication)
9. Stolarski EJ, Koeffler KM, Lotke PA (2003) Aspirin as prophylaxis for thrombophlebitis. Sem Arthroplasty 14

Treatment and Rehabilitation Concepts in Europe

K.E. Dreinhöfer, W. Puhl, M. Flören

Osteoarthritis (OA) is one of the leading causes of pain and disability in the Western World [1]. Over the last 40 years, total hip replacement (THR) has become a successful and widely acclaimed procedure to treat hip arthritis and to restore functional status and quality of life [2]. Due to extensive orthopedic research in improvements of prosthetic materials and design, fixation techniques, implant–tissue interaction and process-optimizing, THR became a highly effective technology with durable long-term results, while being very cost-effective [3].

A variety of surgical approaches are in use for the performance of THR, including anterior, anterolateral, direct lateral, transtrochanteric, and posterior techniques [4–11]. These approaches are typically performed through incisions from 20–30 cm in length and an optimal exposure of acetabulum and proximal femur is guaranteed. Due to excellent results and very low complication rates, these approaches were not yet in need for improvement.

Minimal invasive surgical techniques have been developed and used in orthopedic surgery for cruciate ligament repairs, unicondylar knee replacements and surgical fixation of fractures. Recently, minimally invasive techniques for THA (skin incision <10 cm) have sparked an increased interest among orthopedic surgeons. The modifications include a single abbreviated incision for anterior or posterior approach and a two-incision technique for anterior approach via the femoral neck for cup placement and a posterior approach in the line of the femoral canal for femoral component insertion [12–19]. The premise is to reduce the trauma of surgery while maintaining the perceived high levels of safety, efficacy, and durability of the procedure.

Early results suggest quicker recovery, faster rehabilitation, improved function, better cosmetic appearance, higher patient satisfaction, and better resource utilization by reduced length of hospital stay and lowered costs; however, the patient groups in observation are still small [13–17, 20–22]. On the other hand, there are major concerns about new potential risks due to reduced visualization, resulting in implant malposition, and poor fixation, resulting in compromised long-term results. The potential benefits of a smaller incision need to be balanced against the added operative difficulty, possible new risks, and drawbacks of a new learning curve, associated with minimally invasive procedures.

To become adopted as a standard procedure, the new technique must pass the test of clinical safety, efficacy and durability. A definite answer can only arise from long-term studies. However, today there are no long-term data which compare the durability of hip arthroplasty performed through a minimally invasive approach with conventional THR.

Major variations in the THR rates per head of population can be observed between European countries, as well as variations in the peri-operative regimes used and costs incurred [23]. Evidence-based consensus on the indication for surgical treatment, the most appropriate surgical procedures, optimal peri-operative care regimes and rehabilitation protocols are lacking. This leads to huge variations and potential inequalities in care. Main reasons for this inhomogeneity are differences in the health-care systems, the reimbursement systems and the philosophy behind treatment protocols. Most European countries have a public health system allowing everybody, irrespective of his financial background, to receive a total hip replacement. However, in most countries, the majority of patients has no option to choose between surgeons, operative techniques or implants. Only privately insured patients might have the opportunity to select their surgeon.

In the recent past, in most Western Europe nations the THR treatment process was dominated on the one hand by public health guidelines regulating time of surgery, numbers of procedures per clinic and year, length of hospital stay, and on the other hand by reimbursement unrelated to the implants used and to the fixation technique applied. Therefore, progressive reductions of length of stay or specializations in new but potential expensive techniques in the learning period, was not favorable for the hospital budget [24]. Only recently some countries have introduced DRGs (Diagnosis Related Groups), resulting in payment per procedure and stimulating early discharge from the hospital. However, a quality-related payment or reimbursement for the products used are still not in place.

A comprehensive description of a European treatment and rehabilitation concept is impossible. Different health-care structures and reimbursement systems but also different philosophies, national traditions, cultural differences and marketing activities of the industry have a strong influence on the practice pattern. A descriptive analysis of the THRs implanted is only available in the Scandinavian national registers, some regional THR registers in the UK and some further central European countries [3, 25–28]. There is a huge variety of implant systems available on the market. While in some countries about 80% of all operations are performed using 1 to 5 types of prostheses [29], it is assumed that 120–170 different types of total hip replacements are in use in some of the other countries [30].

In the first three decades of THR operations mechanical loosening and extensive bone losses were the major challenges for the long term success. Substantial changes in implant fixation increased the durability of femoral and acetabular components. Newer cementing techniques on the femoral side including the use of a medullary plug, a cement gun, lavage of the canal, pressurization, centralization of the stem, and reduction in porosity in the cement allowed to reduce stresses in the materials and improved strength of the interfaces with increasing survival rates up to 95% after ten years [31, 32].

Cementless components rely on bone ingrowth into porous or onto roughened surfaces; additionally, several types of calcium phosphate ceramics (often called hydroxylapatite) have been added as coatings to THR surfaces to enhance fixation of non-ingrowth implants to bone [33–35]. Selected cementless femoral components have exhibited clinical success similar to that of cemented components installed with the newer cementing techniques [36, 37]; however, so far the follow-up is much shorter.

On the acetabular side, the cementless components have demonstrated less long-term aseptic loosening compared with the cemented components. Since most prospective and retrospective studies have focused only on specific device designs and techniques, any general comparison of cemented and non-cemented systems should be viewed with caution [38–40].

There are major differences between countries in regard to the philosophy of implant fixation. While in some countries most THRs are implanted without cement (e.g. Austria 85–90%) [41], in others uncemented THRs are uncommon (Norway 14% [42], Sweden 5% [29]). In most countries the decision for an uncemented THR is based on the age and the bone quality. Based on own evaluations, the estimated rates for cemented THR in Europe are 30–50%, for hybrid THR 10–30%, and for cementless THR 20–40%.

Device design and fixation technique have to guarantee load transfer between pelvic bone and femur. Two aspects are important:
1. The contact area between implant and corticalis has to be as large as possible to avoid load peaks,
2. the point of load transfer should be very proximal to reduce bone atrophy due to inactivity.

Today, the standard design for femoral components consist of stem fixation and diaphyseal load transfer [43, 44]. However, recently hip resurfacing has a renaissance and short-stem femoral components are more often in use [45]; so far, due to lack of durable long-term results its use is primarily restricted to some centers.

The main problem in THR unrelated to implant design is aseptic loosening. Most published results are based on single types of prostheses and expert surgeons. In the Swedish THR register some 160 000 cases have been recorded nationwide over the past 20 years. The rate of revisions in this register is low (7.1%) for the cemented group, but considerably higher in the uncemented group (13%).

In revision cases of the femoral component the approach is based primarily on the nature of the remaining bone stock in the proximal femur. In addition, clinical judgment usually takes into account the age and functional demands of the patient. In most cases revision of the femoral component is possible with a cemented stem. However, when there is substantial residual bone stock, non-cemented long-stem high-modular implants, particularly the extensively coated components, are also in use [46–49]. Morselized bone is used in addition to fill defects in the femoral canal or proximal femur.

On the acetabular site, revision strategies depend on the acetabular component, and the presence of adequate bone stock [50, 51]. All types of implants and fixations are in use, often in combination with bone cement, morselized or structural bone graft augmentation [52, 53].

Wear and third-body reaction are still major areas of concern because of resulting implant loosening and failure [54, 55]. In the past, metal to polyethylene articulations have caused catastrophic osteolysis and failure of hip arthroplasties [56, 57]. Newer articulating components (e.g. metal/metal, ceramic/ceramic, ceramic/high-cross-linked polyethylene) are mainly in use with smaller particle sizes and lower wear rates. The decision for different articulation components is on the patient site primarily based on age and demanded and/or expected mobility.

Since length of acute hospital stay has become shorter in the past years, more emphasis is needed to determine the role of preadmission educational programs, as well as appropriate physical therapy and rehabilitation during hospitalization and following discharge.

Post-operative in- or outpatient rehabilitation programs and home-health programs are in use European-wide. They are directed to an early mobilization, gait and balance training as well as muscular restoration. In addition, self-care training and psychological assistance is offered. According to own unpublished evaluations and other sources [30, 41], major regional and cultural differences exist. While in the German-speaking countries the majority of THR patients are discharged to inpatient rehabilitation hospitals for 3–4 weeks, in most of the other health-care systems a combination of in- and outpatient rehabilitation is in use. Inpatient programs seem to be more effective than prolonged hospitalization or outpatient rehabilitation [58]; however, some believe that appropriate home training is at least as good [59]. While the positive influence of a rehabilitation program on short- and mid-term results is proven, the long-term benefits of prolonged therapeutic exercise program for patients who have undergone THR have not been clearly demonstrated to improve mobility or hip stability. There is evidence that hip weakness persists up to 2 years after surgery in the presence of a normal gait. Multiple studies have demonstrated that weakness in the lower extremities is a major risk factor for falls and resulting fractures in the geriatric age group, thus for these patients an extensive rehabilitation seems to be an effective prevention.

Most health-care systems in Europe guarantee easy access to THR for all their people in all regions. The majority of procedures are performed in regional hospitals with 50–300 THR per year and 5–10 orthopedic surgeons; specialized centers with 500–1000 THR or more per year are rare. With demographic changes and more people in the older age groups the number of hip replacements needed will increase. So far, no agreed indication or appropriateness criteria exist that would allow to analyze over- or under-treatment in certain areas and to adjust the appropriate resources.

In regard to introduction of minimally invasive techniques in THR and especially following widespread use, drawbacks of a new learning curve can be expected. All surgeons who are currently performing the new techniques pointed out that these belong into hands of experienced surgeons. Only centers with a high surgical volume can reach the appropriate steady state of the learning curve in a short time. A rapid widespread introduction of minimally invasive approaches might hamper the overall public health due to inappropriate training and inferior results of the less experienced surgeons. For the near future, most hospitals will have to continue with the conventional approaches guaranteeing the long-term success rates of total hip replacements and providing high-quality care to their patients.

References

1. The burden of musculoskeletal conditions at the start of the new millennium. World Health Organ Tech Rep Ser, 2003. 919: i–x, 1–218
2. Murray, D. Surgery and joint replacement for joint disease. Acta Orthop Scand [Suppl], 1998. 281: 17–20
3. Faulkner, A., et al. Effectiveness of hip prostheses in primary total hip replacement: a critical review of evidence and an economic model. Health Technol Assess, 1998. 2(6): 1–133

4. Burwell, H.N., D. Scott. A lateral intermuscular approach to the hip joint for replacement of the femoral head by a prosthesis. J Bone Joint Surg Br, 1954. 36: 104–108

5. Hardinge, K. The direct lateral approach to the hip. J Bone Joint Surg Br, 1982. 64(1): 17–19

6. Harris, W.H. A new lateral approach to the hip joint. J Bone Joint Surg Am, 1967. 49(5): 891–898

7. Iyer, K.M. A new posterior approach to the hip joint. Injury, 1981. 13(1): 76–80

8. Light, T.R., K.J. Keggi. Anterior approach to hip arthroplasty. Clin Orthop, 1980 152: 255–260

9. Smith-Peterson, M.N. Approach to and exposure of the hip joint for mold arthroplasty. J Bone Joint Surg Am, 1949. 31: 40–46

10. Sutherland, R., J.J. Rowe. Simplified surgical approach to the hip. Arch Surg, 1944. 48: 144

11. Watson-Jones, R. Fractures of the neck of the femur. Br J Surg, 1936. 23: 787–808

12. Berger, R.A. Total hip arthroplasty using the minimally invasive two-incision approach. Clin Orthop, 2003 417: 232–241

13. Berry, D.J., et al. Minimally invasive total hip arthroplasty. Development, early results, and a critical analysis. J Bone Joint Surg Am, 2003. 85-A(11): 2235–2246

14. DiGioia, A.M., 3rd, et al. Mini-incision technique for total hip arthroplasty with navigation. J Arthroplasty, 2003. 18(2): 123–128

15. Goldstein, W.M., et al. Minimal-incision total hip arthroplasty. J Bone Joint Surg Am, 2003. 85-A [Suppl 4]: 33–38

16. Kennon, R.E., et al. Total hip arthroplasty through a minimally invasive anterior surgical approach. J Bone Joint Surg Am, 2003. 85-A [Suppl 4]: 39–48

17. Lester, D.K., M. Helm, Mini-Incision posterior approach for hip arthroplasty. Orthopedics and Traumatology, 2001. 4: 245–253

18. Sherry, E., et al. Minimal invasive surgery for hip replacement: a new technique using the NILNAV hip system. ANZ J Surg, 2003. 73(3): 157–161

19. Waldman, B.J. Advancements in minimally invasive total hip arthroplasty. Orthopedics, 2003. 26 [8 Suppl]: s833–836

20. Lester, D.K., L.S. Linn. Variation in hospital charges for total joint arthroplasty: an investigation of physician efficiency. Orthopedics, 2000. 23(2): 137–140

21. Waldman, B.J. Minimally invasive total hip replacement and perioperative management: early experience. J South Orthop Assoc, 2002. 11(4): 213–217

22. Wenz, J.F., I. Gurkan, S.R. Jibodh. Mini-incision total hip arthroplasty: a comparative assessment of perioperative outcomes. Orthopedics, 2002. 25(10): 1031–1043

23. Merx, H., et al. International variation in hip replacement rates. Ann Rheum Dis, 2003. 62(3): 222–226

24. Muller, R.T., N. Schurmann. Cost analysis of hip and knee prostheses as the basis for cost-benefit evaluation. Zentralbl Chir, 2001. 126(1): 55–61

25. Arnold, P., et al. Review of the results of the ARO multicenter study. Orthopäde, 1998. 27(6): 324–332

26. Fitzpatrick, R., et al. Primary total hip replacement surgery: a systematic review of outcomes and modelling of cost-effectiveness associated with different prostheses. Health Technol Assess, 1998. 2(20): 1–64

27. Soderman, P., et al. Outcome after total hip arthroplasty: Part II. Disease-specific follow-up and the Swedish National Total Hip Arthroplasty Register. Acta Orthop Scand, 2001. 72(2): 113–119

28. Puolakka, T.J., et al. The Finnish Arthroplasty Register: report of the hip register. Acta Orthop Scand, 2001. 72(5): 433–441

29. Herberts, P., H. Malchau. Long-term registration has improved the quality of hip replacement: a review of the Swedish THR Register comparing 160,000 cases. Acta Orthop Scand, 2000. 71(2): 111–121

30. Metz, C.M., A.A. Freiberg. An international comparative study of total hip arthroplasty cost and practice patterns. J Arthroplasty, 1998. 13(3): 296–298

31. Callaghan, J.J., et al. Charnley total hip arthroplasty with cement. Minimum twenty-five-year follow-up. J Bone Joint Surg Am, 2000. 82(4): 487–497

32. Harris, W.H. Options for primary femoral fixation in total hip arthroplasty. Cemented stems for all. Clin Orthop, 1997(344): 118–123

33. Head, W.C., D.J. Bauk, R.H. Emerson, Jr. Titanium as the material of choice for cementless femoral components in total hip arthroplasty. Clin Orthop, 1995(311): 85–90

34. Hozack, W.J., et al. Primary cementless hip arthroplasty with a titanium plasma sprayed prosthesis. Clin Orthop, 1996(333): 217–225

35. Overgaard, S., et al. Hydroxyapatite and fluorapatite coatings for fixation of weight loaded implants. Clin Orthop, 1997(336): 286–296

36. Delaunay, C., et al. Grit-blasted titanium femoral stem in cementless primary total hip arthroplasty: a 5- to 10-year multicenter study. J Arthroplasty, 2001. 16(1): 47–54

37. Kim, Y.H., J.S. Kim, S.H. Cho, Primary total hip arthroplasty with a cementless porous-coated anatomic total hip prosthesis: 10- to 12-year results of prospective and consecutive series. J Arthroplasty, 1999. 14(5): 538–548

38. Berger, R.A., et al. Primary cementless acetabular reconstruction in patients younger than 50 years old. 7- to 11-year results. Clin Orthop, 1997(344): 216–226

39. Cautilli, G.P., et al. A prospective review of 303 cementless universal cups with emphasis on wear as the cause of failure. Semin Arthroplasty, 1994. 5(1): 25–29

40. Dunkley, A.B., et al. Cementless acetabular replacement in the young. A 5- to 10-year prospective study. Clin Orthop, 2000(376): 149–155

41. Brodner, W., B. Raffelsberger. Hüft-Total-Endoprothetik in Österreich. Eine bundesweite Umfrage mittels Fragebogen. Orthopäde, 2004. 33(4): 462–471

42. Havelin, L.I., et al. The Norwegian Arthroplasty Register: 11 years and 73,000 arthroplasties. Acta Orthop Scand, 2000. 71(4): 337–353

43. McNamara, B.P., et al. Relationship between bone-prosthesis bonding and load transfer in total hip reconstruction. J Biomech, 1997. 30(6): 621–630

44. Mont, M.A., D.S. Hungerford. Proximally coated ingrowth prostheses. A review. Clin Orthop, 1997(344): 139–149

45. Daniel, J., P.B. Pynsent, D.J. McMinn. Metal-on-metal resurfacing of the hip in patients under the age of 55 years with osteoarthritis. J Bone Joint Surg Br, 2004. 86(2): 177–184

46. Brindley, G.W., R. Adams. Cementless revision of total hip arthroplasty using proximal porous- coated femoral implants. J South Orthop Assoc, 1998. 7(4): 246–250

47. Chareancholvanich, K., et al. Cementless acetabular revision for aseptic failure of cemented hip arthroplasty. Clin Orthop, 1999. 361: 140–149

48. Engh, C.A., W.J. Culpepper, 2nd, E. Kassapidis. Revision of loose cementless femoral prostheses to larger porous coated components. Clin Orthop, 1998. 347: 168–178

49. Mikhail, W.E., et al. Complex cemented revision using polished stem and morselized allograft. Minimum 5-years' follow-up. Arch Orthop Trauma Surg, 1999. 119(5–6): 288–291

50. Dearborn, J.T., W.H. Harris. Acetabular revision arthroplasty using so-called jumbo cementless components: an average 7-year follow-up study. J Arthroplasty, 2000. 15(1): 8–15

51. Garcia-Cimbrelo, E. Porous-coated cementless acetabular cups in revision surgery: a 6- to 11-year follow-up study. J Arthroplasty, 1999. 14(4): 397–406

52. Burssens, P., et al. Acetabular bone stock reconstruction with frozen femoral head allografts and the use of a cementless screw cup in total hip revision surgery. A 5 years' clinical, radiologic and scintigraphic follow-up. Acta Orthop Belg, 1989. 55(1): 38–52

53. Leopold, S.S., J.J. Jacobs, A.G. Rosenberg. Cancellous allograft in revision total hip arthroplasty. A clinical review. Clin Orthop, 2000 (371): 86–97

54. Dai, X., et al. Serial measurement of polyethylene wear of well-fixed cementless metal- backed acetabular component in total hip arthroplasty: an over 10 year follow-up study. Artif Organs, 2000. 24(9): 746–751

55. Elfick, A.P., S.L. Smith, A. Unsworth, Variation in the wear rate during the life of a total hip arthroplasty: a simulator and retrieval study. J Arthroplasty, 2000. 15(7): 901–908

56. Maloney, W.J., et al. Fixation, polyethylene wear, and pelvic osteolysis in primary total hip replacement. Clin Orthop, 1999 (369): 157–164

57. Han, C.D., W.S. Choe, J.H. Yoo. Effect of polyethylene wear on osteolysis in cementless primary total hip arthroplasty: minimal 5-year follow-up study. J Arthroplasty, 1999. 14(6): 714–723

58. Bitzer, E.M., H. Dorning, F.W. Schwartz. Effects of rehabilitation after hip replacement surgery on postoperative complaints regarding the disease and limitation of function. Rehabilitation (Stuttg), 2001. 40(1): 43–49

59. Roos, E.M. Effectiveness and practice variation of rehabilitation after joint replacement. Curr Opin Rheumatol, 2003. 15(2): 160–162

Treatment and Rehabilitation Concepts – Asian Pacific

G.F. Heynen

Introduction

The concept of minimally invasive surgery in orthopedics is not new, and has lead to the whole field of arthroscopic surgery, microdiscectomy in spinal surgery and minimally invasive uni-compartment knee replacement, just to name a few. The idea behind the concept is to minimize the surgical trauma and hence speed the recovery. In hip replacement one of the most confounding problems making minimally invasive surgery difficult is the size and shape of the implants and the long-held traditional view that these can only be inserted via a single large incision giving full exposure to both the acetabulum and the proximal femur.

The drive for minimally invasive surgery, both for the knee and the hip, is early discharge from hospital. Richard Berger's initial claims of day-stay hip replacement galvanized surgeons into an immediate frenzy of interest, but few have been able to consistently reproduce his results. Day-stay surgery is possible for uni-compartmental knee replacement and total hip replacement, but not without significant medical, social and physical therapy back-up to ensure safety. Pain relief in these circumstances is achieved via use of local anesthetic, pain pumps and significant doses of opiates. Is this concept of same day discharge that important, when one or two days as an in-patient means that the patient is more comfortable and not requiring opiates, has had the post-operative therapy and teaching required and feels confident about his mobilization. The drive should be to improve early rehabilitation rate and, above all, to do no harm.

Patient Selection

Patients suitable for minimally invasive surgery select themselves, as by definition they want early discharge and rapid recovery. This is usually with a view towards an earlier gain of independence and ability to return to work.

Patients with high BMI and thick subcutaneous adipose layers tend to make surgery through small incisions very difficult, hence the technique is more suitable for slim patients.

Mini-incision surgery can be utilized for the insertion of any choice of implant, except resurfacing arthroplasty. This includes cemented implants. Two-incision surgery, at present, can only be performed using cementless implants, therefore the anatomy of the hip, that is, acetabular and femoral bone stock, should be considered in terms of patient selection.

Education/Expectation

Because of the direct access the public has to developing technology via Internet and lay press, more patients are expecting and demanding mini-incision surgery. This is on the basis of very limited scientific evidence to back up its efficacy and safety. Initial patient selection involved priming them for early discharge and very much instilling the expectation of early mobilization, in Richard Berger's series. Included in this were aggressive pre-operative rehabilitation and therapy teaching and a program that differed from conventional hip-replacement patients.

We as surgeons are now faced with the increasing demand for these techniques from our patients with every reason from cosmesis to "If it is new it must be better". To meet this demand, it is important for us to familiarize ourselves with these techniques as thoroughly as possible. Most companies offering instruments and methodology of minimally invasive surgery usually provide surgeons with teaching programs, including cadaveric workshops and mentoring programs to help surgeons familiarize themselves with the techniques.

Skepticism is building among surgeons based upon what appears to be significant complications, and the inability to reproduce early single surgical results, and that patients given the expectation of early discharge, even with standard approaches, can achieve this. Mini-incision surgery is clearly a cosmetic procedure in that the deep dissection is very similar to that performed with a standard-size skin incision; two-incision surgery may be "muscle sparing", but the procedure is usually prolonged and technically more difficult than mini- or standard surgery.

The Study

Because of all these questions related to minimally invasive surgery, we devised a randomized prospective study to compare a conventional posterior approach, a mini-posterior approach and a two-incision approach. Parameters compared included operative time, blood loss, hospital stay, complications, early functional return, then radiographic analysis of implant position and, in the future, radiographic interfaces and longevity.

Patients were selected on the basis of being suitable for minimally invasive surgery and cementless implants (◘ Table 4.1). Randomization occurred after the anesthetic, and blinding to some degree was achieved by placing a large occlusive dressing over the proximal thigh and buttock, hiding the wounds. This was left undisturbed for 48 h.

Post-Operative Education and Rehabilitation

The study is a randomized prospective study with full-patient informed consent and ethics approval achieved. Patients, once enrolled, were seen by a physiotherapist

◘ **Table 4.1.** Randomized prospective study comparing conventional posterior approach, mini-posterior approach and two-incision approach

	Two incision	Mini	Standard
Age (yrs)	61	58	59
BMI	26	28	28
HHS	57	54	62
WOMAC	49	44	41
SF-12 (Phys) (Mental)	31	38	37

pre-operatively and the post-operative rehabilitation program reviewed.

Patients are started on their rehabilitation program as soon as muscle control returns after the spinal anesthetic, usually 4–6 h after surgery.

Initial bed exercises including knee flexion, hip flexion and abduction, followed by independent transfers and ability to walk independently are recorded in terms of time, distance and angle depending on the activity. One difficulty encountered with therapists early in the study was the inherent prejudice which restricted them from pushing patients too hard post-operatively and the first day after surgery. This was often awkward with IV lines and catheters in situ. Another problem was the postural hypotension that occurred in most patients for the first 24 h post-operatively.

Patients were judged fit for discharge when they were able to transfer independently, walk at least 100 m, climb stairs, shower and toilet independently, and felt confident that they could manage at home.

In the Australasian health system there is not the same compunction existing to discharge patients by a certain time after surgery. In New Zealand, the average stay after joint replacement in the public sector is 7 days, while in the private system the average is just over 5 days. Patients in the study were enrolled because they wanted early discharge and rehabilitation and did not have the expectation of a certain stay in hospital.

Patients were clinically scored using HHS, also WOMAC and SF-12 Physical and Mental scores were generated. One of the difficulties faced was the lack of an early mobilization or early post-operative functional scoring system, so patients were timed until certain goals were reached.

Importantly, patients were not aware of which procedure was going to be performed, and they were all given the same expectation of early mobilization and discharge. However, this was not the expectation of same day discharge.

Patients were assessed daily as in-patients, at 10 days, 6 weeks, 3 months and 1 year. Plain radiographs are performed post-operatively, at 6 weeks, then 3 months and yearly. At 6 weeks a spiral CT scan is performed of the hip to determine implant positioning and post-operative leg-length discrepancy.

Results

Recruitment continues, but the preliminary results indicate that two-incision surgery is superior in terms of early return of muscle function and on average faster discharge from hospital (◻ Table 4.2). Two-incision patients spent on average just less than 3 days including the day of surgery. No patient was discharged still requiring opiates for pain control. Operative time was however longer in the two-incision group although blood loss was similar (◻ Table 4.3). Pain scores and HHS scores converge, so that by 3 months there is little difference between the groups (◻ Tables 4.4 and 4.5).

Radiographic review showed a trend towards increased acetabular anteversion and abduction as the incision size was reduced and interestingly the patient who dislocated, did so anteriorly and has a measured anteversion angle of 42° on the acetabular side. The patient had a closed reduction and has not gone on to re-dislocate to date. The ability to gauge leg length appeared to be more accurate with the two-incision technique.

Discussion

As surgeons, we should always consider the welfare of our patients first, and therefore make sure that a new technique being introduced is for the right reasons. It appears that two-incision surgery does have some benefit in terms of earlier return of function, but more experience is needed in order to be able to judge it fairly against established techniques. There is a significant learning curve as with any new technique, and compli-

cation rates should be audited to determine the overall safety of the procedure.

My own view is that same-day discharge after surgery does not really achieve anything except giving insurance carriers false expectations of being able to

◻ **Table 4.2.** Study results

Average time (h)	Two incision	Mini	Standard
Knee flexion >45°	5.3	91.1	21.3
Straight leg raise	45.3	117	94.4
Active abduction	6.00	6.15	9.10
Standing	11.40	20.00	6.35
Independent transfers	24.25	78.45	71.10
Stair climbing	68.20	94.3	76.30
Walk >40 m	24.4	48.2	48.00
Discharge	*64*	*98*	*96*

◻ **Table 4.3.** Study results

	Two incision	Mini	Standard
Operative time (min)	85	65	55
Pre-op Hb	138	138	155
Post-op Hb	105	104	110
Complications	1 anterior dislocation	–	1 calcar fracture

◻ **Table 4.4.** Mean Harris hip score

	Two incision	Mini	Standard
Pre-op	56	53	62
6 Weeks	91	84	78
3 Months	98	97	89

◻ **Table 4.5.** Mean pain scores (0–44)

	Two Incision	Mini	Standard
Pre-op	20	19	20
10 days	38	27	27
6 weeks	42	40	37
3 months	44	44	40

curtail costs associated with joint-replacement surgery even further. Intensive and aggressive back-up by health-care professionals is required, and whether it has any long-term benefit or risk in terms of outcome, has yet to be proven.

There is no doubt that more rapid rehabilitation is a realistic goal, achieved by a combination of muscle-sparing surgical techniques and more aggressive pre- and post-operative therapy. By enhancing patient expectations, we have now been able to shorten hospital stay following joint replacement significantly. Thirty years ago, in-patient care often stretched to 3 weeks or more, whereas today approximately 5 days is the average. If by using muscle-sparing techniques we can reduce hospital stay to 1 to 3 days, cosmetically improve the outcome with smaller incisions and shorten the period of recovery and return to function, then this is a reasonable aim. This can be achieved if there is no increase in complications and our accuracy of implant positioning can be maintained along with implant survival.

Conclusions

Patient expectation of a procedure plays an important role in determining outcomes. In total hip replacement, pre-operative teaching including engendering in patients the expectation of early discharge certainly has a significant effect. Reducing the size of the skin incision reinforces this expectation by making patients think of it as less of a procedure. From my own experience and data which is now appearing in our study, two-incision surgery has an advantage over simply smaller incision surgery or standard approaches. The explanation for this is not clear as, technically speaking, two-incision surgery is a significant challenge compared to familiar and conventional approaches. It is likely to be multifactorial including in-situ neck section, use of intermuscular plains and minimizing muscle release, and not placing the leg in extremes of position or aggressively mobilizing the femur by soft tissue release. Computer navigation in hip replacement offers a significant advantage by giving confidence normally only achieved by full surgical exposure and visualization, and in my view, is how two incision and mini-incision surgery will evolve into safer and more accessible procedures in the future.

Part II   The Hip

▼

Principles and History of Total Hip Arthroplasty

W.V. Arnold, R.H. Rothman

❽ "I think the exposure of the acetabulum never gets anything like mine and there have been catastrophic results on the femur ... I absolutely am opposed to its use by beginners but even with experts it is nothing like as good as the lateral exposure." (Professor Sir John Charnley, personal correspondence in reference to the Hardinge approach to Richard H. Rothman)

In 1982 Hardinge published a new surgical approach to total hip arthroplasty [1]. The benefit of this new approach was that it offered improved conditions for implant orientation as well as the correction of leg-length discrepancy. It also avoided the pitfalls of trochanteric osteotomy with its inherent risk of non-union and wire breakage. Technically, the approach was challenged as providing only limited surgical visualization while damaging the nerve supply to the hip abductors as well as placing other neurovascular structures at risk. These criticisms were countered by well-performed studies in the orthopedic literature which established the utility of the approach [2–5]. Despite initial strong criticisms, the Hardinge surgical approach to total hip arthroplasty – and various modifications thereof – has certainly withstood the test of time and is now used routinely for both primary and revision hip arthroplasty.

Today minimally invasive hip arthroplasty is being promoted as a new surgical approach to total hip arthroplasty. Again criticisms of this approach revolve around poor surgical visualization with all of its inherent risks. The comparison to the introduction of past surgical approaches such as that of Hardinge is both a good one and yet at the same time a poor one. Like previous surgical approaches, minimally invasive hip surgery should be judged in terms of the usual standards of hip arthro-

plasty: component positioning, dislocation risk, infection rate etc. Unlike its predecessors, this new surgical approach does not attempt to address some specific surgical shortcoming such as trochanteric non-union or acetabular cup mal-position. Rather the promotion of this technique has revolved around cosmesis and post-operative expediency: shorter hospital stay, less pain, less in-patient rehabilitation, quicker return to function. This is not to say that such goals are poor ones, since all surgeons would promote these benefits for their patients. However, these ends do not justify the means of a new surgical approach if it introduces new problems which are more significant than those encountered with established surgical approaches.

So far there are little peer-reviewed published data regarding minimally invasive hip arthroplasty, particularly when compared with its level of advertisement. The published data available would seem to fall on the side of the minimalists. Berger has recently published his results utilizing a two-incision minimally invasive technique [6]. His study involved 100 cases in which the average patient age was 55 and the average weight was 176 lbs. All of the patients were discharged to home with 75 patients going home the day of surgery. The complication rate was 1% due to one proximal femoral fracture. Radiographic analysis was performed on the first 30 patients and showed 91% of the femoral stems to be in neutral alignment and the average abduction angle of the acetabular component to be 45°. Wenz published data on a series of 124 minimally invasive hip-arthroplasty cases [7]. The approach used involved a modified posterior approach utilizing a single incision. The operation was performed more quickly and with less blood loss when compared with the traditional direct lateral approach. The rates of intra-operative and post-operative complications were comparable. The length of hospital stay was also comparable, although the minimally invasive surgery patients seemed to do better with their post-operative physical therapy. A higher percentage of these patients were also discharged to home.

Studies such as these are quite suggestive but lack the power of a randomized controlled study. In addition, anecdotal non-published data has not always been so supportive. To an outsider this would all seem to appear like the often-repeated cycle of some new idea, struggling to break into an established field. And this is certainly true. However, some relevant background information is needed to clarify this struggle.

Fixing What is not Broken

As with nearly anything touted as an innovation in hip arthroplasty, minimally invasive surgery faces an uphill battle for acceptance. The reason for this is that it must equal or outperform the current impressive standards of total hip arthroplasty. Total hip arthroplasty is currently one of the most successful of all surgeries performed. A recent review [8] has reinforced the low incidence of peri-operative complications encountered in the Medicare population with this surgery (1.0% mortality, 0.9% pulmonary embolus, 0.2% wound infection, 3.1% dislocation). Despite the success of innovations such as the use of cementless components, the fact remains that cemented Charnley prostheses have demonstrated excellent survival rates out to 20 years [9]. Such results are at once extremely satisfying to the orthopedist in terms of providing confidence in what can be offered to patients. These results are at the same time somewhat frustrating to those who wish to put forth what is felt to be a true innovation. All of this is further complicated in that it often takes 5-, 10- and 15-years follow-up to adequately judge the success or failure of any change.

Therefore, any potential innovation in hip arthroplasty is accompanied by a substantial risk. This risk is balanced by the potential benefit of the innovation. In the case of the Hardinge approach, any hip surgeon who has fought with the problem of trochanteric non-union can appreciate the benefit of this approach. A similar argument for minimally invasive hip replacement, in terms of correcting particular surgical shortcomings, cannot yet be made. While the goals of minimally inva-

sive surgery are clear (i.e., better cosmesis and quicker post-operative recovery), the attainment of these goals is less clear. It can be argued that the patient population presented by Berger in his report of his two-incision technique is not the typical patient population for total hip arthroplasty. While the goals of minimally invasive surgery were achieved in this study, these results may not translate so well to those achieved with a more typical elderly-patient population encumbered by their usual medical co-morbidities. Therefore, even if the risk of the operation remained constant, the benefits of the surgery likely do not. Compounding the difficulty in judging the effectiveness of minimally invasive surgery in achieving its stated goals is the undeniable fact that several of these goals are influenced by other disciplines. As an example, improved pain-management techniques may contribute significantly to the successes which are often credited to minimally invasive surgery alone.

Revolutionary?

In many respects the concept of minimally invasive total hip arthroplasty is hardly revolutionary. It makes no pretences towards improving prosthesis fixation or decreasing osteolysis. It contributes nothing towards solving one of the greatest problems in the field; that is, providing younger patients with a lifelong prosthesis. Nonetheless, it is a revolutionary concept in other respects. Today's hip arthroplasty patients have benefited significantly from decades of bio-engineering advances; however, the topics of wear rate, free-radical polymerization and alumina-grain size are rather mundane to the general public. What patients do understand and find revolutionary are promises of shorter hospital stays, less need for in-patient rehabilitation and a quicker return to their daily activities. Understandably, the public excitement over minimally invasive total hip arthropolasty has been tremendous.

Unfortunately, this excitement is often mixed with misinformation. One by-product of the promises of 23-h-hospital stays with a discharge to home has been a lessening of the perception of total hip arthroplasty as major surgery. Another very common misperception is the universality of minimally invasive surgery. Most physicians would agree that the minimally invasive approach becomes tenuous with obese patients. The responsibility falls upon the physician to properly educate patients and temper their expectations with regard to minimally invasive surgery. Surgeons must also remind themselves that the usual medical risks of total hip arthroplasty, such as post-operative myocardial infarction or venous thromboembolism, do not evaporate simply because a patient goes home after 23 h.

Finally, for minimally invasive arthroplasty to truly revolutionize the field of hip replacement it must be broadly applicable. That is, any well-trained orthopedic surgeon specializing in joint replacement should be able to competently perform the procedure. In a practical sense, anything short of this makes minimally invasive surgery more of a dream than a reality for the average patient.

Judging Minimally Invasive Hip Arthroplasty

Although it promises new advances with regard to improved cosmesis and post-operative expediency, minimally invasive hip replacement must be ultimately judged by the same criteria as have previous surgical exposures. These criteria are nothing more than the classic surgical principles of obtaining good visualization, treating tissues in a gentle and atraumatic fashion, avoiding damage to nerves and blood vessels, obtaining absolute hemostasis and performing the surgery in a swift and efficient manner. The achievement of these principles translates into measurable parameters, such as correct component position which minimizes the risk of dislocation. Atraumatic treatment of tissues decreases the risks of infection, heterotopic ossification and postoperative limp. Currently, at our institution we use a lateral Hardinge-type surgical approach for hip arthroplasty. The operation can be performed efficiently with an average operative time of 45 min. Adherence to the surgical principles just described have led to good results with minimal complications: 0.4% neurovascular injury, 0.2% dislocation rate, 0.4% infection rate. It is not obvious that minimally invasive hip arthroplasty presents any particular advantage in achieving any of these surgical goals. Using the minimally invasive approach, good visualization of the acetabulum is more difficult to achieve, thereby increasing the risk of poor component positioning. Because of the smaller working space, great care must be taken to not traumatize soft tissues by vigorous retraction. Care needs to be taken in reaming the acetabulum and broaching the femur in order to insure that the skin edges of the incision are not damaged. Repeated contact of surgical instruments with damaged skin edges during these procedures risks pulling skin flora into the operative wound.

These obvious increased risks have not simply been ignored in minimally invasive surgery. The two-incision approach incorporates the use of fluoroscopy to compensate for visual deficits in placing the acetabular component. With this technique, Berger has reported good results with component placement [6]. Others are trying to take advantage of the emerging technology of computer navigation in a similar way to improve the more limited visualization inherent in minimally invasive surgery. Specifically, DiGioia et al. [10] reported on 33 mini-incision cases in which computer navigation was employed. They found no difference in the acetabular cup alignment in the mini-incision technique compared with that obtained using a traditional posterior approach. Overall, the cup alignment for both groups was within 5° of the preoperatively planned alignment of 45° of abduction and 20° of flexion. While the use of additional technology may allow for the maintenance of good component placement, it is not clear that similar advantages are obtained in minimizing neurovascular injury. Also it is important to appreciate that good cup placement can still be obtained even if poor techniques of acetabular reaming are done. For example, an acetabulum can be over-reamed with significant damage done to the anterior or posterior column, although the radiographic appearance of the cup placement may be excellent. At the time of revision surgery this can become a major problem which could have been easily avoided during the primary procedure.

Other modifications introduced for minimally invasive hip replacement have also included the introduction of new instrumentation which is meant to facilitate the procedure and minimize the risks of soft-tissue trauma. Some of this new instrumentation is clearly beneficial; however, it also represents an area where the marketplace has collided with a surgical innovation. As a new surgical approach, minimally invasive surgery provides some promotional advantage for surgeons. However, the approach itself offers little advantage to orthopedic companies because it employs no new special prosthetic components. Where companies have capitalized on this new technique has been in promoting new instrument systems that are "essential" to performing this new approach. Unlike in the case of new prosthetic components, where there is usually at least some available supportive biomechanical data, these new instrument systems are being rigorously promoted while there is still relatively little data or experience to support their effectiveness. Clearly, the surgeon needs to maintain a certain level of healthy skepticism to evaluate which of these new company-driven "improvements" are truly necessary. Unfortunately, it has been the aggressive commercialization of minimally invasive surgery which has turned many orthopedists against it.

Conclusions

In conclusion, minimally invasive hip arthroplasty represents nothing more than the introduction of new surgical approaches into the field of hip replacement. At its best, minimally invasive surgery is a true revolution which can potentially benefit a significant number, albeit not all, hip arthroplasty patients. If so, it deserves its current attention and should be offered as a real alternative to traditional total hip arthroplasty. It should be capable of being performed competently by any well-trained hip arthroplasty surgeon. At its worst, minimally invasive surgery is the latest in a long litany of promised innovations which have failed to advance the field. The only way to judge minimally invasive hip arthroplasty is to perform well-controlled unbiased multicenter trials with adequate and appropriate follow-up. In the meantime, surgeons need to provide their own honest self-assessment of whether minimally invasive hip arthroplasty in their hands can deliver benefits without undue risks to patients. This is nothing more than a reaffirmation of the old surgical adage *primum non nocere*.

References

1. Hardinge K (1982) The direct lateral approach to the hip. J Bone Joint Surg 64B: 17–19
2. Minns RJ, Crawford RJ, Porter ML, Hardinge K (1993) Muscle strength following total hip arthroplasty: a comparison of trochanteric osteotomy and the direct lateral approach. J Arthroplasty 8: 625–627
3. Mulliken BD, Rorabeck CH, Bourne RB, Nayak N (1998) A modified direct lateral approach in total hip arthroplasty: a comprehensive review. J Arthroplasty 13: 737–747
4. Horwitz BR, Rockowitz NL, Goll SR, Booth RE, Balderston RA, Rothman RH, Cohn JC (1993) A prospective randomized comparison of two surgical approaches to total hip arthroplasty. Clin Orthop 291: 154–163
5. Simmons C, Izant TH, Rothman RH, Booth RE, Balderston RA (1991) Femoral neuropathy following total hip arthroplasty: anatomic study, case reports, and literature review. J Arthroplasty 6: S59–S66
6. Berger RA (2003) Total hip arthroplasty using the minimally invasive two-incision approach. Clin Orthop 417: 232–241
7. Wenz JF, Gurkan I, Jibodh SR (2002) Mini-incision total hip arthroplasty: a comparative assessment of perioperative outcomes. Orthopedics 25: 1031–1043
8. Mahomed NN, Barrett JA, Katz JN, Phillips CB, Losina E, Lew RA, Guadagnoli E, Harris WH, Poss R, Baron JA (2003) Rates and outcomes of primary and revision total hip replacement in the United States medicare population. J Bone Joint Surg 85A: 27–32
9. Schulte KR, Callaghan JJ, Kelley SS, Johnston RC (1993) The outcome of Charnley total hip arthroplasty with cement after a minimum twenty-year follow-up. The results of one surgeon. J Bone Joint Surg 75A: 961–975
10. DiGioia III AM, Plakseychuk AY, Levison TJ, Jaramaz B (2003) Mini-incision technique for total hip arthroplasty with navigation. J Arthroplasty 18: 123–128

Traditional Approaches to the Hip

Direct Anterior Approach to the Hip

F. Rachbauer, M. Nogler

The first descriptions of the anterior approach to the hip are attributed to Sprengel (1878), Bardenheuer (1907), Depuy de Frenelle (1924) and Larghi. Smith-Peterson (1917, 1949) has improved and revived the interest in this approach, which he utilized for his technique in mold arthroplasty [1–4]. Nearly all surgery of the hip joint may be carried out through this approach, or separate parts can be used for different purposes.

The whole iliac wing and the hip joint can be approached by the iliac portion of the incision. It is especially used for access to the anterolateral part of the femoral head and neck. It permits a direct access to the acetabulum and frees the superior part of the femur without extensive detachment of the gluteal muscles from the iliac wing or without tenotomies of the outer rotators. Letournel and Judet (1974) described an iliofemoral approach which allows surgical extension to laterally expose the anterior and posterior pelvic columns [2, 4].

The inferior part of the approach, denominated as Hueter-Schede, does not even need any muscular detachment besides the eventual dissection of the tendinous origin of the rectus femoris muscle [2, 3].

The anterior approach gives safe access to the hip joint and ilium by exploiting the internervous plane between the sartorius and the tensor fasciae latae muscles. Its is used for

- Open reduction of congenital dislocations of the hip
- Pelvic osteotomies
- Excision of tumors of hip and pelvis
- Total hip arthroplasty
- Hemiarthroplasty
- Resurfacing arthroplasty
- Synovial biopsies.

Technique

The patient is placed supine on the operating table. To free the posterior border of the iliac wing put a small pad under the affected buttock to push the affected hemipelvis forward. The whole lower extremity is prepared to allow manipulation of the leg and the hip during the intervention.

Identify the anterior superior iliac spine, which is subcutaneous and easily palpable in thin patients. The groove between the tensor fasciae latae and sartorial muscle is easily found below the anterior superior iliac spine. In obese patients, when covered by adipose tissue, you can locate it more easily if you bring your thumbs up from distal.

The iliac crest serves as a point of origin and insertion for the gluteal and the tensor fasciae latae muscles and can be palpated subcutaneously.

The skin incision starts in the middle of the iliac crest, but for a larger approach the starting point can also be set more posteriorly. The incision follows the crest approximately 2 cm distal to prevent painful adhesions of the scar to the bone. It proceeds to the anterior superior iliac spine and from there is vertically curved down the thigh heading toward the lateral border of the patella. (◻ Fig. 6.1).

The approach uses an internervous plane between the femoral nerve and the superior gluteal nerve. It lies superficially between the sartorial and the tensor fasciae latae muscles, the deep dissection uses the plane between the rectus femoris and the gluteus medius and minimus muscles.

The superficial and the profound fasciae lateral to the sartorial muscle are incised on the medial border of the tensor fasciae latae muscle. The lateral cutaneous

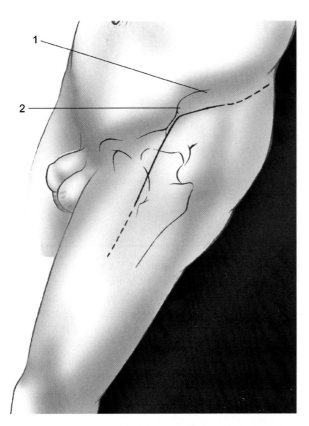

Fig. 6.1. The skin incision runs parallel to the iliac crest and proceeds to the superior iliac spine where in vertically curves down the thigh heading toward the lateral border of the patella. *1* iliac crest; *2* anterior superior iliac spine

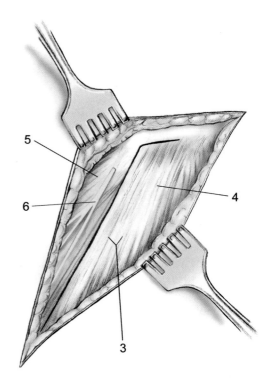

Fig. 6.2. The lateral femoral cutaneous nerve pierces the deep fascia close to the intermuscular interval between the tensor fasciae latae and the sartorius. Incise the facia on the medial side of the tensor fasciae latea and retract the sartorius with the lateral femoral cutaneous nerve superomedially and the tensor fasciae latae inferolaterally. *3* fascia lata; *4* fascia overlying tensor fasciae latae; *5* fascia overlying sartorius; *6* lateral femoral cutaneous nerve

femoral nerve, which pierces the deep fascia just below the anterior superior iliac spine, is identified and shifted with the sartorial muscle (■ Fig. 6.2). Staying within the fascial sheath of this muscle will protect you from damaging the lateral femoral cutaneous nerve because the nerve runs over the fascia of the sartorius. It should be noted that the nerve may as well lie lateral to the sartorial muscle. Retract the sartorius upwards and medially and the tensor fascia latae downwards and laterally.

The anterior part of the tensor fasciae latae muscle is subperiostally detached from the iliac wing where it is fibrously attached to the iliac crest. This can be performed in an avascular zone as it is not necessary to cut muscle fibers. Following detachment of the tensor fasciae latae, there is a good view on the gluteus medius muscle and the rectus femoris muscle, which contrasts

by its tendineous appearance from the neighboring muscles.

With a periosteal elevator, strip the periosteum with the attachments of the gluteus medius and minimus muscles from the lateral surface of the ilium. Control bleeding from the nutrient vessels by packing the interval between the ilium and the reflected muscles with gauze sponges. Individual bleeding points can be controlled by the application of bone wax.

Now carry the dissection through the deep fascia of the thigh and between the tensor fasciae latae laterally and the sartorius and rectus femoris medially. Clamp and ligate the ascending branch of the lateral femoral circumflex artery, which lies 5 cm distal to the hip joint.

Identify the origin of the rectus femoris muscle (■ Fig. 6.3). The rectus femoris originates with its direct head from the anterior inferior iliac spine, and the

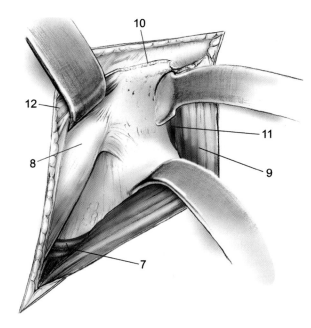

Fig. 6.3. Following subperiostal detachment of the tensor fasciae latae from the iliac wing identify the origin of the rectus femoris muscle (direct and reflected head). The ascending branch of the lateral femoral circumflex artery, which lies 5 cm distal to the hip joint has to be clamped or ligated. *7* ascending branch of lateral femoral circumflex vessels; *8* rectus femoris with its direct and reflected head; *9* tensor fasciae latae; *10* detachment of tensor fasciae latae at iliac crest; *11* gluteus medius; *12* sartorius

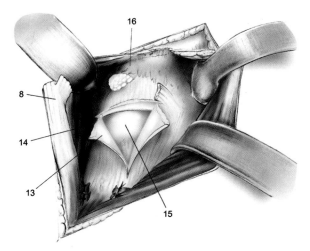

Fig. 6.4. Following detachment of the rectus femoris from both its origins bluntly separate the iliopsoas muscle from the capsule medially and retract the gluteus muscle laterally. Now the hip joint capsule is fully exposed and can be incised. *8* rectus femoris; *13* capsule of the hip joint; *14* psoas muscle; *15* femoral head; *16* anterior inferior iliac spine

reflected head from the superiolateral lip of the acetabulum and the anterior capsule of the hip joint. The reflecting head is intimate with the capsule and has to be split from the capsule of the adjacent hip joint. Detach the rectus femoris from both its origins and retract it medially. Retract the gluteus medius laterally.

The iliopsoas muscle is also separated from the capsule by blunt dissection and held aside. Then the whole anterior aspect of the hip joint is exposed.

The capsule of the hip joint is now exposed. Inferomedially, you can see the iliopsoas as it approaches the lesser trochanter: retract it medially. The iliopsoas is often partly attached to the inferior aspect of the hip joint capsule and must be released from it.

Inferolaterally, the shaft of the femur lies under cover of the vastus lateralis. Adduct and fully externally rotate the leg to put the capsule on stretch; incise the hip joint capsule as the surgery requires. The capsule is longitudinally incised following the axis of the femoral neck, and transversally dissected parallel to the acetabular roof. In order to anteriorly dislocate the hip, the capsule has to be opened as wide as necessary and may be excised as well as a part of the acetabular labrum (**◘** Fig. 6.4). Dislocate the hip by external rotation and adduction.

Dangers

The lateral femoral cutaneous nerve usually leaves the pelvis by passing deep to the lateral end of the inguinal ligament about 1 cm medial to the anterior superior iliac spine. The nerve then splits into anterior and posterior divisions approximately 5 cm below the anterior superior iliac spine and continues distally to innervate the skin over the lateral aspect of the thigh. Alternatively, the nerve may be absent, with a branch from the femoral nerve arising below the inguinal ligament, or it may be replaced by the ilioinguinal nerve.

The nerve should be preserved when you incise the fascia between the sartorius and the tensor fasciae latae. If the nerve is cut, this may lead to the formation of a painful neuroma and may produce an area of diminished sensation on the lateral aspect of the thigh (meralgia paresthetica).

The variability of the course of the lateral femoral cutaneous nerve suggests that during any operative approach to the iliac crest or inguinal region, awareness that it may cross the surgical site is the only way to prevent injury to this nerve.

The ascending branch of the lateral femoral circumflex artery crosses the operative field, running proximally in the internervous plane between the tensor fasciae latae and the sartorius. Ligate or coagulate it when you separate the two muscles.

Extensile Procedures

The skin incision may be extended posteriorly along the iliac crest to expose the iliac bone.

To extend the approach distally, lengthen the skin incision downward along the anterolateral aspect of the thigh. Incise the fascia lata in line with the skin incision; underneath lies the interval between the vastus lateralis and the rectus femoris. To expose the shaft of the femur you will have to split muscle fibers in this interval. You may as well use the interval between the vastus lateralis muscle and the intermuscular septum.

The approach can be as well extended to visualize the inner and outer wall of the pelvis for pelvic osteotomy. Gently strip the muscular coverings from the bone at the level of the origin of the reflected head of rectus using blunt instruments. This dissection will lead you into the sciatic notch. Take great care to stay close to the bone, since the sciatic nerve is also emerging through the notch. Following detachment of the rectus femoris from the anterior inferior iliac spine, carefully lift off the iliacus muscle from the inside of the pelvis. Proceed by blunt dissection until the greater sciatic notch is reached and both instruments are in contact with each other and with the bone of the sciatic notch. This allows sufficient visualization of the entire thickness of the pelvis to permitting an accurate osteotomy.

For exposure of the posterior column detach the insertion of the glutei from the greater trochanter. This can be performed either by dividing this insertion with a knife or preferably by a trochanteric osteotomy. Pay attention to the superior gluteal nerve and artery which emerge through the greater sciatic notch and serve the gluteus medius and minimus muscles. Do not stretch these vessels unless you risk thrombosis that may lead to massive muscle necrosis. Part of the posterior column of the acetabulum and the lateral aspect of the iliac crest are now exposed.

To access the inner part of the iliac wing until the sacroiliac joint, subperiosteally lift off the iliacus muscle after detachment of the origins of the abdominal muscles from the iliac crest.

References

1. Bauer R, Kerschbauer F, Poisel S (1990) Operative Zugangswege in Orthopädie und Traumatologie. Vorderer Zugang zum Hüftgelenk. Thieme, Stuttgart, New York pp 117–118
2. Calandruccio R (1992) Voies d'abord de la hanche. In Roy-Camille R, Laurin CA, Riley Jr LH (eds): Atlas des chirurgie orthopédique, Tome 3 Membre inférieur. Masson, Paris, Milan, Barcelona, Bonn, pp 65–70
3. Crenshaw AH (1987) Campbell's Operative Orthopaedics. Surgical approaches. Mosby, St. Louis, Washington DC, Toronto, pp 58–59
4. Hoppenfeld S, deBoer P (1994) Surgical Exposures in Orthopaedics; The anatomic approach; Chapter Eight; The Hip & Acetabulum. JB Lippincott, Philadelphia, pp 323–341
5. Weber M, Ganz R (2002) Der vordere Zugang zu Becken und Hüftgelenk. Modifizierter Smith-Petersen-Zugang sowie Erweiterungsmöglichkeiten. Operat Orthop Traumatol 14:265–279

Modified Direct Lateral Approach

V. Krebs, E. Sladek, A. Baddar, W. Barsoum, L.S. Borden

Introduction

The direct lateral approach provides a number of distinct advantages over the others approaches most commonly used. It allows for excellent exposure of the acetabulum and femur with the option for extension in revision and complex primary cases. The advantages of the direct lateral approach include: preservation of the posterior capsule, a dislocation rate <1% and a low incidence of sciatic nerve injury. Its main drawbacks are a reported increased risk of heterotopic ossification and superior gluteal nerve injury with resultant abductor weakness and limp.

Evolution of the Lateral Approach

The direct lateral approach and numerous modifications have become popular since the 1982 publication by Hardinge; the technique combined in a reproducible manner specific technical points of exposures described by Kocher, McFarland and Osborne, and Bauer. Hardinge described a gluteal sparing technique that splits the muscle anterior and inferior, preserving the proximal insertion. The Hardinge technique did not describe handling of the gluteus minimus muscle detachment and reattachment to the trochanter. A modification of the Hardinge direct lateral approach used and taught by the senior author for the past 15 years is subsequently described. The modifications limit disruption of the abductor mechanism, preserve the tissue integrity, allow wide femoral and acetabular exposure and result in an anatomic tissue repair. The modified direct lateral approach is appropriate for all primary and revision cases, and can be easily extended in complicated situations. Limited skin incisions less than 10 cm can be performed in thin patients, but difficulties can arise in muscular or obese individuals, given the fact that this is a muscle-splitting procedure.

Technique

Operating Room

No specific modifications to the operative setting are needed for the procedure. A beanbag or pegboard positioner is used on a standard operating-room table. The use of laminar flow and surgical hoods is dependent on the surgeon's preference and availability.

Instruments

A standard hip tray including a variety of sharp and blunt Hohmann retractors, Cobra retractors, and a Charnley self-retractor are preferred for this procedure. In general, no gross modifications to the oscillating saw, acetabular reamers or broach handles are necessary to perform this approach, although offset acetabular reamer handles and acetabular insertors are helpful.

Positioning

This approach is performed in a lateral decubitus position, and is dependant on knowledge of the patient and the pelvic orientation prior to sterile preparation and draping. Alignment and stability of the pelvis are vital to cup orientation, and can be achieved using a variety of stabilization methods, including, but not limited to, a peg board, kidney rests or a vacuum positioning bag. The pegboard is an easy and reproducible method for achieving pelvic stability. Four pegs are placed in the following order:

1. anterior inferior peg at the level of the pubic symphysis,
2. posterior peg at the level of the lumbosacral junction,
3. anterior peg at the level of the xyphoid process,
4. posterior peg at the level of the inferior scapular angle.

Skin Incision

The incision can range from 6–15 cm, and depends on the patient's body habitus; length is directly proportional to the depth of the trochanter. A straight or curvilinear incision centered over the tip of the greater trochanter is used (◘ Fig. 6.5). The proximal portion curves posteriorly while the distal portion extends longitudinally in line with the anterior margin of the femur. With the leg flexed 90°, the incision will become a straight line, and the trochanter should remain centralized. The proximal incision in flexion exposes of the femoral canal, while the distal portion allows acetabular preparation in extension. Awareness of this relationship ensures proper incision mapping and can limit length. In obese patients, a more anteriorly placed incision improves exposure, decreases the need for additional retraction, and also limits the need for a lengthy incision.

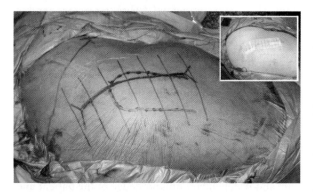

◘ **Fig. 6.5.** Skin incision and superficial landmarks

Superficial Muscle Dissection

After dissection through the subcutaneous tissues, the fascia lata is exposed and split in line with its fibers posteriorly over the tip of the greater trochanter. The distal end runs along the anterior border of the femur, and the proximal extent in line with the fascial lines and muscle fibers of the gluteus maximus. The appearance of this fascial dissection is that of a lazy "S" shape. The abductor muscles are now centered in the operative field, and the bursa is released to expose the proximal portion of the vastus lateralis. A Charnley self-retractor can be placed with the anterior blade deep to the fascia and the posterior blade above the fascia in the subcutaneous adipose, both at the level of the greater trochanter.

Deep Muscle Dissection

The gluteus medius proximal muscle split is started at the junction between the middle and anterior third of the greater trochanter in a palpable raphe and extends in line with muscle fibers proximally; the bulk or proximal 2/3 of the medius is left attached to the greater trochanter (◘ Fig. 6.6). Care must be taken to avoid splitting the gluteus medius too superiorly as this may injure the most inferior branch of the superior gluteal nerve which is located approximately 3–4 cm proximal to the tip of the greater trochanter. The incision is then carried out distally along the tendinous portion along the gluteus-medius insertion into the vastus lateralis. A tendinous cuff should be left on both the greater trochanter and free muscle flap to allow for later repair. The superficial vastus fascia should be split in the line of the anterior femur approximately 3–4 cm distally to the inferior insertion of the gluteus medius. A tagging stitch at the superior portion of the tendinous remnant of the gluteus medius can be used for retraction as it is released from the underlying gluteus minimus muscle and anterior capsule through an adipose tissue plane. In severely contracted or revision situations this plane may not be easily defined. A straightened cobra retractor is then placed inferior to the capsule.

The gluteus minimus insertion is then identified approximately 1.4 cm medial to the gluteus medius insertion along the anterior trochanteric ridge. A longitudinal incision should be made through the minimus and capsule at the superior aspect of the greater trochanter, traveling vertically and superiorly in line with the muscle fibers to the posterior superior corner of the acetabulum (◘ Fig. 6.7). It is important that this incision is properly placed since it will be critical for acetabular and femoral exposure, as well as for later

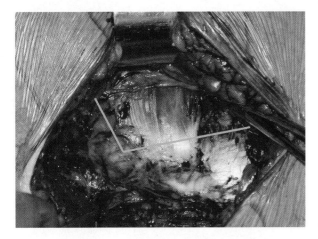

◘ **Fig. 6.6.** The gluteus medius proximal muscle split at the junction between the middle and anterior third of the greater trochanter

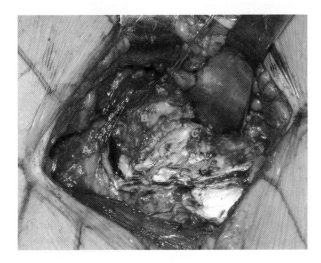

◘ **Fig. 6.7.** Incision and reflection of the gluteus minimus with underlying capsule. A longitudinal incision starting at the superior aspect of the greater trochanter traveling vertically and superiorly in line with the muscle fibers to the posterior superior corner of the acetabulum. A=Gluteus Medius. B=Gluteus Minimus. C=Inferior capsule and femoral neck

repair. The minimus incision/release requires gentle retraction of the remaining anterior edge of the gluteus medius as excessive retraction can lead to heterotopic ossification within the muscle. A second capsular incision is then made horizontally along the inferior border of the minimus along the femoral neck from the trochanter to the acetabular rim. The minimus and capsule between these two splits should then be elevated off the femoral neck and reflected anteriorly. The inferior capsule can be removed in its entirety if contracted, or retained if compliant for later repair. The hip is dislocated with a combination of forward flexion and gentle external rotation. If the hip does not dislocate with gentle manipulation, then the superior capsular split and the inferior excision of the capsule should be revisited. Failure to release a contracted anterior capsule can result in a difficult dislocation and may increase the risk for fracture of the proximal femur in patients with osteoporotic bone.

Femoral Exposure

With firm but gentle adduction, flexion and external rotation, the head may be placed within the surgical field. Cobra retractors are then placed around the femoral neck to protect the underlying soft tissues while the neck cut is made, and the posterior impinging osteophytes are removed. Any remaining inferior capsule that is tethering the femur can be released to facilitate exposure and to prevent anterior soft-tissue impingement.

Preparation of the femoral canal can occur before or after acetabular preparation, but in our opinion is more easily performed afterwards. With the hip flexed, adducted and externally rotated, the foot and lower leg are placed in a sterile leg bag. The femoral canal is then accessible through the proximal portion of the incision (◘ Fig. 6.8). One retractor should be placed behind the greater trochanter to keep the skin and fascia lata retracted while a second retractor is placed around the anterior portion of the neck cut to retract the psoas muscle and anterior soft tissues. The posterior retractor should be placed prior to externally rotating the femur in order to avoid inadvertent placement of the retractor on the sciatic nerve. This exposure allows the final preparation of the femur, using reamers and broaches under direct visualization.

6.2

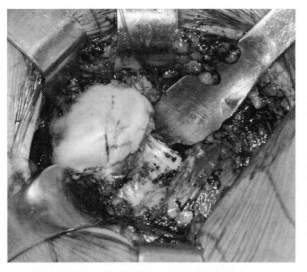
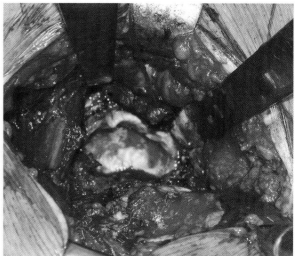

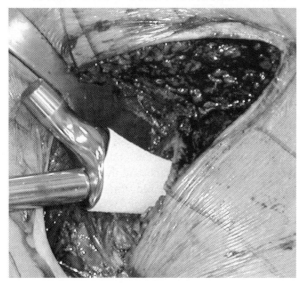
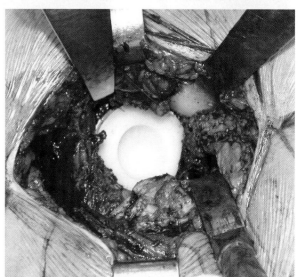

◾ **Fig. 6.8.** Femoral exposure

◾ **Fig. 6.9.** Acetabular exposure

Acetabular Exposure

Acetabular exposure is typically accomplished using a combination of Hohmann retractors. A blunt Hohmann can be placed posteriorly and inferiorly around the edge of the acetabulum just posterior to the insertion of the transverse acetabular ligament. This retractor will create leverage on the osteotomy to move the femur distally and out of the way. This maneuver is critical for acetabular exposure and works best with the leg in a slightly flexed and externally rotated position. It is important that this retractor is placed directly on bone and not posteriorly where it could potentially injure the sciatic nerve. A sharp narrow Hohmann retractor is placed beneath the minimus and capsular sleeve at the most superior position of the acetabulum between the margin of the labrum and the superior capsule. This retractor can be tapped into the ileum, freeing the assistant's hands. If necessary, a third blunt Hohmann can be carefully placed over the anterior medial edge of the

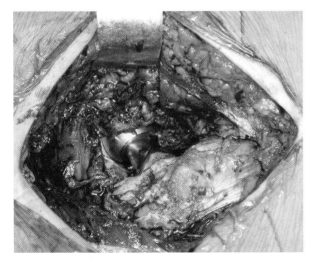

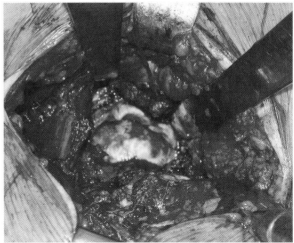

Fig. 6.10. Final component orientation

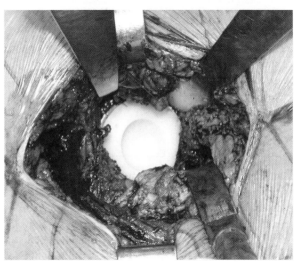

acetabulum and retracted gently to avoid injury to the femoral nerve and artery. The labrum is excised circumferentially, and the transverse acetabular ligament is retained unless it compromises exposure or reamer access.

Acetabular reaming (■ Fig. 6.9) can then be undertaken in a straightforward manner under direct visualization. The retractors should not interfere with the reamer and cause an undesired deflection. After preparation of the socket, trials or final components can be placed. Orientation of the components is dependent on stable and appropriate patient positioning, performed at the start of the case, and bony landmarks (■ Fig. 6.10). Acetabular osteophytes should also be removed to prevent impingement; the posterior inferior osteophytes are most critical as they can create anterior instability. The cleared ischium is also an excellent landmark for proper acetabular flexion.

Fig. 6.11. Gluteus minimus muscle and superior joint capsule repair to the anterior portion of the greater trochanter with trans-osseous monofilament absorbable suture. A=Drilling for repair. B=Minimus reattachment. C=Final anatomic repair

Wound Closure

Proper closure is critical for implant stability and restoration of muscular anatomy. After final hip reduction, the remaining anterior superior portion of the joint capsule and the overlying gluteus minimus muscle are re-attached to the anterior portion of the greater trochanter with trans-osseous monofilament absorbable suture (■ Fig. 6.11). As these are pulled and tied snug, the leg will need to be brought into slight abduction and internal rotation to take tension off the repair. The longitudinal split up the minimus and capsule should also be repaired to the remaining cuff of capsule and muscle just under the attached edge of the gluteus medius. The medius is then repaired as a separate layer by bringing the tagged corner to its anatomic position, and then suturing the cuff of tendon to the remnant on the antero-lateral trochanter (■ Fig. 6.12). Suturing the overlying fascia, avoiding deep stitches

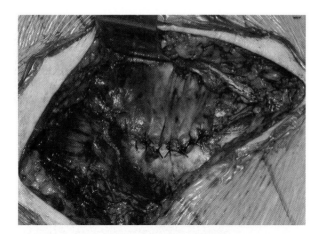

Fig. 6.12. Gluteus medius repair, suturing the cuff of tendon to the remnant on the antero-lateral trochanter

that will damage the muscle, closes the proximal split in the medius. The fascia lata, subcutaneous tissue and skin are then closed. In most cases a drain is not required.

Challenges

The direct lateral approach is an extremely versatile approach. It allows direct visualization of both the acetabulum and femur during preparation. It can be readily extended distally along the femur to allow for cabling, strut grafting, plating etc. as may be needed in more complex or revision cases. It has an inherently low risk of dislocation or nerve palsy. The greatest concern has been over abductor weakness, but with appropriate tissue-handling and repair of both the gluteus minimus and gluteus medius it can be avoided.

Inadequate removal of the inferior capsule as well as an inadequate longitudinal split along the superior-posterior portion of the capsule are the two biggest impediments to acetabular exposure. Retraction of the femur out of the field of the acetabulum can be particularly difficult if a portion of the inferior capsule remains. The sciatic and femoral nerves are at minimal risk as long as retractor placement is done carefully and with a good understanding of the anatomical position of these nerves.

References

1. Barber TC, Roger DJ, Goodman SB, Schurman DJ (1996) Early outcome of total hip arthroplasty using the direct lateral vs the posterior surgical approach. Orthopedics 19(10): 873–875
2. Masonis JL, Bourne RB (2002) Surgical approach, abductor function, and total hip arthroplasty dislocation. Clin Orthop 405: 46–53
3. DeWal H, Su E, DiCesare PE (2003) Instability following total hip arthroplasty. Am J Orthop 32: 377–382
4. Hedlundh U, Hybbinette CH, Fredin H (1995) Influence of surgical approach on dislocations after Charnley hip arthroplasty. J Arthroplasty 10(5): 609–614
5. Hewitt JD, Glisson RR, Guilak F, Vail TP (2002) The mechanical properties of the human hip capsule ligaments. J Arthroplasty 17(1): 82–89
6. Kennon RE, Keggi JM, Wetmore RS, Zatorski LE, Huo MH, Keggi KJ (2003) Total hip arthroplasty through a minimally invasive anterior surgical approach. J Bone Joint Surg Am 85-A [Suppl 4]: 39–48
7. Madsen MS, Ritter MA, Morris HH, Meding JB, Berend ME, Faris PM, Vardaxis VG (2004) The effect of total hip arthroplasty surgical approach on gait. J Orthop Res 22(1): 44–50
8. Masonis JL, Bourne RB (2002) Surgical approach, abductor function, and total hip arthroplasty dislocation. Clin Orthop 405: 46–53
9. Masterson EL, Masri BA, Duncan CP (1998) Surgical approaches in revision hip replacement. J Am Acad Orthop Surg 6(2): 84–92
10. Morrey BF, Adams RA, Cabanela ME (1984) Comparison of heterotopic bone after anterolateral, transtrochanteric, and posterior approaches for total hip arthroplasty. Clin Orthop 188: 160–167
11. Mulliken BD, Rorabeck CH, Bourne RB, Nayak N (1995) The surgical approach to total hip arthroplasty: complications and utility of a modified direct lateral approach. Iowa Orthop J 15: 48–61
12. Navarro RA, Schmalzried TP, Amstutz HC, Dorey FJ (1995) Surgical approach and nerve palsy in total hip arthroplasty. J Arthroplasty 10(1): 1–5
13. Nezry N, Jeanrot C, Vinh TS, Ganz R, Tomeno B, Anract P (2003) Partial anterior trochanteric osteotomy in total hip arthroplasty: surgical technique and preliminary results of 127 cases. J Arthroplasty 18(3): 333–337
14. Parker MJ, Pervez H (2002) Surgical approaches for inserting hemiarthroplasty of the hip. Cochrane Database Syst Rev. (3): CD001707
15. Robinson RP, Robinson HJ Jr, Salvati EA (1980) Comparison of the transtrochanteric and posterior approaches for total hip replacement. Clin Orthop 147: 143–147
16. Weeden SH, Paprosky WG, Bowling JW (2003) The early dislocation rate in primary total hip arthroplasty following the posterior approach with posterior soft-tissue repair. J Arthroplasty 18: 709–713
17. White RE Jr, Forness TJ, Allman JK, Junick DW (2001) Effect of posterior capsular repair on early dislocation in primary total hip replacement. Clin Orthop 393: 163–167
18. Woolson ST, Rahimtoola ZO (1999) Risk factors for dislocation during the first 3 months after primary total hip replacement. J Arthroplasty 14: 662–668
19. Zimmerma S, Hawkes WG, Hudson JI et al. (2002) Outcomes of surgical management of total HIP replacement in patients aged 65 years and older: cemented versus cementless femoral components and lateral or anterolateral versus posterior anatomical approach. J Orthop Res 20: 182–191

An Extensile Posterior Exposure for Primary and Revision Hip Arthroplasty

C.S. Ranawat, V.J. Rasquinha, A.S. Ranawat, K. Miyasaka

Introduction

The posterior approach to the hip joint has enjoyed varying degrees of popularity among orthopedic surgeons over the past 125 years. There is general agreement that the posterior approach offers the advantages of reduced blood loss, early post-operative recovery and a reduced hospital stay [1, 2]. The main arguments against the use of posterior approach are an increased risk of dislocation following hip replacement surgery [2–8], difficulty in component orientation and inadequate visualization of the acetabulum [9, 10].

The senior author has been using the posterior approach for total hip arthroplasty for over 25 years in the performance of more than 4000 hip arthroplasties, in the context of both primary and revision hip arthroplasty. The senior author alternatively used the transtrochanteric and anterolateral approaches for exposures during the seventies and early eighties. Over the years, the technique has evolved to maximize the exposure without jeopardizing soft-tissue stability. The most important factor in avoiding many of the problems blamed on the posterior approach was to obtain an extensile acetabular exposure without interfering with the abductor mechanism or performing an unnecessary trochanteric osteotomy. This would allow the surgeon to place the components in the proper orientation with respect to the bony anatomy.

This paper outlines the specific steps, so far not described in the literature, to improve acetabular exposure by anterior mobilization of the proximal femur. Data is also presented on 100 consecutive patients to assess the reproducibility of component placement in cemented total hip replacement surgery.

Technique

After induction of hypotensive, epidural anesthesia, the patient is placed in the lateral position with the affected hip facing up. A special fracture table with sacral and pubic posts, and a back support is used to secure the patient in the desired position. The table allows intraoperative tilting of the patient towards the surgeon to facilitate acetabular reaming.

The skin incision is a gentle curve centered over the greater trochanter. It extends distally for 5–10 cm along the posterior part of the femoral shaft and proximally the same distance but angled posteriorly by about 40° heading towards the posterior superior iliac spine (◘ Fig. 6.13). The fascia is incised in the line of the incision and the gluteus maximus muscle is split in the proximal part of the incision in the direction of its fibers. A Charnley retractor is used to retract the fascial and muscle edges.

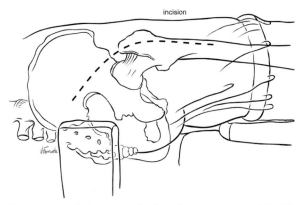

◘ **Fig. 6.13.** Right hip prepped in lateral position on hip table with proposed posterolateral incision

Gentle internal rotation of the hip exposes the posterior border of gluteus medius, which is retracted by an angled Hohmann retractor. All the short external rotators from the piriformis to the quadratus femoris are visualized at this stage. The tendon of gluteus maximus is identified at the distal corner of the incision. It is released (completely if necessary) with diathermy, preserving a stump of 2–3 mm at its insertion for future re-suturing (Fig. 6.14). An ink marking is made on the posterior soft tissues and femoral shaft at the level of quadratus femoris to facilitate accurate approximation during closure. The quadratus femoris is released from its insertion at the posterior margin of the vastus lateralis. A posterior sleeve, consisting of the short external rotators and the capsule, is released from the bony surface of the posterior aspect of the femoral neck with diathermy (Figs. 6.14 and 6.15). A trapezoidal soft-tissue flap based medially on the pelvis is developed where the capsule is closely adherent to the rotator muscles (see Fig. 6.15, Fig. 6.16). The proximal limb is located above the superior border of the piriformis tendon while the distal limb is located below the inferior border of the inferior gemellus muscle. This capsular sleeve extends from the 11 o'clock- to 7 o'clock position for the right hip. The posterior soft-tissue sleeve consists of the gluteus maximus tendon and the short external rotators, including the quadratus femoris, gemellus inferior, obturator internus, gemellus superior and piriformis, in the caudal-cephalad direction. Care

should be exercised to maintain the dissection close to the bone in order to avoid the branches of the circumflex vessels and to obtain the maximum length of soft tissue needed for repair.

An Aufranc retractor is inserted into the space created at the acetabular notch in a rent in the inferior capsule. A Steinman pin is inserted into the infra-cotyloid groove of the acetabulum and held vertically against the bone. A locator mark is made on the greater trochanter for future reference for the leg-length measurement. The position of the limb is identified when

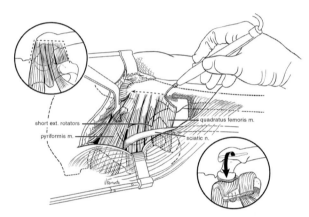

 Fig. 6.15. Exposure continues with release of the quadratus femoris muscle, followed by release of the short external rotators and capsule as one contiguous flap. Note the outline of the trapezoidal capsulotomy in the upper inset

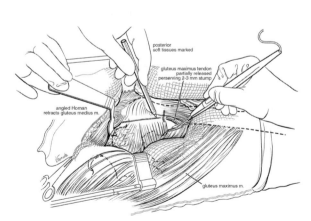

 Fig. 6.14. The same hip after exposure of the posterior structures of the hip. Note the partial release of the insertion of the gluteus maximus tendon

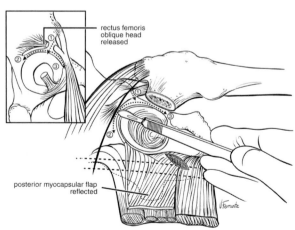

 Fig. 6.16. The hip has been dislocated and the femoral head osteotomized to expose the acetabulum. Note the release of the reflected head of the rectus femoris which allows for anterior mobilization of the femur and placement of the curved C-retractor

6.3

this mark is being made. This position is in slight adduction, flexion and internal rotation. With the knife, the femoral attachment of the gluteus minimus and the superior capsule are detached from the femoral neck. Abduction of the hip facilitates this release maneuver. The hip is dislocated posteriorly by flexion, adduction and internal rotation. The distance from the center of the head to the top of the lesser trochanter is measured for future reference. The neck is osteotomized as required. If the patient has significant anterior soft-tissue tightness or a pre-operative flexion contracture, the limb is rotated internally and the anterior capsule is partially or completely released close to the anterior surface of the femoral neck from the intertrochanteric crest.

A double angled C-shaped retractor is inserted in front of the anterior acetabular wall to retract the proximal femur anteriorly. A Steinman pin is inserted in the supra-acetabular region to retract the gluteus medius. An Aufranc retractor is placed below the acetabular notch, which retracts the inferior soft tissues and facilitates hemostasis. A right-angled Hohmann retractor is inserted behind the posterior edge of the acetabulum, inside the posterior capsule and rotator muscle flap but outside the labrum. The sciatic nerve is well protected in this position. The antero-lateral capsule and the reflected head of the rectus femoris is released from the anterior and antero-superior border of acetabulum from the 11 o'clock position to the antero-inferior iliac spine (□ Fig. 6.16). The double-angled retractor is repositioned at this site in the space created by the release of the rectus femoris origin. The femur is now positioned into slight abduction, flexion and neutral rotation to further facilitate a global exposure of the acetabulum (□ Fig. 6.17). The substance of the rectus femoris tendon and iliacus muscle protects the femoral nerve from this retractor. Tilting the patient towards the surgeon facilitates the visualization of the acetabulum.

The inside of the transverse acetabular ligament, which corresponds to the mark on the inter-teardrop line on the radiograph, is identified. The superior bony landmark on the acetabulum corresponding to the 45 degree angled line on the radiograph is also identified. The redundant acetabular labrum is excised in a global fashion so as to gain a complete view of the bony anatomy of the opening of the acetabular bony socket. The acetabulum is reamed in a progressive and concentric fashion. The initial reamer is directed medially in order

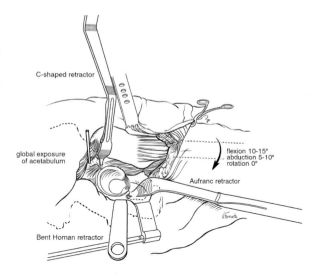

□ Fig. 6.17. Exposure of the acetabulum with a C-retractor anteriorly, a Steinmann pin superiorly, an Aufranc inferiorly, and a bent Hohmann retractor posteriorly

to obtain the desired medialization of the socket onto the true floor of the acetabulum. The socket is reamed in 2 mm increments until the cancellous bone of the pubis and ischium comes into view. Care is taken to maintain the reaming of the acetabular socket in a concentric manner in order to avoid the creation of an eccentric bony socket. This is of great importance in re-creating the optimal hip center and has a major bearing on the biomechanics of the implanted hip arthroplasty. An acetabular trial of the same outer diameter as the last acetabular reamer used is placed to assess the adequacy and concentricity of the reamed socket as well as to gain information about the desired angle of anteversion and angle of inclination of the socket (□ Fig. 6.18).

Component orientation is assessed by alignment of the trial to the bony landmarks of the socket and the previously described correlation of these landmarks on the pre-operative radiographs. Multiple keyholes are made to a depth of 5–8 mm using a high-speed burr in order to facilitate optimal macro- and microlock of the cement into the cancellous bone. The acetabular socket is thoroughly lavaged with pulsed irrigation and dried in order to create the ideal bone-cement interface. This is facilitated by well-controlled hypotensive anesthesia.

The prepared cement mass in a semi-viscous state is placed into the dry bony bed of the acetabular socket

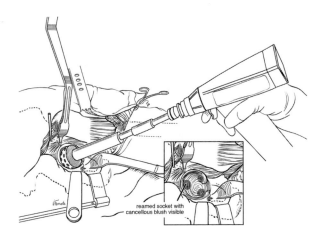

reamed socket with
cancellous blush visible

Fig. 6.18. Concentric reaming of the acetabulum can now be performed in an unimpeded fashion

and pressurized with a latex pressurizer. Attention is focused on the maintenance of a dry cement interface. The polyethylene socket is implanted into the cement mass under steady pressure in the optimal alignment and anteversion as previously assessed with respect to the bony landmarks. Minor adjustments are made if desired, and the excess cement is removed. The socket is maintained under steady pressure until the cement has cured.

For the femoral preparation, the femur is rotated internally, adducted and flexed. A broad neck retractor elevates the proximal femur into full view. An Aufranc retractor is placed inferiorly beneath the lesser tuberosity and a right-angled Hohmann retractor is placed in the abductor mass between the gluteus medius and minimus to expose the neck area in its entirety. A pilot hole is created in the postero-lateral aspect of the cut surface of the neck, using a high-powered burr. The canal is identified with a canal finder. A straight rod is inserted in the canal to a depth of 180 mm to identify the center of the femoral canal. A combination reamer is used to remove overhanging trochanteric bone in order to permit femoral broaching in the neutral plane of the femoral canal. The proximal femur is prepared using sequential broaches with attention directed to the desired anteversion and adequate broaching of the lateral wall in order to attain the ideal alignment of the femoral implant in the neutral axis of the femur.

A trial reduction is performed using the appropriate broach and trial head. The coplanar position is identified by appropriate internal rotation of the femur to provide an estimate of the combined anteversion of the femoral and acetabular components. The distance from the lesser trochanter to center of the head and the offset are noted and compared against similar measurements that were made prior to the osteotomy of the femoral head. The leg lengths are evaluated after the trial hip reduction, by introducing the Steinman pin in the infra-cotyloid groove and the difference between the previously placed mark on the greater trochanter and the Steinman pin is measured. The aim is to equalize or increase the leg length by 2–5 mm. The anterior soft-tissue tension is also evaluated by an objective evaluation of the resistance to passive external rotation of the femur. One should be able to bring the proximal femur passively within one finger's breadth from the ischial tuberosity. The length and tightness of the tensor fascia lata is evaluated utilizing Ober's test. All anterior osteophytes must be removed to eliminate bony impingement of the neck of the trial broach which may predispose to hip instability.

The issues of limb lengths and soft-tissue tension can be appropriately addressed by adjustments to the implant seating, head–neck length modularity and soft-tissue releases, including the iliotibial band and anterior capsule release as required.

After the trial reduction, the desired femoral prosthesis and head is assembled. The femoral canal is plugged at the measured distance using the appropriately sized cement restrictor. The femoral canal is thoroughly lavaged, using pulse irrigation, and dried and packed with ribbon gauze in a retrograde manner. The cement is prepared by vacuum mixing and loaded into a cement gun. The femur is confirmed to be dry by final suction of any fluid at its base. The cement is implanted into the femur when it has reached the ideal consistency in retrograde fashion. The cement is pressurized into the cancellous bony interstices, using the cement gun and a proximal femoral seal. The exudation of marrow and fat from the neck of the femur is considered a sign of optimal pressurization. The cement interface is dried and the femoral component is implanted into the cement mass with consideration given to the anteversion and the neutral alignment of the component along the axis of the femur. The excess cement is removed and the implant is impacted to the desired level, utilizing the previously measured lesser trochanter to center of the head distance. The hip is reduced after the cement has cured and the acetabular component is confirmed to be devoid of any debris. The limb length is confirmed before commencement of the closure.

Suturing the gluteus maximus tendon to its insertion and the quadratus femoris to the posterior aspect of the shaft with non-absorbable thick sutures performs the closure (◘ Fig. 6.19). The posterior capsulo-muscular flap is sutured by non-absorbable osseous sutures to the depth of piriformis fossa at the base of the femoral neck. Sutures passed through drill holes near the posterior edge of greater trochanter are used to secure the posterior flap (◘ Fig. 6.20). The fascia lata is sutured with interrupted and continuous sutures to attain a watertight closure.

Extension of the exposure for revision hip replacement surgery and some difficult primary cases is achieved by releasing a part of the gluteus medius, minimus and vastus lateralis along with the anterior capsule as one sleeve from the anterior surface of the femoral neck. This approach utilizes the modification of the direct lateral approach as described by Hardinge. This anterior sleeve is elevated to the level of the lesser trochanter distally and beyond the acetabulum superiorly and allows easier anterior translation of the trochanter to visualize the acetabulum completely. At the conclusion of the case, the closure of this anterior release is again performed, using non-absorbable interrupted sutures as a continuous layer.

Material and Methods

A retrospective radiographic review was performed of 100 consecutive cemented primary total hip replacements for which adequate quality pre-operative and one-month post-operative anterior-posterior (AP) pelvis radiographs were available. All the procedures were performed using the posterior approach described in the technique section. Patients were excluded if they had previously sustained a fracture of either hip, if they had undergone hip-replacement surgery on the opposite hip, or if they had any condition other than osteoarthritis which significantly affected the bony architecture of either hip (e.g., hip dysplasia). All the patients underwent unilateral cemented total hip replacement with modern cementing technique, using a single type of implant.

All the radiographs of 100 patients were evaluated independently by two observers to assess the restoration of hip center of rotation and femoral component alignment. The axis of the femoral prosthesis relative to that of the femoral canal was measured on the AP pelvis radiographs and was considered mal-aligned if it differed by 3° or more.

The location of the pre-operative center of rotation was determined by identifying the center of the bony arc of the acetabulum visualized on the AP pelvis radiograph. When acetabular bony deficiency was present, the center of rotation was placed at the location where it

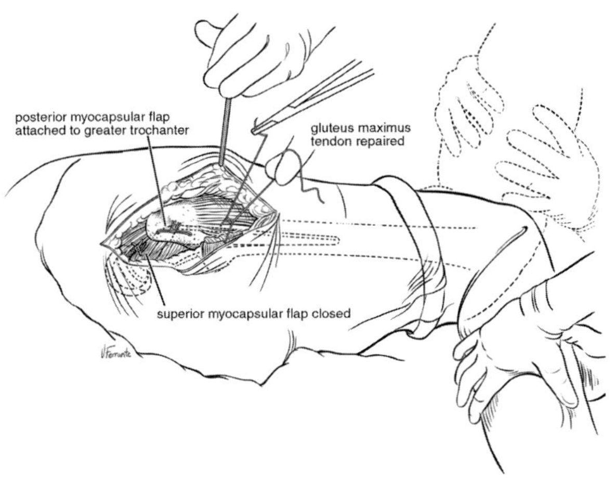

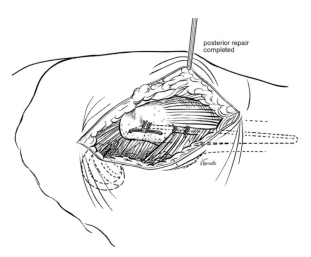

◘ **Fig. 6.19.** The trapezoidal posterior flap of capsule and short external rotators are now repaired through drill holes passed through the greater trochanter. Note the repair of the superior capsule proximally and the repair of the gluteus maximus and quadratus femoris distally

◘ **Fig. 6.20.** Appearance of the posterior approach to the hip after final repair would have been had the bony deficiency not existed. Its horizontal and vertical distance from the inferior and medial borders of the ipsilateral radiographic teardrop recorded the location of the center of rotation. The line tangent to the inferior edges of both teardrops defined the horizontal axis. The post-operative center of rotation was defined as the center of the prosthetic femoral head. The horizontal and vertical distance from the teardrop similarly recorded its location.

Leg-length differences were estimated using the AP pelvis radiographs. The leg-length difference was defined as the difference in the perpendicular distances from the inter-teardrop line to the center of the ipsilateral and contralateral lesser trochanters. The center of the lesser trochanter was utilized because its location varies less with femoral rotation than does the superior or inferior edge of the lesser trochanter. This method of leg-length measurement presumes that the remainder of both limbs below the lesser trochanter is equal in length and that no pelvic obliquity exists.

Results

The femoral alignment was graded as neutral by the two observers in 88% and 89% of the cases, respectively. The stem was classified as being in 3° or more of valgus in 9% and 10%, respectively. Both observers agreed that two of the stems were positioned in 3° of varus.

Averaging the two observers' measurements, the post-operative center of rotation of the hip joint was elevated a mean of 1.0 mm (±2.5 mm) and medialized 4.2 mm (±3.6 mm) compared to the pre-operative center of rotation. The hip center was raised >5 mm in 7%, but was never elevated >9 mm. It was medialized >10 mm in 7% of the cases.

Pre-operatively, the leg length on the involved side was shorter than the contralateral leg by an average of 2.5 mm ±5.5 mm. Post-operatively, the involved leg was lengthened so that it was longer than the opposite leg by 3.3 mm ±4.7 mm. In 73% of the cases, the leg-length difference after surgery was 5 mm or less. Post-operatively, the operated leg was longer than the opposite side by >5 mm in 26%, with a difference of 6–10 mm in 20 cases and 11–18 mm in 6%. In 5 of these cases, the involved side was longer by >5 mm both pre-operatively and post-operatively, but the length was not altered >5 mm by surgery. In one case, the operated leg was shorter than the opposite side by >5 mm post-operatively. In that case, the involved extremity was shorter pre-operatively as well and surgery actually lengthened the leg by 3 mm. Also, in no case did the surgery result in the operated extremity being shortened by >5 mm.

Discussion

From the time Langenbeck initially described it in 1874, the posterior approach to the hip joint had mainly been used for hip-infection treatment [11–13]. Kocher and Osborne modified it, respectively, to improve the exposure and to avoid the trochanteric osteotomy in face of infection [11–14]. The credit for introducing this approach to North America is usually attributed to Gibson, who used it extensively for non-infection cases like cup arthroplasty, slipped femoral epiphysis management and hip-fracture treatment [11]. He, however, released the gluteus medius and minimus from the greater trochanter and dislocated the hip anteriorly by externally rotating the hip. In the fifties, many surgeons used the posterior approach and many variations were reported. Horwitz described an approach for the treatment of fractures of femoral neck [15]. Marcy and Fletcher used a similar technique for hemiarthroplasty of the hip joint [16]. In both techniques, the gluteus maximus is split along its fibers and the external rotators are sharply detached from the femur. Moore described his variation with an inferiorly placed incision, which later became famous as the "Southern approach" [17, 18]. This provided a good exposure of the femur for the purpose of a hemiarthroplasty, but was limited in the amount of acetabular exposure it offered. None of these approaches gave any special attention to the exposure of the acetabulum or to the repair of the capsule and external rotators.

As total hip arthroplasty became more frequently performed, the stability of the artificial hip joint became an important issue. McFarland and Osborne in 1954 and later Scheck in 1973 reported variations of the anterior approach based on the observation that the gluteus medius and vastus lateralis form a continuous cover over the greater trochanter [19, 20]. They advised reflecting the gluteus medius and vastus lateralis as a continuous layer from the greater trochanter and releasing the gluteus minimus from its trochanteric attachment. They preserved the small external rotators and dislocated the hip anteriorly.

Several surgeons in the United States developed the posterior exposure for the purpose of total hip arthroplasty and addressed the risk of posterior dislocation of the hip with the preservation of the gluteus medius and minimus. Lack of attention to the posterior repair was prevalent until recently [21, 22]. The increased incidence of hip dislocation following the posterior approach was published [1–5] with dislocation rates of 3–9.5% [5, 8, 23]. To address this problem, various methods were suggested to improve the posterior stability following a posterior approach. Iyer suggested oblique osteotomy of posterior part of greater trochanter with the attached posterior muscles and capsule [24]. He re-attached the osteotomized fragment with cerclage wires and demonstrated good stability against posterior directed forces in a cadaveric study. Shaw performed a limited clinical study, utilizing a similar approach wherein he fixed the posterior partial trochanteric osteotomy with two screws [25]. These techniques, using a partial osteotomy of the greater trochanter, add to the complexity of the approach, increase the blood loss and may involve an increased risk of heterotopic ossification. The efficacy of these modifications has not been well documented. Headley et al. suggested using osseous repair of the posterior soft tissues to the posterior edge of greater trochanter [26].

In our approach, the combined posterior soft-tissue flap (capsule and external rotators together) gives good posterior stability when it is sutured to the depth of piriformis fossa. During fixation, the inferior angle of this trapezoidal flap is brought posteriorly and upwards, thus augmenting the posterior stability. The secured repair has allowed us to start early ambulation of the patients from the first post-operative day.

Another factor, which has been mentioned in the literature about the drawbacks of the posterior approach, is the difficulty in the assessment of the correct orientation of the components due to the lateral position of the patient. An increased rate of dislocation has been partly attributed to the suboptimal orientation of the acetabular and femoral components when the posterior approach has been utilized [9, 10]. The inability of a surgeon to orient the components depends directly upon the three-dimensional comprehension and visualization of the bony anatomy. This in turn depends upon the adequacy of the exposure. The combination of key steps in our technique facilitates a global visualization of the acetabulum. These previously undescribed steps include:

1. Near complete release of gluteus maximus tendon from posterior femur;
2. release of anterior and lateral capsule from its acetabular attachment in the antero-superior region;
3. release of the reflected head of rectus femoris tendon from its origin at the anterior inferior iliac spine;
4. release of the anterior capsule from the femoral neck;
5. placement of the anterior "C" retractor and positioning of the femur appropriately.

The combination of these steps allows appropriate anterior retraction of the femur. As a result of the complete visualization of all the bony boundaries of the acetabulum, the orientation of the component is significantly facilitated. The data of the 100 consecutive patients confirms that the anatomic placement of acetabulum and femur can be reproduced with predictable accuracy. The position of the patient on the table is not used to position the component, instead the orientation of the acetabular cup is achieved with respect to the visible bony landmarks that are correlated with the landmarks assessed on the pre-operative radiograph. This permits tilting of the patient towards the surgeon and makes for easier reaming and implantation during surgery.

The extensile posterior approach described herein provides wide exposure of both the acetabulum and proximal femur nearly obliviating the need for transtrochanteric approaches that might otherwise be deemed necessary in severely contracted hips.

References

1. Roberts J, Fu FH, McClain E, Ferguson A (1984) A comparison of posterolateral and anterolateral approaches to total hip arthroplasty. Clinical Orthop 187: 205–210
2. Robinson R, Robinson HJ Jr, Salvati E (1980) Comparison of transtrochanteric and posterior approach for total hip replacement Clinical Orthop 147: 143–147
3. McRay R (1987) Practical orthopaedic exposures. Churchill Livingston, New York
4. Ritter MA (1976) Dislocations and subluxations after total hip replacement. Clinical Orthop 121: 92
5. Woo RYG, Morrey BF (1982) Dislocations after total hip arthroplasty. J Bone Joint Surg 64A: 1295
6. Carlson DC, Robinson HS (1987) Surgical approaches for primary total hip arthroplasty. Clinical Orthop 222: 161
7. Lewinnek GE, Lewis JC, Tarr R (1978) Dislocations after total hip arthroplasty. J Bone Joint Surg 60A: 217

8. Vicar A, Coleman C (1984) A comparison of antero-lateral transtrochanteric and posterior approaches in primary total hip arthroplasty. Clinical Orthop 188: 152

9. Hovelius L, Hussenius A, Thorling J (1977) Posterior versus lateral approach for hip arthroplasty; Acta Orthop Scand 48: 47–51

10. Patiala H, Lehto K, Rokkanen P, Paavolainen P (1984) Posterior approach for total hip arthroplasty. Arch Orthop Trauma Surg 102: 225–229

11. Gibson A (1950) Posterior exposure of the hip joint. J Bone Joint Surg 32B: 183

12. Acton RK (1988) Surgical approaches to the hip. In: Tronzo RG (ed) Surgery of the hip joint, Vol 1. Springer, New York

13. Pellegrini VD Jr, McCollister Evarts C (1990) Surgical approaches to the hip joint. In: McCollister E (ed) The surgery of musculoskeletal system, vol 3. Churchill Livingston, New York, pp 2735–2756

14. Osborne RP (1930/31) The approach to the hip joint: A critical review and a suggested new route. Br J Surg 18: 49

15. Horwitz T (1952) Postero-lateral approach in the management of basilar neck, inter-trochanteric and sub-trochanteric fractures. Surg Gynaec Obstetricc 95: 45

16. Marcy GH, Fletcher RF (1954) Modification of the postero-lateral approach to the hip for insertion of femoral head prosthesis. J Bone Joint Surg 36A: 142

17. Moore AT (1957) The self locking metal hip prosthesis J Bone Joint Surg 39A: 811

18. Hunter SC (1986) Southern hip exposure. Orthopaedics 9: 1425–1428

19. McFarland B, Osborne G (1954) Approach to the hip joint: A surgical improvement on Kocher's method. J Bone Joint Surg 36-B: 364–367

20. Scheck M, Gordon RB, Glick JM (1973) The Kocher–McFarland approach to the hip joint for prosthetic replacement. Clinical Orthop 91: 63–69

21. Sarmiento A, Zych GA, Latta L, Tarr RR (1979) Clinical experience with titanium alloy hp prosthesis: a posterior approach. Clinical Orthop 144: 166–173

22. Pellicci PM, Bostrom M, Poss R (1998) Posterior approach to total hip replacement using enhanced posterior soft tissue repair. Clinical Orthop 355: 224–228

23. Carlsson AS, Gentz CF (1977) Post-operative dislocations in Charnley and Brunswick total hip arthroplasty. Clinical Orthop 125: 177

24. Iyer KM (1981) A new posterior approach to the hip joint. Injury 13: 76–80

25. Shaw JA (1991) Experience with modified posterior approach to the hip joint. A technical note. J Arthroplasty 6: 11–18

26. Hedley AK, Hendren DH, Mead LP (1990) Posterior approach to the hip joint with complete posterior capsular and muscular repair. J Arthroplasty 5 [Suppl]: S57–S66

6.3

Minimally Invasive Approaches to the Hip

Direct, Anterior, Single-Incision Approach

M. Krismer, M. Nogler, F. Rachbauer

Description of the Approach

The approach is intended to allow for the implantation of a standard total hip prosthesis by the use of standard instruments. Cemented as well as non-cemented implants can be used with this approach. However, the implantation process is facilitated with standard instruments that have undergone slight modification. In any minimally invasive approach the use of straight cup and stem inserters, straight cement-plug inserters and straight rigid reamers and broaches require more soft-tissue mobilization, which can cause excessive tension on these structures. Therefore, the use of instruments specifically developed for this approach is recommended.

The entire procedure is performed using a single-incision anterior approach. In a modified Smith-Peterson anterior technique, the gluteal muscles remain attached to the ileum, using a safe intermuscular and inter-nervous plane to gain direct, unimpeded access to the hip capsule. The capsulotomy is performed using an H-shaped incision and retained. The femoral neck is then osteotomized with two parallel cuts. After removal of the bony disc created by this maneuver, the femoral head can be easily removed without significant soft tissue distraction. Mobilization of the capsule from the femur and the placement of the specially designed retractors permit direct access to the femoral canal in the anterior approach by elevating the femur out of the wound. After implantation of the acetabular and femoral components and relocation of the femoral head in the acetabulum, the capsulotomy is closed to decrease the risk of dislocation.

Patient Selection

The direct anterior approach can be safely and adequately performed in over 95% of patients who undergo a total hip arthroplasty. Although obesity is not a contraindication because the anterior peri-incisional subcutaneous fat is usually not very thick, evaluation of each patient's anatomy is suggested. However, it is also recommended to start the use of this approach with "ideal" patients, those with relatively thin anterior musculature and fat, and then proceed to the more difficult cases. In addition to the usual contraindications for hip arthroplasty, there are additional specific contraindications for the direct anterior approach:

Absolute contraindications:

- **Destruction of the proximal femur:** In the case of a per-trochanteric fracture or metastatic disease of the proximal femur, elevation of the femur out of the wound cannot be adequately accomplished.

Relative contraindications:

- **Morbid obesity:** The decision, if this means a BMI index of 30 or more, is entirely dependent on the experience of the surgeon.
- **Decreased range of motion:** If the hip joint is excessively stiff and range of motion is decreased, mobilization of the soft tissue to access the joint may be more difficult. This parameter is also dependent on the experience of the surgeon.
- **Difficult and concomitant procedures:** If additional procedures are necessary, e.g. the removal of a plate or of a dynamic hip screw, revision cases, or central dislocation of the hip, a degree of mobilization greater than that achieved with the anterior approach may be required.

Operative Technique

Equipment of the Theatre, Position of the Surgeon

A standard operating theatre can be used, without any special requirements. It is necessary to use additional devices for illumination, and a head-mounted lamp for the surgeon is sufficient.

The operation is conducted with the surgeon in the standing position on the side of the affected hip and the first assistant above or cranial to that position. The second assistant stands on the opposite side. During stem preparation, the surgeon and the first assistant can change places as necessary. The scrub nurse is positioned at the foot of the operating table.

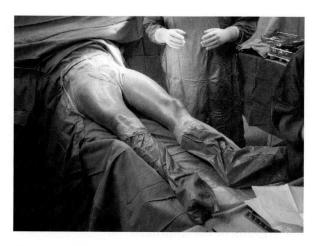

☐ **Fig. 7.1.** Position of the patient on the operating table after draping with both legs draped free

Specialized Instruments

Retractors. To facilitate retraction and visualization, each instrument should be bent at the level of the skin as they exit from the wound, and the bend should approximate 90°. Fortunately, the thickness of soft tissue in the area of the approach does not demonstrate a high degree of variability. Even very obese patients do not have a thick subcutaneous fat layer in the area of this approach; otherwise it would be difficult for them to sit. Typically, one size of retractors is sufficient to handle patients of varying body habitus.

Oscillating Saw. A standard-size saw is too bulky in this minimally invasive approach. A small electric oscillating saw permits an osteotomy with adequate visualization.

Curved Acetabular Reamer Handle and Cup Inserter. They are not necessary, but the curvature of the instruments reduces the pressure and tension exerted on the skin.

Curved Broach Handle, Intra-Medullary Plug Inserter and Stem Holder. Without these curved instruments, femoral canal preparation and stem implantation may be impossible. In cemented stems, a curved or flexible intramedullary plug inserter is necessary.

Patient Position

The patient is placed in the supine position on the operating table without any support placed under the pelvis. Draping of the pelvis and both legs is required to accom-

modate the leg positioning used during the procedure. Preparation of the femoral canal requires a position where the operative leg is placed in external rotation and adduction behind the opposite leg (known as the figure-4 position). The draping of the legs must be sufficiently flexible to permit such movement. The anus and genitals are covered by a drape, and after prepping, both legs are placed in impervious sterile stockings up to the proximal aspect of the patella. A bilateral self-adhesive hip drape is used to cover the trunk and the genitals. Both anterior superior iliac spines (ASIS) remain uncovered to permit identification of the anatomic landmarks used during cup positioning. A self-adhesive drape is placed on each leg in order to fix the position of the drapes. After draping, the index hip is fully flexed to verify proper draping (☐ Fig. 7.1).

Pre-Operative Planning

It is important to perform thorough pre-operative planning. For the acetabulum, the depth of reaming with relationship to the acetabular fossa must be determined. The acetabular fossa can be clearly recognized on pre-operative X-rays and intra-operatively in the acetabulum. If it is planned to ream deeper, the relation between the reamer and the acetabular rim can be determined as soon as the reamer has reached the fossa. Then the distance between the acetabular rim and the end of the reamer can be determined, which will diminish with further reaming. Also the approximate size of the implant can be determined.

The resection plane of the femur should be determined using the junction between the neck and trochanter and the lesser trochanter as landmarks. The size of the implant is important, as well as the distance between stem shoulder and the tip of the greater trochanter, in order to determine reconstruction of the leg length.

Skin Incision

The success of this approach is dependent on the exact positioning of the skin incision. The intermuscular space can easily be palpated. This space is formed by the muscles medial to the approach – the sartorius and femoral rectus which originate from the ASIS and the AIIS (anterior inferior iliac spine) – and the muscles lateral to the approach – tensor fasciae latae and medial gluteus – which originate from the lateral surface of the iliac wing. Abduction and external rotation of the hip will lateralize the lateral musculature and decrease tissue tension in the intermuscular space, facilitating palpation.

The incision starts two finger breadths below the ASIS and follows the intermuscular space. A skin incision placed too medial can cause damage to the lateral femoral cutaneous nerve. An incision placed too lateral will reduce this risk as well as the pressure on the skin during femoral preparation (Fig. 7.2). Alternatively, a skin incision parallel to the inguinal skin fold will result in a better cosmetic result and make the approach to the femoral canal easier on the surgeon and the soft tissues. However, this incision will cross the branches of the lateral femoral cutaneous nerve, and place undue tension on these branches resulting in a high likelihood of paresthesias of the anterior and lateral skin of the thigh. If patients wish to receive this optimal scar with regard to cosmetics, the increased risk of nerve damage must be discussed pre-operatively with the patient.

The length of the skin incision depends on the expected size of the acetabular component (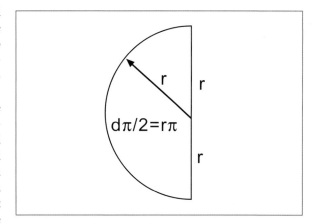 Fig. 7.3). The skin can also be stretched, but the more the skin is stretched, the more likely a wound-healing problem will result. Ideally, there is an optimal balanced solution with regards to the goal of minimal damage to the patient with minimal incision length.

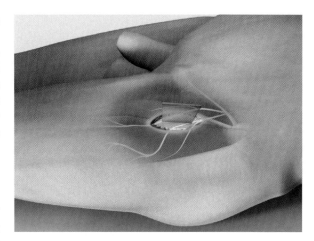

Fig. 7.2. Skin incision in relation to the sartorius and tensor fasciae latae muscle originating at the ASIS. The incision starts between both muscles about two finger breadths below the ASIS. The branches of the lateral femoral cutaneous nerve must be preserved

Fig. 7.3. Calculation of the length of skin incision. A hemispherical cup inserted as shown in the figure requires a circumference of $U = 2\,r + r\pi$. The same circumference can be created by a longitudinal incision of the length $L = (2\,r + r\pi)/2$. For following cup diameters the corresponding incision lengths are 44–57 mm, 54–69 mm, 64–82 mm. With an error of only 3% the formula L = cup diameter + cup diameter/4 can be applied, e.g. for a 54 mm cup: L = 54 + 54/4 = 67.5 mm incision length

Muscle Dissection

After dissection of subcutaneous fat, which is normally quite thin, the fascia appears in the incision. Palpation of the structures is repeated at this point and the fascial separation is made at the site of the intermuscular space or

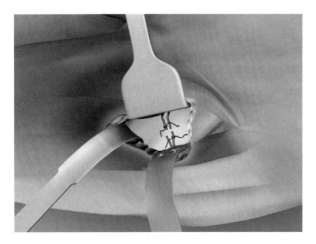

Fig. 7.4. The deep layer of muscles (rectus and medial gluteal muscle) is retracted. The lateral circumflex vessels appear in a fat layer covering the capsule and are ligated and resected

The capsulotomy is carried out using an H-shaped incision. This step starts with a longitudinal incision of the capsule anterior and longitudinal to the femoral neck. Then, the proximal incision is completed along the acetabular rim. The labrum or remnants of it are resected as well. It is not recommended to expose the space between the medial capsule and the psoas tendon, because bleeding can occur. The third incision is placed at the attachment of the capsule to the femur at the intertrochanteric line.

The joint is now exposed and by rotating the leg, a clear view can be achieved. The femoral neck is prepared with a Cobb, and the medial inferior and lateral proximal retractors are removed and repositioned on the medial and lateral aspect of the femoral neck inside the capsule. It is recommended that optimal femoral neck exposure is accomplished, especially the posterior aspect, to facilitate removal of the femoral neck disc as described below.

is slightly lateralized to provide greater protection of the lateral femoral cutaneous nerve. The fascia is split with either a scissors or by blunt finger dissection. The intermuscular space can be easily developed by blunt dissection until the capsule can be palpated. This preparation should be completed without force in order not to damage the lateral circumflex vessels within the operative field. A blunt retractor is placed laterally on the capsule proximal to the greater trochanter. A second retractor is placed around the greater trochanter. The medial musculature is retracted out of the field. The capsule is exposed and the lateral circumflex vessels are either cauterized or ligated, depending on the size of the vessel (◘ Fig. 7.4).

Capsule Preparation and Femur Mobilization

With a Cobb elevator, the space between the rectus and vastus intermedius muscles on the one hand, and the femur on the other hand is prepared, and then a third Hohmann retractor is placed just proximal to the lesser trochanter on the medial side of the femoral neck. Then, the reflected head of the rectus, which forms a second anterior layer of the capsule close to the acetabular rim, is cut with the cautery. The origin of the rectus from the AIIS, however, remains intact. The Cobb is used again to prepare the space between the origin of the rectus tendon above, and the capsule and superior acetabular rim below.

Removal of the Femoral Head

The femoral neck is osteotomized with two parallel cuts, using a small oscillating saw, producing a bone disc. This disc, approximately 1 cm thick, is removed first to facilitate the removal of the femoral neck prior to removal of the femoral head through this minimally invasive incision. This procedure not only makes removal of the femoral head easier but also reduces the risk of a femoral or sciatic nerve lesion due to reduced tension on the nerve during the dislocation procedure.

The cranial osteotomy is completed first, otherwise the proximal bone fragment would move excessively, followed by the second osteotomy which should be placed exactly where the femoral neck resection was planned. A 40°- to 45°-resection plane can be determined easily under direct visualization of the neck from the anterior field. The greater trochanter as well as the lesser trochanter can be palpated with a forceps. The femoral neck-bone disc is mobilized, using a Cobb elevator, and removed, using a blunt forceps. Then, the femoral head is removed, using an elevator or a corkscrew instrument (◘ Fig. 7.5).

If the surgeon encounters any difficulty removing the femoral head, the proximal capsular incision may need to be enlarged or remaining labrum may be restricting the extraction. In some cases, removal of anterior osteophytes or a thickened femoral head ligament may be required. At this point, the femur is usually sufficiently mobile so that it can be rotated in both

7.1

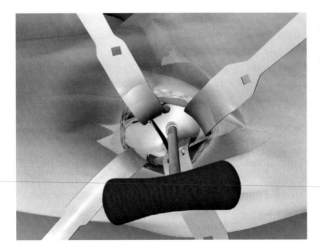

Fig. 7.5. After an H-shaped capsulotomy, two retractors are placed around the femoral neck, one retractor in front of the acetabulum and the other below the greater trochanter. Two cuts with an oscillating saw create a femoral neck disc which can then be removed. By this procedure, enough space is created to remove the femoral head

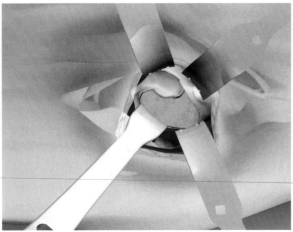

Fig. 7.6. With four retractors placed around the acetabulum, the exposure of the surgical field compares favorably to traditional open approaches

directions, the posterior attachments of the capsule to the femur can be resected and the femoral head can be removed from the field.

Cup Preparation

After removal of the femoral head, satisfactory exposure of the acetabulum is facilitated through the use of four properly placed retractors (Fig. 7.6):

- Medial anterior – the retractor on the superior acetabular rim. The previously cleared capsule permits the surgeon to easily place this retractor.
- Medial posterior – the retractor is placed either behind an osteophyte or the medial rim of the acetabulum, behind the transverse ligament.
- Lateral anterior – the retractor lies at the anterolateral acetabular rim.
- Posterior – the double-pronged retractor is placed with the tips behind the posterior rim of the acetabulum. As the posterior capsule has not been resected, it may be necessary to fashion a small rent in the capsule at this location to permit satisfactory capture of the retractor.

The acetabular fossa is cleared of soft tissue and osteophytes, and acetabular cysts are bone-grafted. Reaming is conducted with a curved or cranked reamer handle. Caution should be taken not to press the reamer too much against the posterior wall. The fossa is the best landmark for determining the depth of preparation during reaming. After reaming, the cementless cup is press-fit into position. In those cases in which a cemented cup is implanted, the bony bed is prepared in accordance with third-generation cementing techniques, including the use of anchor holes, pulsatile lavage and cement pressurization.

Stem Preparation

The capsular attachment to the femur has already been resected and should be re-checked to ensure appropriate femoral mobility. The proximal femur is elevated out of the field with a bone hook so that the greater trochanter is pulled laterally and anterior. The leg is placed in a figure-4 position, in 90° external rotation and slight adduction. Excessive adduction places undue stress on the medial gluteal muscle. A modified straight femoral elevator is placed behind the greater trochanter. The retractor is pressed down with caution to avoid excessive pressure on the greater trochanter which is levered out of the wound. The retractor is placed lateral to the iliac bone and the space in front of the retractor forms a working canal for stem preparation. Two retractors are placed lat-

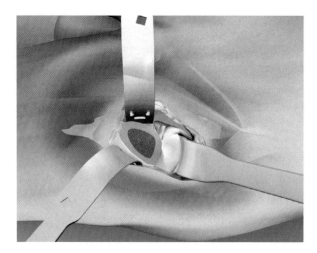

Fig. 7.7. The femur is pulled out of the wound with a bone hook. A specially designed retractor is placed behind the greater trochanter. This retractor is kept in an oblique direction and compresses and protects the soft tissue during preparation of the femur. Two additional retractors keep the soft tissue medial and lateral, respectively

eral and medial to the femur, so that the resection plane is completely free as depicted in ◘ Fig. 7.7. If the femur is not mobile enough, especially when the leg is positioned in a figure-4 position, the internal obturator tendon can be incised. This step is usually sufficient, so that all the other external rotators, including the piriformis and all gluteal muscles, can remain intact.

The further stem preparation is completed as is done in a traditional approach. The femoral canal is opened with a sharp trochar and broaching is completed as recommended for the particular prosthesis to be implanted. Relocation of the hip with a trial head on the broach, determination of leg length, verification of a satisfactory stem position, assessment of the stability of the construct through a range of motion, dislocation and stem implantation and relocation are completed as with the traditional approach.

Wound Closure

After relocation of the femoral head in the acetabulum with the final implants, a full range of motion is performed to verify the stability of the construct and to ensure that there is no soft-tissue interposition between the cup and the head. Capsular closure can be completed with two or three strong stitches. Wound drainage

can be placed in front of the capsule. The fascia is sutured with running sutures while avoiding the branches of the lateral femoral cutaneous nerve. The subcutaneous tissue is closed with interrupted sutures and the skin is closed with a subcuticular suture.

Challenges

Femoral mobilization is critical to provide sufficient access to the femoral canal during preparation of the canal for implantation. The proximal femur must be positioned anteriorly with slight adduction. There are three major potential obstacles to satisfactory mobilization:

Capsule. The capsule can be thought of as a fibrous tube which has some rigidity due to the three-dimensional arrangement of its fibers. This rigidity is accentuated with the scarring that accompanies an arthritic hip joint. As long as capsular fibers remain intact, the proximal femur will rotate around the intact fibers. Mobilization of the femur anteriorly is therefore combined with a more medial and cranial position. This mobilization is facilitated with resection of all of the anterior, medial and lateral capsular attachments to the femur. Those capsule fibers which are attached to the acetabular rim can remain relatively intact with only the anterior portion of the H-shaped capsulotomy being necessary.

External Rotators. The external rotation of the figure-4 position stretches these structures, and anterior displacement of the femur will produce additional medialization of the proximal femur. We have found that the internal obturator tendon can be an impediment to femoral mobilization. The orientation of the other external rotators has not been found to significantly hinder the anterior movement of the femur.

Gluteal Muscles. Usually, these muscles do not hinder femoral mobilization. A femoral elevator can be placed behind the greater trochanter for appropriate positioning while the gluteal muscles are preserved.

Risks and Sources of Complications

The **lateral cutaneous femoral nerve** (LCF nerve) enters the thigh medial to the ASIS and typically divides into 4 or 5 branches. The branches demonstrate variability, therefore there is no zone for the skin incision that is completely safe. However, the more lateral the skin inci-

7.1

sion is located, the less likely is the risk of a nerve lesion. We recommend a longitudinal skin incision, slightly lateral to the entrance to the intermuscular space. If a branch of the nerve is detected, it is sometimes possible to mobilize the branch and to suture a layer of subcutaneous fat tissue around the mobilized and displaced branch, in order to protect it against pressure during the further procedure. On rare occasions, the course of one of the branches crosses the operating field and must be ligated and cut. The consequence of a lesion of the LCF nerve is either a neuropathy or anesthesia in an area of the anterior or lateral thigh, or both. Anesthesia is usually not a long lasting problem; the patient becomes accustomed to it. In neuropathy, infiltration of the nerve can help. The **femoral nerve** is well protected by the sartorius, the rectus and iliopsoas muscles. The **sciatic nerve** is out of the surgical field and is not endangered.

In patients with significant osteoporosis, the femoral retraction during canal preparation could result in a fracture of the greater trochanter which, if small, could be ignored or could be fixed with the use of two cables through the same approach.

Salvage Procedures

Femoral stem fissure: A fissure of the femoral shaft can also be addressed by the use of circumferential cables. If the fissure continues distal to the incision, an additional skin incision 8 cm in length and placed laterally is more sensible than to lengthen the original approach. The vastus muscles form a thick layer of muscles, which gets thicker the more the anterior incision is extended caudal.

Minimally Invasive Single-Incision Anterior Approach for Total Hip Arthroplasty – Early Results

F. Rachbauer, M. Nogler, E. Mayr, M. Krismer

Introduction

The concept of less invasiveness has become an established aim of all surgeons in the orthopedic community. Various attempts have been made to discover the most suitable technique for minimally invasive hip arthroplasty [1–3]. Even though there is no universally accepted definition of minimal invasiveness, its focus is clearly to minimize soft-tissue trauma and accelerate soft-tissue regeneration [4].

Before the promise of reducing soft-tissue trauma can be fulfilled, the surgeon must get through three different layers: the skin, the muscles and the joint capsule, not to mention nerves and vessels within in order to exposure the hip joint. An optimal approach should therefore deliver a short skin incision, omit muscle splitting and/or detachment and preserve the joint capsule.

To reach this goal, several issues have to be addressed. First, the skin incision should be kept as short as possible. Next, there should either be none or as little muscle splitting and detachment as possible. The joint capsule should be preserved and there should be an unrestricted view onto the acetabulum and the entrance into the femoral medullary canal.

We hypothesized that a single-incision anterior approach for hip arthroplasty could uphold the premises of minimal invasiveness. Further on, we wanted to know whether this approach can be safely performed und whether there are possible advantages compared to traditional approaches. In the following, we present the data on our single-incision direct anterior approach for total hip arthroplasty.

Patients

One hundred consecutive patients who underwent total hip arthroplasty via the minimally invasive single-incision anterior approach were prospectively followed for at least 12 weeks. No exclusion criteria were applied, neither weight, height, age, gender, previous hip surgery nor secondary osteoarthritis. We enrolled 52 female and 48 male patients, median age was 65.6 years. Total hip arthroplasty was performed on 50 right and 50 left hips. A body mass index (BMI) >30 was found in 19 patients, BMI 25–29.9 in 35 patients, BMI 18.5–24.9 in 43 and BMI <18.5 in 3 patients.

Five patients suffered from osteoarthritis secondary to avascular necrosis of femoral head, and two patients had osteoarthritis secondary to dysplasia. One patient had osteoarthritis secondary to juvenile septic arthritis of hip joint. Three patients had undergone surgery for dysplasia of the hip (one Chiari pelvic osteotomy, one Ganz pelvic osteotomy, one intertrochanteric varus osteotomy). Two patients had non-displaced medial fractures of the femoral neck.

Surgical Technique

The patients were placed in the supine position on the operating table. This created a predictable stability. No sandbags were used to push the hip forward. The anterior superior iliac spine was palpated and the gap between the tensor fasciae latae and the sartorius muscle identified. The incision started 3–4 cm distal to the anterior superior iliac spine and followed the anterior border of the tensor fasciae latae muscle. The length of skin incision was approximately as long as half the circumference of the cup to be inserted. We carefully dissected down through the subcutaneous fat, making sure to avoid cutting the lateral femoral cutaneous nerve. Next, the deep fascia on the medial side of the tensor fasciae latae was incised. The anterior capsule of the hip could then be identified by blunt dissection. A blunt-tipped curved special retractor was placed laterally around the capsule, overlying the neck of the femur, and a special sharp-tipped curved retractor was placed around the innominate tubercle of the greater trochanter. The sartorius muscle was retracted medially. Care had to be taken not to pull too hard in order to avoid the risk of bleeding from the ascending branches of the lateral femoral circumflex vessels. These vessels were carefully suture ligated or electrocoagulated.

The medial capsule of the femoral neck which is covered by the rectus femoris muscle and fatty tissue was bluntly exposed. The rectus femuris muscle was medially retracted by a sharp-tipped curved special retractor. The rectus femoris originates from two heads: the direct head from the anterior inferior iliac spine, and the reflected head from the superior lip of the acetabulum as well as the anterior capsule. The origin between these two heads had to be transected. Then the hip was slightly bent and the sharp-tipped curved retractor was placed from the anterior rim of the acetabulum medial to the origin of the rectus femoris at the anterior inferior iliac spine. The exposed hip joint capsule was incised using an H-shaped capsular incision. Next, the curved retractors were placed within the hip capsule. The capsule was detached at the inter-trochanteric line as far to the medial and lateral side as possible, thereby clearing the junction between the anterior surface of the neck and the shaft. The lesser trochanter and the junction between femoral neck and greater trochanter were palpated to facilitate orientation for osteotomy of the neck (■ Fig. 7.8).

The femur was rotated into a neutral position and the femoral neck cut with an oscillating saw according to pre-operative templating with the patient's radiographs. The level of the femoral cut varied, depending on the anatomy of the femoral neck. A corkscrew extractor was screwed in and the head removed. Occasionally, the head had to be fragmented and removed in piecemeal fashion. The retractor was left on the anterior acetabular rim in place and the others were removed.

The sharp-tipped curved retractor was placed around the transverse acetabular ligament which was sometimes ossified and part of an inferior osteophyte. A second sharp-tipped curved retractor was placed on the

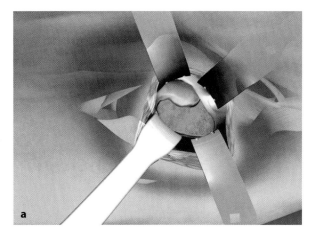

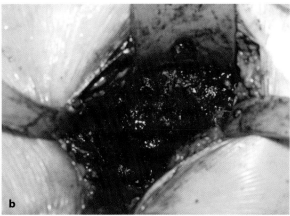

■ **Fig. 7.8. a** Sketch illustrating the view of the acetabulum during the minimally invasive single-incision anterior approach. **b** Patient, female, 72 years, view of the acetabulum during the minimally invasive single-incision anterior approach

lateral ilium and a two-pronged acetabular retractor inserted under the bony rim of the inferior acetabulum. Next, the remnants of the acetabular labrum were excised and the depth of the acetabular fossa defined. Any overhanging osteophytes were excised and synovectomy performed. No capsulectomies were performed.

Since acetabular exposure was excellent and the position of the pelvis could be easily palpated on the table, orientation by direct visualization proved quite simple. Soft tissues were removed from the acetabulum with curettes and rongeurs. The acetabulum was reamed down to the subchondral bone, using angulated reamers designed to protect soft tissue. Cemented as well as cementless cups were used. From this anterior position, it was easy to

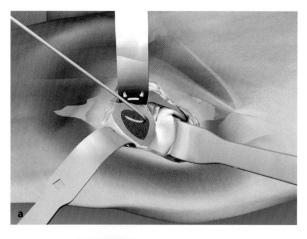

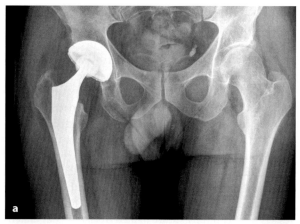

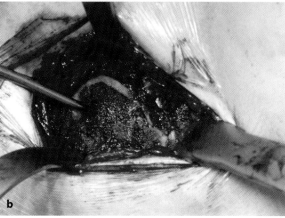

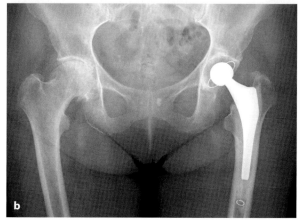

Fig. 7.9. **a** Sketch illustrating view of entry into the femoral canal during the minimally invasive single incision anterior approach. **b** Patient, male, 57 years, view of the entry of the femoral canal via minimally invasive single-incision anterior approach

Fig. 7.10. **a** Patient, male, 43 years, osteoarthritis secondary to avascular necrosis of the femoral head, minimally invasive total hip arthroplasty utilizing a cementless technique. **b** Patient, female, 73 years, primary osteoarthritis, minimally invasive total hip arthroplasty utilizing a cemented technique

establish the exact anteversion which was kept at approximately 15–20° and corresponded to normal anatomy.

A bag was placed under the proximal thigh and the entrance of the medullar channel was brought to the level of skin incision by pulling the calcar up with a hook (◘ Fig. 7.9). Then capsulotomy was performed at the greater trochanter. The two-pronged femoral retractor was placed around the greater trochanter and the femur externally rotated and positioned in a figure-4 position. If necessary, the tendons of the internal obturator and gemelli had to be released near their insertion on the medial side of the trochanter. In such instances, no reattachment was carried out. Following this, rasping of the femoral shaft was started, using angulated rasps. After determining the proper size, a permanent, either cemented or cementless, prosthesis was inserted into the femur. After final reduction, capsular repair was performed using reefing sutures and reattachment at the acetabular rim.

The Accolade femoral system was used in 59 patients and the ABG II cemented femoral system in 41 patients. The Trident acetabular system using a crosslink polyethylene inlay was implanted in 66 patients, an All-poly cup was used in the other 34 patients. Implantation technique was cementless in 52 patients (◘ Fig. 7.10a), cemented in 28 (◘ Fig. 7.10b) and hybrid in 20 patients.

The choice of implantation technique was based on subjective estimation of bone quality during surgery.

Results

Median and mean (SD) operating time was 105 (±33) min (range 61 to 270 min). The learning curve showed a decline in the moving average (10 patients) from 125 to 86 min (◘ Fig. 7.11).

Three intra-operative complications occurred, but were not considered to be caused by the surgical approach: one perforation of the inner cortex of the osteoporotic acetabulum, one avulsion of the tip of the greater trochanter and one fissure of the proximal shaft. The perforation of the inner cortex of the acetabulum was treated by an enforcement ring through the same approach. The tiny trochanteric fragment was excised since it was considered too small for reattachment. The

fissure went unnoticed intra-operatively until subsidization became apparent on post-operative radiograph, upon which revision surgery was performed by the anterior approach. The Accolade femoral component was exchanged for a cemented ABGII prosthesis and the proximal femoral stem was secured by cerclage through the same approach.

Blood was collected in the cell saver for 93 patients. Median (mean, SD) re-transfused blood was 160 ml (200±210) range 0–900 ml. Collected blood was given in 61 patients, in 32 patients the amount of collected blood was considered too little to justify re-transfusion. In addition, 23 patients received autologous and 3 patients homologous transfusions with an average of 113 ml (0 to 5 erythrocyte blood concentrates). Blood loss was assessed, using the methods of Rosencher et al. [13]. When compared to their results on primary 1122 hip replacements with a median blood loss of 1944 ml (SD ±1165 ml), the blood loss of a median 1566 ml (SD ±1041 ml) calculated for our sample was 25% less. This difference is highly significant ($p < 0.01$).

Naproxen was given for 14 days to prevent heterotopic ossification and additionally served as pain medication. Post-operative opioids were given routinely on the day of operation. On the first post-operative day, however, opioid therapy was only necessary in five patients.

Despite prophylaxis, one patient developed extensive, motion-limiting heterotopic ossification. There were no dislocations or nerve palsies. One patient developed thrombosis of the fibular vein.

Patients were discharged from the hospital an average of 4 days earlier than patients receiving standard conventional total hip arthroplasty (reduction of 36%). Delayed wound healing, located at the distal edge, occurred in three patients, and was due to the fact that only straight reamers were available at the beginning of the study. Nevertheless, no revision surgery was needed, since all wounds healed by granulation and epithelialization within 4 weeks.

One case of deep infection evolved during the first 3 months; the patient refused to undergo revision surgery at our department.

The WOMAC score was assessed before and 6 weeks after surgery. Seventy-eight patients had completed the WOMAC score at the 6-week follow-up. An improvement could be deduced from the median score (mean ± SD) of 43 (43.8±19.2) to 90.4 (87.9±11.6). The median (mean ± SD) pain sub-score at 6-week follow-up was 97 (90.3±15.6).

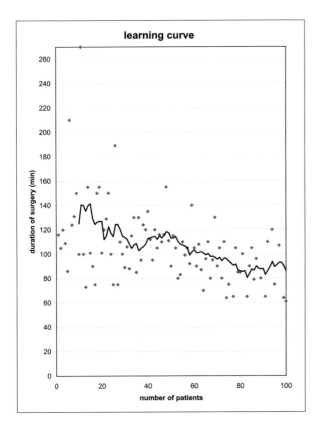

◘ Fig. 7.11. Dot plot of operating times and trend curve (learning curve) based on the moving average of 10 patients

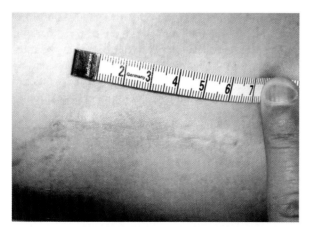

Fig. 7.12. Patient, female, 61 years, scar at 6-week follow up

At the 6-week follow-up, scars measured a median (mean, SD) of 6.75 cm (7.09±1.66) in length, ranging from 4.5 to 11.5 cm. Scar length was 83% (87±19.4) of half the circumference of the cup. Photographs of the scars (□ Fig. 7.12) were available in 68 patients and were assessed according to Beausang et al. [10]. Based on these images, the median scar quality was rated as 5.9 points (5.7±1.4) range 4.05 to 9.45 on a scale of 4 (best) to 24 (worst). On a scale of 0 to 100%, this converted to a median of 8.8% (9.4±1.4%), range 0 to 30.

At the 3-month follow-up, there were no leg-length discrepancies >1 cm in 97 patients. A leg-length inequality of >1 cm and <2 cm was seen in three patients. In two of these three patients, the leg-length discrepancy was the same as before surgery, thus there was only one case of true elongation.

Radiographs were assessed at 3-month follow-up. The median inclination angle was 44.1° (43.5±6.34), range 31°–58°. Median alignment of the femoral component was 0° (0.6° varus ±1), range 3° valgus to 5° varus. There was one case of subsidization, which was due to a fissure of the proximal femur and had to be revised. Four patients expressly complained of numbness in the lateral thigh.

Discussion

The aim of minimal invasive surgery is to reduce soft-tissue trauma and thereby operative blood loss, postoperative pain, and hospitalization time while speeding post-operative recovery and improving the cosmetic appearance of the surgical scar [4]. To properly prevent soft tissue trauma, minimal invasiveness must apply to skin, muscles, joint capsules and to the nerves and vessels contained therein.

Minimally invasive hip arthroplasty using an anterior approach can be accomplished through an incision about half the size of the cirumference of the cup to be inserted. As exceedingly small incisions tend to be stretched during the procedure, the length of the post-operative scar is the only valid measure.

The anterior approach has been reputed to produce unfavorable scars. This statement is not consistent with our own observations and experience. There is only one truly intermuscular and internervous plane of dissection to access the hip joint, and it lies anteriorly between the tensor fasciae latae and sartorius muscle and gluteus medius/minimus and rectus femoris muscles [14–17]. Anatomically, all other classical approaches to the hip, e.g. anterolateral, lateral, posterior and medial, are either intermuscular or internervous.

With our minimally invasive single-incision direct anterior approach for total hip arthroplasty, perfect exposure of and view onto the acetabulum can be expected. The presumption was that, through a small incision, it would be impossible to sufficiently lever out the femur to implant the femoral component and that visibility would be insufficient. This attitude has led to double-incision approaches and the use of fluoroscopy [1]. In our judgment, there is no need for a second incision or muscle splitting. Nevertheless, exposure of the entrance of the medullar canal demands meticulous detachment of the capsule on the femur, eventually involving partial tenotomies of the obturator internus and gemelli tendons. For this purpose, good anatomical knowledge of muscle attachments on the greater trochanter is mandatory [18–20]. In addition, special retractors facilitate the maneuver.

Moreover, these double approaches were restricted to slim and non-athletic patients. We have successfully implanted hip prostheses via a single incision by the minimally invasive approach even in very obese persons who tend to have less fat in the flexion crease overlying the hip joint. Capsular repair by the minimally invasive single-incision anterior approach is a feasible procedure.

Both cemented and cementless devices can be used on the acetabular side as well as on the femoral side. Acetabular reaming and cup placement may be facilitated by the use of curved reamers and inserters. Special broach handles and stems make broaching and femoral component implantation substantially easier. Radiographic evaluation provide no evidence of any differences in implant position compared to our records on classical exposures. There was no need for the use of an image intensifier.

There is no mystery to the minimally invasive single-incision anterior approach, although it is imperative to use special instrumentation, such as the retractors, reamers, broach handles and inserters discussed above. In addition, the design of some prostheses is obviously more suitable for this technique than others. The procedure is associated with less pain for the patient who can be ambulated earlier. The need for blood transfusions is usually low.

We did not observe any dislocations, there were no nerve palsies, although four patients reported hypesthesia on the lateral side of the femur indicative of partial laceration of femoral cutaneous nerve.

In conclusion, minimally invasive hip arthroplasty by the single-incision anterior approach is a safe procedure that allows correct placement of acetabular and femoral implants. The exposure is facilitated by the use of special retractors, reamers, broachers and inserters; implantation is made easier with specially designed prostheses. The proposed technique can reduce peri-operative blood loss, post-operative pain, and hospitalization time; it speeds up post-operative recovery and leads to small, cosmetically satisfactory surgical scars. We encourage the conduct of comparative prospective randomized studies to fully evaluate outcomes and benefits.

References

1. Berger RA (2003) Total hip arthroplasty using the minimally invasive two-incision approach. Clin Orthop 417: 232–241
2. Kennon RE, Keggi JM, Wetmore FS, Zatorski LE, Huo MH, Keggi KJ (2003) Total hip arthroplasty through a minimally invasive anterior surgical approach. J Bone Joint Surg 85-A [Suppl 4]: 39–48
3. Di Gioia III AM, Plakseqchuk AY, Levsion TJ, Jaramaz B(2003) Mini-incision technique for total hip arthroplasty with navigation. J Arthroplasty 18: 123–128
4. Goldstein WM, Branson JJ, Berland KA, Gordon AC (2003) Minimal-Incision total hip arthroplasty. J Bone Joint Surg 85-A [Suppl 4]: 33–38
5. Garrow JS, Webster J (1985) Quetelet's index (W/H^2) as a measure of fatness. Intern J Obesity 9: 147–153
6. Bellamy N, Buchanan W, Goldsmith CH, Campbell J, Stitt LW (1988) Validation study of WOMAC: A health status instrument for measuring clinically important patient relevant outcomes to antirheumatic drug therapy in patients with osteoarthritis of the hip and the knee. J Rheumatol 15: 1833–1840
7. Aszmann OC, Dellon ES, Dellon AL (1997) Anatomical course of the lateral femoral cutaneous nerve and its susceptibility to compression and injury. Plast Reconstr Surg 100: 600–604
8. De Ridder VA, de Lange S, Popta Jv (1999) Anatomical variations of the lateral femoral cutaneous nerve and the consequences for surgery. J Orthop Trauma 13: 207–211
9. Murata Y, Takahashi K, Yamagata M, Shimada Y, Moriya H (2000) The anatomy of the lateral femoral cutaneous nerve, with special reference to the harvesting of iliac bone graft. J Bone Joint Surg 82-A: 746–747
10. Beausang E, Floyd H, Dunn KW, Orton CI, Ferguson MWJ (1998) A new quantitative scale for clinical scar assessment. Plast Reconstr Surg 102: 1954–1961
11. Bierbaum, BE, Hill C, Callaghan JJ, Galante JO, Rubash HE, Tooms RE, Welch RB (1999) An analysis of blood management in patients having a total hip or knee arthroplasty. J Bone Joint Surg 81-A: 2–10
12. Helm AT, Karski MT, Parsons SJ, Sampath JS, Bale RS (2003) A strategy for reducing blood transfusion requirements in elective orthopaedic surgery. Audit of an algorithm for arthroplasty of the lower limb. J Bone Joint Surg 85-B: 484–489
13. Rosencher N, Kerkkamp HEM, Macheras G, Munuera LM, Menichella G, Barton DM, Cremers S, Abraham IL (2003) Orthopaedic Surgery Transfusion Hemoglobulin European Overview (OSTHEO) study: blood management in elective knee and hip arthroplasty in Europe. Transfusion 43: 459–469
14. Calandruccio R (1992) Voies d'abord de la hanche. In : Roy-Camille R, Laurin CA, Riley Jr LH (eds) Atlas des chirurgie orthopédique, tome 3 membre inférieur. Masson, Paris Milan Barcelone Bonn, pp 65–70
15. Crenshaw AH (1987) Campbell's Operative Orthopaedics, 7th edn. Surgical approaches. Mosby, St. Louis Washington DC Toronto, pp 58–59
16. Hoppenfeld S, deBoer P (1994) Surgical exposures in orthopaedics, 2nd edn. The anatomic approach; chapter 8: The Hip and Acetabulum. JB Lippincott, Philadelphia, pp 323–341
17. Weber M, Ganz R (2002) Der vordere Zugang zu Becken und Hüftgelenk. Modifizierter Smith-Petersen-Zugang sowie Erweiterungsmöglichkeiten. Operat Orthop Traumatol 14: 265–279
18. Pfirrmann CWA, Chung CB, Theumann NH, Trudell DJ, Resnick D (2001) Greater trochanter of the hip: attachment of the abductor mechanism and a complex of three bursae – MR imaging and MR bursography in cadavers and MR imaging in asymptomatic volunteers. Radiology 221: 469–477
19. Beck M, Sledge JB, Gautier E, Dora CF, Ganz R (2000) The anatomy and function of the gluteus minimus muscle. J Bone Joint Surg 82-B: 358–363
20, Williams PL, Warwick R, Dyson M, Bannister LH (1989) Gray's Anatomy, 37th edn. The Femur. Relations and attachments. Churchill Livingstone, Edinburgh London Melbourne New York, pp 435–439

The Direct Anterior Approach

K.J. Keggi, R.E. Kennon

Introduction

The anterior approach is the most direct route into the hip and has been described by many authors. It was advocated for hip arthroplasties by Smith-Petersen more than 60 years ago and well described by Lowell and Aufranc in 1968 [1–3]. It was shown to be feasible in total hip replacements in the 1970s [4].

We have been using this approach for more than 30 years through a modified shorter Smith-Petersen incision in over 6000 primary and revision hip replacements [5–8]. Even though it is possible in thin patients with small acetabulums to perform the operation through a very short incision (5 cm, with proximal and distal instrument portals), it has always been our belief that the clinical success of the anterior approach is primarily based on the sparing of the major hip muscles, their innervation and their function. The entry into the hip is muscle splitting and through an "internervous line" between the muscles innervated by the femoral and superior gluteal nerves. We think of it as an anterior Muscle Sparing Approach (MSA™) that can be used in all types of patients and could also be called minimally invasive.

The hip capsule is easily exposed and, once excised, allows exposure of the femoral neck and head in their anatomical position. After the removal of the femoral head, the acetabulum is visualized and easily prepared for prosthetic replacement. If properly mobilized and brought up into the wound, the femur is also easily prepared and replaced, but this requires understanding of the muscles, tendons and ligaments that have to be released from the proximal femur. Some specially designed instruments may also be required.

The femoral replacement has been simplified by modular components which do not require major muscle releases and femoral mobilization. The variety of modular components also allows better reconstitution of the patient's hip anatomy. The body of the prosthesis is inserted through a second proximal incision. The shoulder and neck components are introduced through the main anterior incision and are then affixed in situ to the main portion of the prosthesis.

Techniques

General Exposure and Acetabulum

The patient is in the supine position with a small sand bag or radiolucent rolled towels under the sacrum to slightly tilt the pelvis away from the operating table (⬛ Fig. 7.13). The leg is draped free. The iliac crests, the thighs, the patellae, the medial malleoli and the feet are visible or palpable throughout the procedure which facilitates the orientation of the prosthetic components and the estimation of the leg lengths. We frequently perform bilateral hip arthroplasties, and the supine position allows this to be done without repositioning or redraping during the case [9, 10].

The incision is made from a point just distal to the anterior superior iliac spine to what is estimated to be the midpoint of the anterior intertrochanteric line (⬛ Fig. 7.14). Its length depends on the patient's size, the subcutaneous fat and/or the muscle mass. We try to make it as short as possible but will not hesitate to extend it if indicated for proper exposure and component placement.

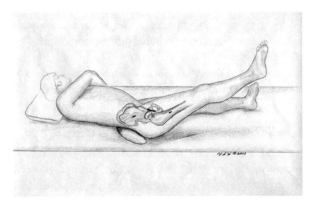

Fig. 7.13. The supine position facilitates the orientation of the prosthetic components and the estimation of the leg lengths and also has the advantage of allowing bilateral procedures without repositioning or redraping. There is no need for fluoroscopy or special operating tables

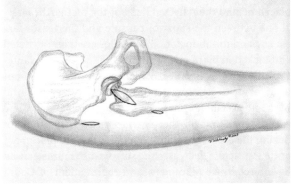

Fig. 7.14. The incision is made from a point just distal to the anterior superior iliac spine to the mid-point of the anterior intertrochanteric line, with or without the use of accessory proximal and distal stab wounds

Even though the skin will stretch slightly, the length of the incision is also dictated by the size of the femoral head that has to be removed, and by the acetabulum that has to be inserted. If indicated, the incision can be extended distally and curved along the lateral thigh down to the knee if necessary in femoral fractures, femoral grafting or other complex shaft procedures [11–13]. If greater acetabular exposure is needed, it can be curved proximally along the anterior border of the iliac crest.

Another advantage of the anterior approach is access to the abdomen. It can be draped free, should there be concern about vascular, intestinal and bladder injuries in complex revisions or acetabular reconstructions. In case of an intra-pelvic or abdominal catastrophe, rapid access to the injured structures may mean the difference between life and death.

Once the subcutaneous fat has been dissected, the tensor fascia lata is identified and split along its anterior margin. The thin strip of muscle and fascia left medially protects the lateral femoral cutaneous nerve and allows better wound closure.

The anterior hip capsule is visualized and the reflected head of the rectus femoris is elevated from the underlying capsule by blunt or sharp dissection (Fig. 7.15). The ascending branch of the lateral femoral circumflex artery is identified and coagulated. The main transverse portion of the lateral circumflex artery and vein is identified and protected if possible. If more exposure is

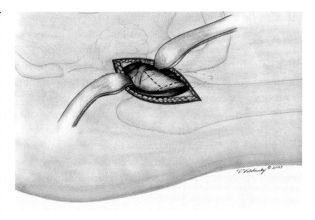

Fig. 7.15. The tensor fascia lata is split along its anterior margin. The anterior hip capsule is identified, and the reflected head of the rectus femoris is elevated from the underlying capsule

needed, they are transected and controlled by coagulation, clips or ligatures. In the case of resurfacing arthroplasties where the blood supply to the femoral neck and head is critical, these vessels must be protected with maximum care [14].

For many years we have used Cobras as the retractors of choice, but the Omni Tract self-retaining retractor (Arthro-Tract Retractor System, Omni-Tract Surgical, St. Paul, Minnesota), fixed to the operating table by a rigid post, now gives us better exposure and stabilizes the operative field (Fig. 7.16). The medial blade is placed behind the reflected head of the rectus, the lateral one between the superior capsule and the tensor fascia lata and the abductors. The blades are then ratcheted and locked in place giving an excellent view of the anterior hip capsule. If properly placed, these blades do not need to be repositioned during the capsular, femoral neck and acetabular phases of the operation and in some cases, depending on the patient's size and/or implant during the entire procedure. This single rigid placement of the retractors decreases the soft-tissue trauma caused by the repetitive placement, and replacement of Cobra retractors definitely decreases intra-operative bleeding and may decrease overall blood loss.

Once exposure has been achieved, a complete anterior capsulectomy is performed. At various times we have tried to perform the acetabular replacement with capsular incisions only, but have abandoned them for the sake of better exposure. A tight contracted anterior capsule can also be a contributing factor to posterior dislocations. There are advocates of capsular incision preservation and repair, but the operation is easier and probably safer with the excisional approach. The excision of the capsule may cause some more bleeding, but the bleeding tissues can be coagulated. Following the capsulectomy, Cobra retractors, when used, are now placed in the capsule with their tips under the femoral neck, but the rigid, well-placed Omni Tract retractor now gives excellent neck exposure without any change in the position of the blades. The leg is placed in a neutral, anatomical position, and the bony landmarks of the proximal femur can be identified by direct visualization or palpation. The cut of the femoral neck is determined by templating the X-rays prior to the operation and can be duplicated with relative ease on the visualized base of the femoral neck without dislocation. In severe deformities and contractures of the hip, a preliminary subcapital osteotomy can be done to place the femur in the anatomical position for the final neck cut. The position of the femoral cut varies, according to the anatomical configurations of each femur, but should be distal enough to allow neutral placement of the prosthesis in the medullary canal. The cut is completed, and the femoral head is removed with a skid and/or corkscrew device. The acetabulum is prepared with large curettes and basket reamers. The true medial wall is exposed in order to fully medialize the acetabular prosthesis and to recreate as much as possible the patient's normal center of rotation.

If the patient is large and bulky, it may be necessary to extend the incision distally or to retrograde standard straight acetabular reamers through a distal stab wound in order to get the desired 40–45° varus/valgus acetabular angle and the 15–20° of anteversion. The basket reamer and acetabular prosthesis can be attached in the main incision after inserting the shaft through the distal stab wound (❑ Fig. 7.17). A dog-leg acetabular reamer may obviate the need for this particular step, but the stab wounds have been helpful and facilitated this surgery in patients as large as 450 lbs. Our experience and results in

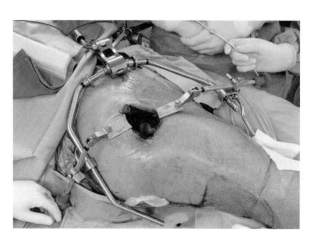

❑ **Fig. 7.16.** We have used cobra retractors for many years, but a self-retaining retractor (Arthro-Tract Retractor System, Omni-Tract Surgical, St. Paul, Minnesota) fixed to the operating table by a rigid post now gives us excellent exposure and stabilizes the operative field

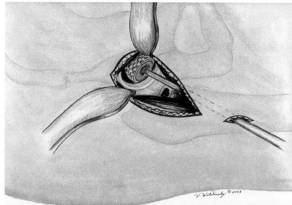

❑ **Fig. 7.17.** If the patient is large, it may be necessary to extend the incision distally or to retrograde the reamers through a distal stab wound in order to get the desired varus/valgus acetabular angle and anteversion

obese patients have been excellent, and we do not hesitate to perform total hip arthroplasty in these weight-challenged individuals [15]. The acetabular preparation and insertion is relatively easy since it is done under direct vision.

For non-cemented prostheses the bony acetabulum is usually under-reamed by 2 mm. It is over-reamed by 2–3 mm to achieve an even cement mantle in the cemented ones. The non-cemented metal acetabulums or shells are impacted into the bone, and in the majority of cases are stable without additional dome screws. The ceramic or polyethylene liners are then placed in the metal shells. Standard techniques are used to cement an all-polyethylene prosthesis if needed. All acetabular osteophytes are removed to allow maximum motion and to remove any possible fulcrum points that may contribute to post-operative dislocations. The posterior medial osteophytes must be handled with special care due to their proximity to the sciatic nerve.

The acetabular angles are determined by looking at the pre-operative X-rays, by examining the acetabulum, by palpating the iliac crests and by visualizing the position of the entire leg in its relationship to the acetabulum and pelvis. There are advocates of fluoroscopy or navigational systems to determine exact acetabular angles, and this is easily applied in this supine position on a radiolucent table, but with experience such aids may not be necessary and we have only used them rarely for teaching purposes.

Femoral Monoblock Prosthesis

Mobilization and exposure of the proximal femur is imperative for the safe and proper insertion of the monoblock femoral component. It is achieved in a stepwise manner.

The lateral blade of the Omni Tract retractor can be left in place or adjusted for modular femoral components, but in most monoblock prostheses it is removed and the leg is placed in external rotation. In thin and loose hips it may be possible to deliver the proximal femur in the anterior wound by using a bone hook placed around the lesser trochanter. Next, a pointed cobra-like trochanteric retractor or one of the long-handled straight or slightly curved ribbon retractors can be placed under the greater trochanter to lever the femur into an accessible position.

If femoral mobilization is difficult, a partial or complete posterior capsulectomy can be done. If necessary, the external rotators can be released from their insertion in the trochanteric fossa. The piriformis tendon can also be transected. The foot of the operating table can be dropped to extend the femur. There are recent advocates of the anterior approach who routinely do their total hip replacements on a "fracture table" that allows distraction and extension of the leg for access to the proximal femur, but we have performed our more than 6000 total hip replacements on regular operating tables. As a last resort, a trochanteric "fold-back" or "slide" osteotomy is possible, but this has been rarely necessary in the past 10 years [16]. A release or Z-plasty of the iliopsoas is another extreme step to achieve femoral exposure in complex primary or revision cases. The last two steps have been rare in our hands. In most cases, a partial release of the posterior capsule and short external rotators from the greater trochanter, as the femur is externally rotated and levered or pulled up into the wound, has been sufficient. We have never repaired these posterior releases and continue to have excellent functional results and a low dislocation rate of 1.3% in a consecutive series of 2132 primary total hips. During these soft-tissue releases the posterior circumflex vessels must be controlled, if at all possible, prior to their transection. If the capsule and rotator tendons are cut slowly, the vessels are easily visualized and coagulated. If they retract, the process is somewhat more difficult and may require traction on the leg for exposure of the bleeding vessels. The sciatic nerve is medial and posterior to the area of the tendon releases and has not been a problem.

Once the femur is mobilized and exposed, it is rasped to accept the prosthesis to be used. Curved anterior "Keggi" rasps facilitate this procedure (☐ Fig. 7.18a). These rasps have been available through several orthopedic manufacturers (Howmedica, Zimmer, Smith-Nephew-Richards). In non-cemented devices where precise reaming of the femoral canal is required, the reamers are passed through a proximal stab wound or "second incision" (☐ Fig. 7.18b). This stab wound or second incision is in line with the greater trochanter and the long axis of the femur close to the iliac crest. It cannot be posterior since a posterior incision can misguide the reamers, broaches and implants to the sciatic nerve. The reamer is inserted through the thin triangular fascia between the posterior proximal portion of the tensor fascia lata and superior border of the gluteus maximus muscles. It then passes lateral to the medius and minimus, anterior medial to the maximus and posterior to the tensor fascia lata muscles. It is once more in an "internervous" line between the superior and inferior gluteal nerves. It passes through the greater trochanteric insertion of the gluteus medius or between the medius and the piriformis on its way into the proximal femur.

After the preliminary reaming of the medullary canal, the bent anterior hip rasp can be used to complete the femoral preparation through the main incision. Straight rasps with long handles are also available for preparation of the femur through the stab wound or second incision described above. Even though it is possible to insert the monoblock prosthesis through the second proximal incision, our preference is to mobilize the femur and to insert the prosthesis through the main incision when using nonmodular systems. If the various releases described previously are not sufficient to insert the femoral component, a release of the tensor fascia lata from its origin along the anterior portion of the iliac crest is done, but this has rarely been necessary. Both non-cemented and cemented devices can be used (◘ Fig. 7.19).

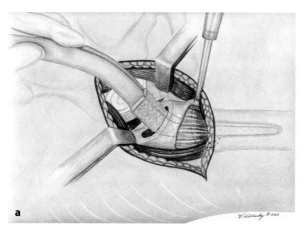

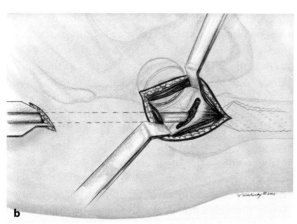

◘ Fig. 7.18. a Curved anterior "Keggi" rasps facilitate this procedure. Since the 1970's, this modification has been the only change from standard instrumentation for routine, cemented monoblock total hip replacements. **b** The reamers are passed through a proximal stab wound in non-cemented devices where precise reaming of the femoral canal is required. Modular femoral stems can also be inserted through this stab wound without the need for a posterior capsular release to mobilize the femur

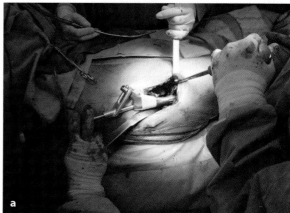

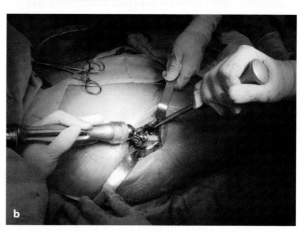

◘ Fig. 7.19. a A non-cemented prosthesis is impacted into place. Newer modular systems allow the femoral component itself to be passed through the proximal stab wound. **b** A cemented prosthesis is cemented into place. The determination of whether to use a cemented or noncemented femoral component is made based on the patient's physiologic age and bone quality

We seek neutral anteversion of the neck and use trial heads to determine the final head height. Leg lengths are assessed by palpation of the iliac crests, patellas and medial malleoli. In less than 5% of our cases there may be a minor leg-length discrepancy (1.5 cm or less). As a rule, we are more concerned about hip stability than a minor leg-length discrepancy.

Pre-operative implant selection may be necessary to reproduce the patient's anatomy and hip stability without leg lengthening. In the past 10 years there has been a greater variety of monoblock prostheses to accommodate individual femurs, but the process becomes easier with modular hips that allow greater range of neck shaft angles, varus, valgus offset, etc. The stability of the hip is tested with trial prostheses and again at the end of the operation with the permanent components.

On occasion, since the late 1980's we have passed monoblock prostheses through the proximal incision, but our experience with this method has not been positive since the neck and/or collar of the devices tend to get caught in the abductor muscles. It has been easier with a press-fit collarless stem (Zweymuller), but we have had some tense moments with some of the cemented monoblock implants that have to pass through the muscles as the intramedullary cement is starting to set. For monoblock femoral prostheses we prefer the insertion through the main anterior incision with an appropriate posterior capsular release to mobilize the femur.

Femoral Modular Stems

Even though we continue to use some monoblock prostheses, since 2002 the majority of our hip replacements have been done with modular femoral components. The primary reasons for this have been the ease of their insertion and the variety of proximal neck configurations that provide for the more accurate reconstruction of the proximal femur, soft-tissue balancing, and leg-length adjustment.

We have been using three different devices of this type (Apex Modular™ Cementless Stem, OTI R-120™ and Cremascoli-Wright Medical™).

The body or intra-femoral portion of these devices is inserted into the femur after appropriate reaming and broaching through the proximal (second) incision. The femoral preparation and the insertion of the component itself does not require the extensive soft-tissue releases

necessary for the safe insertion of the monoblock prosthesis. The posterior circumflex vessels do not present a problem. Even though trial components are available, the modularity of the proximal portion of the prosthesis makes them unnecessary in most cases.

The proximal component or shoulder and neck of these implants has to be small enough for insertion into the body of the femoral portion through the anterior incision (◘ Fig. 7.20). Two of our implants (OTI R-120™ and the Cremascoli-Wright Medical™) are simply femoral necks and are easy to insert into the femoral stems. The Apex Modular™ device is the shoulder and neck of the prosthesis and is somewhat more difficult to assemble, but it has extremely solid fixation to the body of the prosthesis and a variety of neck configurations.

It is the variety of neck configurations of all of these prostheses that allows better reconstruction of the patient's femoral anatomy. Varus, valgus, anteversion and retroversion can be dealt with, and this has the potential of a better clinical result.

The modular femoral components made the anterior approach to hip replacement safer and easier to teach. The modularity also allows for the salvaging of femoral components inserted with improper version. If the femoral component is in excessive retroversion, the neck can be inserted in anteversion, creating a neutral acceptable position.

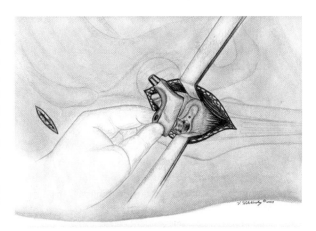

◘ Fig. 7.20. Modular prosthesis designs facilitate minimal incisions by reaming and then inserting femoral stem components through the proximal stab wound. These systems also allow a greater range of neck shaft angles, varus, valgus, offset and leg lengths than traditional monoblock femoral components

The other major advantage of the modular femoral components is that the neck can be removed if it should be necessary to reposition the acetabulum during the primary procedure, or to revise it secondarily if there should be a failure of the device. With the neck component out of the way, the acetabular revision is easier and does not necessitate the removal of the entire femoral component. After the acetabular revision, a different neck may be necessary and can be used without problems.

Conclusions

The anterior approach for total hip replacement is done with the patient in a supine anatomical position which allows better orientation of the prosthetic components. It is also a physiological approach since it accesses the hip through internervous planes and spares the major muscles. Finally it can be done in all patients with incisions short enough or long enough to achieve proper implant position without major complications. It can be as short as 5 cm but more often is 6–10 cm in length with or without proximal and distal accessory incisions or stab wounds for acetabular and femoral preparation.

The acetabular insertion is simple and the femoral portion of the operation has been simplified by modular components inserted through a second incision. With proximal and distal extensions of the incision, it can be used in all revisions, with the additional advantage that anterior revision surgery avoids significant scar tissue and the sciatic nerve.

A recent analysis of 2132 of our consecutive primary hips done through this approach revealed low rates of intra and peri-operative complications, short operative times, low blood loss and a few dislocations [6, 7]. We also reviewed 468 consecutive revision arthroplasties with few complications [8]. We continue to use this adaptable approach for all primary and revision hip arthroplasties as well as hemiarthroplasties for hip fractures. If properly performed, the anterior approach is physiological, muscle sparing and minimally invasive.

References

1. Smith-Petersen MN. A new supra-articular subperiosteal approach to the hip joint. Am J Orthop Surg 15: 592–595, 1917
2. Watson-Jones R. Fracture of the neck of the femur. Br J Surg 23: 787, 1935
3. Lowell JD, Aufranc OE. The anterior approach to the hip joint. Clin Orthop 61: 193–198, 1968
4. Keggi K, Light TR. Anterior approach to total hip arthroplasty. Scientific Exhibit, American Academy of Orthopaedic Surgeons. Las Vegas, NV, 1977
5. Keggi KJ, Huo M, Zatorski LE. Anterior approach to total hip replacement: Surgical technique and clinical results of our first one thousand cases using non-cemented prostheses. Yale Journal of Biology and Medicine 66: 243–256, 1993
6. Kennon RE, Keggi JM, Keggi KJ et al. Anterior approach to total hip arthroplasty. Scientific Exhibit, American Academy of Orthopedic Surgeons. New Orleans LA, 2003
7. Kennon RE, Keggi JM, Wetmore RS, Zatorski LE, Huo MH, Keggi KJ. Total hip arthroplasty through a minimally invasive anterior surgical approach. J Bone Joint Surg 85-A: 39–48, 2003
8. Kennon RE, Keggi JM, Keggi KJ et al. Anterior approach THA – beyond the minimally invasive approach. Scientific Exhibit, American Academy of Orthopedic Surgeons. San Francisco, CA, 2004
9. Lorenze M, Huo MH, Zatorski LE, Keggi KJ. A comparison of the cost effectiveness of one-stage versus two-stage bilateral total hip replacement. Orthopedics 21: 1249–1252, 1998
10. Weintein MA, Keggi JM, Zatorski LE, Keggi KJ. One-stage bilateral total hip arthroplasty in patients > or = 75 years. Orthopedics 25: 153–156, 2002
11. Huo MH, Cox M, Zatorski LE, Keggi KJ. Oblique femoral osteotomy in cementless total hip arthroplasty: a prospective consecutive series with minimum 3 year follow-up. J Arthroplasty 10: 319–327, 1995
12. Huo MH, Keggi KJ. Periprosthetic femoral fracture treatment with an intramedullary extension sleeve. J Orthopaedic Techniques 2: 191–196, 1994
13. Huo MH, Elliot AJ, Keggi KJ. Periprosthetic infection in total hip replacement: management with temporary prostheses and antibiotic impregnated cement between stages. J Orthopaedic Techniques 2: 93–102, 1994
14. Hendrikson RP, Keggi KJ. Anterior approach to resurfacing arthroplasty of the hip: a preliminary experience. Connecticut Medicine 47: 8–12, 1983
15. Dicaprio MR, Huo MH, Chan PS, Zatorski LE, Keggi JM, Keggi KJ. Total hip arthroplasty in the obese. American Academy of Orthopaedic Surgeons, Annual Meeting, San Francisco, CA, March 2001
16. Fulkerson JP, Crelin ES, Keggi KJ. Anatomy and osteotomy of the greater trochanter. Arch Surg 114: 19–21, 1979

Anterolateral Mini-Incision Surgical Technique

M. Austin, W.J. Hozack

Introduction

Total hip arthroplasty is perhaps the most successful operation of the 20th century – this must be foremost in the mind of the surgeon who is considering the various alternative techniques to "traditional" hip-replacement approaches. The orthopedic surgery community of the 21st century must be careful not to change too radically or too quickly an operation with such a proven track record.

To be considered minimally invasive, any total hip-arthroplasty approach must lessen the impact of surgery on the patient's quality of life and disruption of daily routine. Serious complications, such as nerve injury, leg-length discrepancy, dislocation and fracture must be minimized. The surgeon must pay attention to reducing surgical time in order to minimize blood loss, contamination leading to infection, and phlebitis. Minimally invasive does not mean just a small incision but refers more importantly to what goes on beneath the skin. The emphasis is on gentle exposure that minimizes overall muscle trauma. Although some exposures do not require removal of any muscle insertions, these indirect exposures can severely bludgeon the muscle and have the potential to create maximal trauma (invasion).

Mini-incision surgery requires careful patient selection and education. Patients must have realistic expectations consistent with their body habitus. It is essential that the surgeon discuss the benefits of small incision surgery balanced with the ultimate goal of accurate component positioning, minimal risk of complication and maximal potential for durable result.

Surgical Technique

Rationale

The antero-lateral mini-incision approach is a modification of the standard approach developed and used at Rothman Institute Orthopaedics over the past 20 years. The incision length is shortened, and therefore modified techniques and specialized equipment are required to maximize direct visualization without the need for fluoroscopy. Direct visualization of the bony anatomy of the hip is critical to a successful technical result.

The patient is positioned in the supine position. This allows simple and very accurate leg-length measurement, without the use of calipers or pins, by simply palpating the malleoli. Acetabular orientation is simplified without concern over intra-operative pelvic shift. The surgeon can directly palpate the anatomic landmarks of the pelvis (anterior superior iliac spines, pubic symphysis) and have an easier appreciation of the three-dimensional anatomy of the acetabulum. It is well documented that the antero-lateral approach has a lower dislocation rate than the other approaches (Maisonis, Bourne). The posterior capsule is retained to minimize post-operative restrictions and speed early recovery.

Instrumentation and Prosthetic Choice

Three special acetabular retractors have been designed to facilitate exposure (🔲 Fig. 7.21). One retractor is fitted with a fiberoptic light to improve visualization of the acetabulum (🔲 Fig. 7.22). Special acetabular compo-

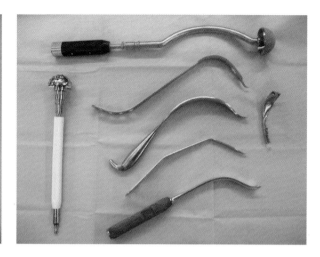

Fig. 7.21. Acetabular retractors

Fig. 7.23. Low profile Trident® (Stryker Howmedica Osteonics, Allendale, NJ) acetabular component impactors

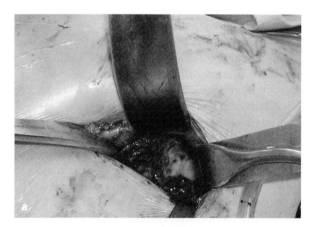

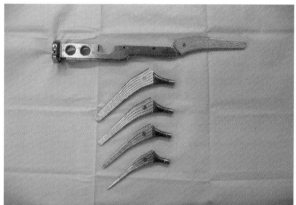

Fig. 7.24. Low profile broach handle

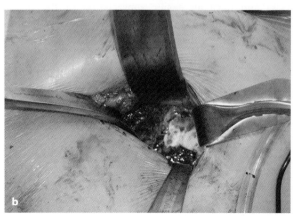

Fig. 7.22. a Acetabular visualization without fiberoptic lighting. **b** Acetabular visualization with fiberoptic lighting

nent impactors ease insertion of the final component (Fig. 7.23). The special femoral retractors consist two double-footed retractors. The broach handles have been modified for ease of insertion through a smaller incision (Fig. 7.24). The trial instruments have snap-on heads with a special insertion device to aid in head-neck trials. Low-profile component insertion handles and head impactors have been designed. This special instrumentation has been consolidated into a single-equipment tray (Fig. 7.25) available from Stryker Orthopedics (Mahwah, NJ). Finally, component selection is important. A system must be selected which facilitates component positioning through a small incision. This particular system must have proven clinically success, yet be extremely simple and quick to prepare the bone and implant the prosthesis (again minimizing the overall trauma to the patient). A proximally coated tapered titanium-alloy prosthesis is utilized to minimize long-term bone loss associated with distal fixation stems.

Technique to Minimize Incision Length

Overall incision length will vary from 8–12 cm depending upon patient weight, local adipose thickness, muscle mass, flexibility and anatomy. The initial incision should extend from the anterior third of the tip of the greater

trochanter to a point several centimeters distal, along the diaphysis of the femur (◘ Fig. 7.26). This initial incision can be extended proximally (for femoral exposure) or distally (for acetabular exposure) as needed. The initial incision is made through skin down to the level of the fascia. At this point the fat tissue is dissected bluntly off the fascia to maximize the visualization of the fascia. The skin and subcutaneous tissue can then be mobilized in any direction throughout the procedure to maximize visualization.

Surgical Approach

The initial incision is made to the level of the fascia, as described above. The fascia is then split just anterior to the most lateral aspect of the greater trochanter. The anterior and posterior aspect of the gluteus medius muscle is identified. The anterior third of the gluteus medius, the entire gluteus minimus, and the anterior half of the hip capsule are elevated anteriorly in one flap. The femoral head is then dislocated and the neck osteotomized. This gentle exposure limits trauma to the muscle belly, yet closure of this flap is readily obtained (◘ Fig. 7.27). The superior capsule is incised along the posterior aspect of the gluteus minimus, and the infero-medial capsule is incised with care not to divide the iliopsoas tendon. This technique – capsular incision rather than capsular excision – maximizes exposure and stability and minimizes the potential for leg-length discrepancy. It also allows the patient full, unrestricted activity immediately after the surgery.

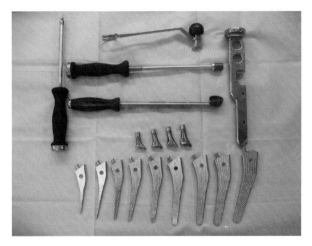

◘ **Fig. 7.25.** Accolade™ Femoral Hip System modified instruments (Stryker Howmedica Osteonics, Allendale, NJ)

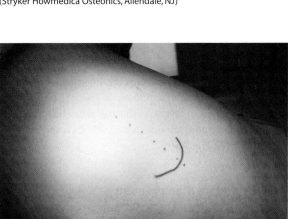

◘ **Fig. 7.26.** Planned incision with the greater trochanter marked

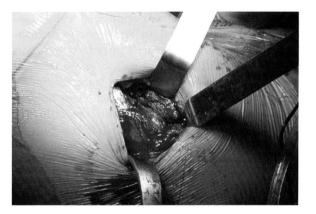

◘ **Fig. 7.27.** Split of the gluteus medius, with minimal trauma, prior to repair

Acetabular retractors are placed in the following sequence: anterior, superior, inferior. The anterior cobra retractor is placed with the hip flexed so as to relax the anterior neurovascular structures, allowing safe placement of this retractor. The superior retractor is best positioned at the 10:00 position on a right hip (2:00 on a left hip). The initial inferior retractor is a double-angle type and is best placed on the ischium as medial as possible. The medial capsular structures are placed on stretch by this retractor. The medial capsule is then incised, taking care not to violate the iliopsoas tendon. The visualization of the acetabulum is then assessed and, if deemed suboptimal, the double-angle is replaced with a double-footed retractor placed as medial as possible onto the ischium. At this juncture, the surgeon should be able to visualize the entire periphery of the acetabulum prior to reaming (■ Fig. 7.28).

The surgeon should identify all the landmarks important for acetabular positioning including the anterior and posterior columns, anterior and posterior walls, cotyloid fossa, and the acetabular notch prior to reaming. The reaming should progress sequentially so that a hemisphere is created that is medialized and so that the inferior edge of the cup is at the level of the teardrop. Great care must be taken not to aggressively ream away walls or columns. Proper placement of the acetabular retractors protects the skin from damage by the reamers, regardless of incision size. The cup is generally under-reamed by 1 mm so as to obtain a press-fit. The acetabular component is then inserted under direct visualization. Screws are generally not needed. At this point, a trial liner or the actual liner may be impacted into place.

Femoral exposure requires externally rotation and adduction of the leg. A double-footed retractor is placed posterior to the femur and another double-footed retractor is placed lateral to the femur to facilitate broaching (■ Fig. 7.29). Properly placed, the retractors will minimize soft-tissue and muscle injury from the instruments. If the femur cannot be adequately exposed for broaching despite appropriate leg and retractor positioning, the incision must be extended proximally. The entire cortical rim of the proximal femur must be exposed to properly assess version, axial stability and rotational stability, and for early detection of fracture, should it occur, during the femoral preparation and component insertion. The starter reamer is used to open the canal and then the femur is sequentially broached. Elimination of all but the small starter reamer mini-

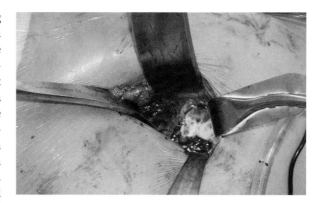

■ **Fig. 7.28.** Acetabular exposure. Note the excellent view provided by this approach which allows accurate component insertion under direct visualization

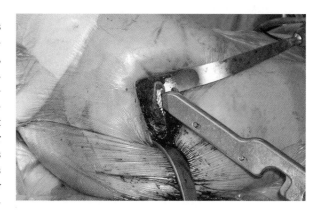

■ **Fig. 7.29.** Femoral exposure. Note that the entire circumference of the proximal femur is visualized

mizes the potential for trauma to the gluteus medius muscle. The broach serves as a trial and a special head-neck insertion device is available to make trial reduction easier. After testing for stability, impingement, leg length and offset, the final component is then inserted. The incision is closed in layers, with careful attention paid to repair of the gluteus medius tendon. The closed incision is pictured (■ Fig. 7.30).

Post-Operative Management

Patients are not required to use bracing, hip precautions or restricted weight bearing. The morning after surgery, the Foley catheter and all intravenous medications and fluids are discontinued. Physical therapy is given twice daily, but the patient is encouraged to be out of bed as much as possible. Oral pain management consists of oxycodone for the inpatient stay and for discharge. The pain management is supplemented by non-steroidal anti-inflammatory medication. The patient is discharged to home on the second or third post-operative day based solely on progress in therapy. The patient uses a walker on the first day, is discharged with crutches and progresses to a cane by 2 weeks.

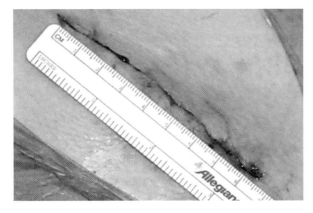

◻ **Fig. 7.30.** Closed small-incision total hip arthroplasty

Conclusions

The antero-lateral mini-incision technique for total hip arthroplasty balances the desire for less invasive surgery with the requirement of adequate visualization. It is a modification of an existing, successful method that emphasizes gentle soft-tissue dissection and excellent exposure. The initial incision may be extended as needed to improve direct visualization and subsequent accurate component positioning. Specialized instrumentation has been developed to facilitate the success of this technique.

Posterior Approach for MIS with Image-Free Computer-Assisted Navigation

L.D. Dorr, A.G. Yun

Introduction

This chapter will describe the technique of the posterior mini-incision of average 8 cm length. Sixty percent or more of total hip replacements in the United States are performed through the posterior approach. Therefore, it only makes sense that the majority of surgeons will need to initially learn to perform MIS THR through a posterior approach. Most will not go beyond this approach to an intermuscular one because the posterior mini-incision operation satisfies the needs of most patients. Gait studies have always shown better function post-operatively, at least in the first 6 months, in patients with a posterior rather than an anterior approach [1].

In this chapter the use and benefits of image-free computer navigation will also be described. The advantage of the computer is the precision it provides the surgeon in decision-making during the operation. Most of the anxiety of the surgeon during a hip-replacement operation is whether or not the components are correctly placed and the biomechanical reconstruction (leg length and off-set) is optimal. The computer provides precise information to enable these decisions. With image-free computer navigation the additional operating time approximates 15 min.

The Process of Posterior MIS THR

The satisfaction of patients with MIS operations has been, in part, because of the improvement for the patient of the process of the entire surgical experience. Pre-operative education, anesthesia, and pain management, as well as post-operative rehabilitation combined with a less invasive operation have improved patient outcomes

[2]. Patient interest has been fueled by the entire process and not just that their body image is less injured by a small incision.

The improved process of THR has permitted patients to go home easily within 48 h – and often the same day with the Berger two-incision operation and process [2]. Of greater importance than early hospital discharge is that this new process permits the patient to achieve part-time return to work within 7–10 days. It also minimizes the time off work for the spouse or family of the patient. Our patients, excluding those with laboring occupations, returned to some hours of work at one week post-operative. The necessity for a patient to go to a rehabilitation ward after the operation has almost disappeared with our incidence decreasing from 40% to 2%. The cost savings to medicine and to society can be appreciated.

The process of the operation begins with pre-operative education which is conducted as a pre-operative class. This class educates the patient and his/her family to the hospital course and expectations, the implants to be used, the physical therapy to be received, the anesthesia to be used, and the nursing protocols. Therefore, the patients "know the routine" prior to coming to the hospital, and they expect to go home within 48 h unless medically this is not safe. Of equal importance is that the families expect this also and prepare for this timing of discharge.

Anesthesia is best done by regional techniques of epidural or short-term spinal anesthesia [2]. We prefer epidural anesthesia to decrease the prevalence of spinal headache and permit maintenance of the epidural for 24 h in patients who have bilateral total hip replacements. The important fact is that *no* narcotics are used in the epidural or spinal. We use Ropivacaine (Astra Zeneca,

Washington, DE) only. The avoidance of epidural narcotics and intravenous narcotics prevents post-operative nausea, dizziness, and emesis. This avoidance of intravenous narcotics may be the single most improvement in patient treatment for this operation because it prevents physical depression of the metabolism of the patient and the mental depression that then accompanies the physical symptoms of lethargy, dizziness, and emesis. The patient is unconscious during the operation by the infusion of propofol (Astra Zeneca, Wilmington, DE) which, when withdrawn, allows the patient to be wide awake in the post-anesthesia recovery room. This further allows the patient to be walking with physical therapy within 4 h of the operation. Oral anti-inflammatory and narcotic medications are administered one hour pre-operatively to the patient and the oral narcotics are given preemptively post-operatively [2]. By including the preemptive medications through the first two nights, the patients are able to sleep, which improves their performance with physical therapy, and their mental attitude, during the day or two of hospitalization.

Post-operative rehabilitation is simplified in this THR process. Patients are allowed to be full weight-bearing with a single crutch or cane, even when the implants are non-cemented, because implant stability and muscle function permit this. We use the anatomic porous replacement stem (APR, Zimmer, Warsaw, IN) which is anatomic and has inherent stability by design. Many other stems also permit immediate full weight-bearing post-operatively. Motivated patients with unilateral hip disease, and without medical comorbidities, can usually walk 1 mile within 2 weeks with a cane. The improvement for a patient is week by week during the first 3 months and then becomes month by month for the next 3–6 months.

Registration for Computer Navigation

Computer navigation requires data acquisition of the orientation of the pelvis in space so that this information is known while the operation is being performed. This is accomplished by registration of the anterior-posterior (AP plane) of the pelvis from which the computer software can determine the orientation of the acetabulum and acetabular component within the pelvis. The registration is done by first attaching a registration guide to the pelvis using of pins through the pelvic crest. With the infrared light-emitting diode markers (silver balls which will be called the light guide) positioned for the optical camera, the pelvis is registered by touching the pointing probe (probe) to the two anterior superior iliac spines (ASIS) and the pubis near the pubic tubercles (◘ Fig. 7.31). This registration is image-free which means that it does not require pre-operative CT scan or fluoroscopy.

After registration of the AP plane, the patient is positioned laterally and secured with thoracic and pelvic supports (◘ Fig. 7.32). The posterior supports are touched by the probe to register the position of the spine so that the software can measure the tilt of the pelvis. The pelvic tilt affects the anteversion of the cup and therefore the software will calculate the adjusted anteversion position of the cup based on the pelvic tilt. The

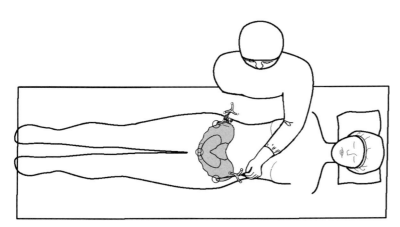

◘ **Fig. 7.31.** Pelvic tracking device in place and AP plane of pelvis registered by anterior superior iliac spines and pubis.

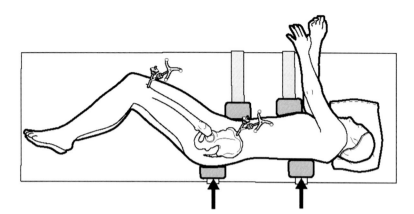

Fig. 7.32. Patient supported in lateral position with pelvis and femoral tracker in place. Posterior supports are used to register pelvic tilt (arrows)

pelvis is often tilted posteriorly when the patient is in the lateral position whereas it is tilted anteriorly when the patient is supine on the operating table. It is apparent that the knowledge of the tilt is critical to measuring the correct cup anteversion within the pelvis.

Once the skin preparation and draping has been completed, the femoral registration device is fixed. This is a 4.5 mm screw which is drilled into the distal lateral femur. A sleeve slides over the screw which has the light guide attached for registration of the femur (see **Fig. 7.32**). This sleeve is slotted so that it can be removed during the surgery and precisely replaced for measurements when they are performed. By registration of the femur, the computer will be able to tell the surgeon the anteversion of the femoral component, as well as the leg length and the off-set of the hip reconstruction.

This entire registration process of the pelvis and femur requires ten minutes of time in addition to the skin preparation and draping. However, the knowledge of component position and of the biomechanical reconstruction replaces several minutes of decision-making for the surgeon when using manual methods.

Technique

To accomplish this MIS operation with ease of technique and protection against excessive soft-tissue tension, specialized tools, including retractors, reamers, and implant holders, are needed. Several features are required for these instruments. Long handles are a necessity for the retractors to allow retraction with little soft-tissue tension, to keep the assistants' hands and bodies clear of the wound and the operating surgeon, and to allow the assis-

tant to hold multiple retractors which minimizes the number of assistants needed.

The acetabular retractors are shown in **Fig. 7.33** and are numbered in the order they are used at surgery, which is not the order in which they are presented in this descriptive explanation of the operation. A unique retractor (retractor #7) for the posterior capsule that has a long tip to engage the cortical bone of the cotyloid notch (just below the transverse acetabular ligament), and a paddle that sits on the ischial bone and protects

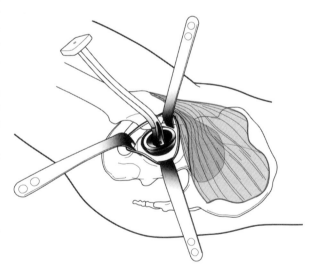

Fig 7.33. Acetabular exposure with retractor #5 at the top, retractor #4 at the lower right, and retractor #7 at the lower left. The curved reamer is placed into the acetabular cavity and it shows how the angle of the reamer permits reaming without the reaming impinging on the distal wound edge. The curved acetabular cup holder is shown during placement of the cup and illustrates how the curved holder allows the cup to be placed without the wound affecting the cup holder

the sciatic nerve as it retracts the posterior capsule, is key to complete exposure of the acetabulum. The retractor used to displace the femoral bone anterior to the acetabulum is named the "snake-retractor" (retractor #5) and was designed by Dr. Chit Ranawat (Lennox Hill Hospital, New York, NY). It has a point which is engaged on the anterior ilium, just lateral to the anterior-inferior spine, to give secure fixation for the retractor. It also has a radius of curvature which gives great leverage to retract the femur anteriorly without damage to the bone. By not placing an anterior retractor against the anterior wall of the acetabulum, both the wall is protected from breakage and the femoral nerve does not have tension on it. A posterior-superior retractor (retractor #4) has a point which can be pounded into the bone to stabilize it as it retracts the posterior-superior capsule and small external rotators.

The femoral retractors are also designed to maximize exposure of the cut surface of the femoral neck for preparation of the femur without excessive retraction force (Fig. 7.34). A new "jaws" retractor (retractor #8) was designed with a radius of curvature and a long handle which will effectively elevate the cut surface of the femoral neck into the wound by retracting the posterior-superior flap of the wound. The posterior-superior retractor for the acetabulum (retractor #4) is placed around the cut femoral neck under the quadratus

femoris muscle to protect this muscle, and expose the medial cortex of the neck, during femoral preparation. The anterior skin and gluteus maximus muscle must be retracted from overhanging the greater trochanter. A trochanteric reamer (retractors #9 and #10) has two parts, which can be joined by a linking tool. Retractor #9 is for the overhanging gluteus maximus and skin, while retractor #10 is for the gluteus medius muscle. Both are not always necessary depending on the thickness of skin and fat and of the position of the gluteus medius and/or maximus muscles.

Soft-Tissue Exposure

The surgical technique being described is performed through an incision that is posterior to the greater trochanter (Fig. 7.35). The patient is in the lateral decubitus position and supported at the pelvis and at the chest so that there is complete stability of the body position (see Fig. 7.32). The site of the incision is absolutely critical. This incision must be on the posterior border of the trochanter, for if it is anterior to that, an extension of the incision will be necessary to provide completion of the operation. The length of the incision is proximally at the tip of the greater trochanter to distally at the level of the vastus tubercle of the femur. Therefore, the length of the incision can be changed according to the height of the patient. Very tall patients would have a longer length of their trochanter and therefore a longer incision. The best length of the skin incision is 8 cm which provides the best visual exposure for the surgeon and the assistants. An incision of 5–6 cm of the skin reduces the ability of the assistant to visualize the oper-

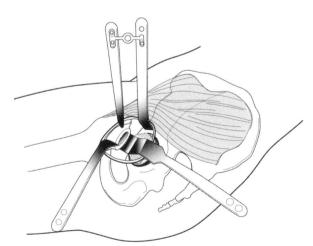

Fig 7.34. Femoral exposure with retractor #8 at the lower right, retractor #4 under the quadratus muscle, and around the medial neck at lower left, retractor #9 (more distal) and #10 (more cephalad) retracting the gluteus maximus and gluteus medius muscles. (These retractors can be joined by a link)

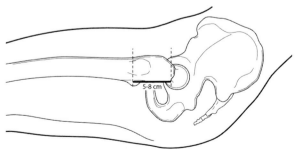

Fig. 7.35. The incision must be made along the posterior border of the greater trochanter

ation. Furthermore, this shorter skin incision does not give benefit to the patient. The length of the muscle incision, which can almost always be kept at 6 cm, is of greater importance to the function of the patient and does not change the attitude of the patient toward the cosmesis of the surgery.

The incision is made through the skin and the sub-cutaneous tissue and 6 cm of gluteus maximus muscle fibers adjacent to the posterior edge of the greater trochanter. Following the initial skin incision, the remainder of the exposure is done with an electro-cautery Bovey. The leg is then turned into internal rotation with the knee kept in the center of the table (and on top of the lower leg). It is important *not* to let the knee drop over the side of the table because this puts too much tension on the soft-tissue structures in the posterior hip. With the leg in this position the separation between the gluteus medius muscle and the gluteus minimus muscle is divided with the surgeon's finger. This can easily be found by identifying the piriformis tendon and then sliding the finger under the gluteus medius and on top of the gluteus minimus. The gluteus medius muscle by retractor #2 is retracted from the gluteus minimus muscle. The gluteus minimus muscle is then incised to the pelvic bone beginning 3 cm superior to the attachment of the piriformis tendon because the superior edge of the acetabulum is 3 cm proximal to the piriformis tendon. The incision is continued as a single flap distally to the proximal edge of the quadratus muscle and then the capsule is divided beneath the quadratus muscle, leaving the quadratus muscle intact (◘ Fig. 7.36). In some patients, the most superior attachment of the quadratus muscle to the trochanter must be released for 2–3 mm to relax the muscle enough that the capsule underneath it can be incised.

Once the hip is dislocated, a retractor (retractor #3) is placed around the femoral neck underneath the quadratus femoris muscle to both retract the quadratus femoris muscle from the femoral neck and to protect the sciatic nerve. The level of the femoral neck cut most often needed to recreate the off-set, and leg length for a patient is 2 cm below the distal edge of the femoral head. This can be determined by pre-operative templating, but has held to be true through our experience with hundreds of these hip replacements. Previously, we used the lesser trochanter to determine the level of femoral neck cut, but with retention of the quadratus femoris muscle this is not possible and this new technique has proved to

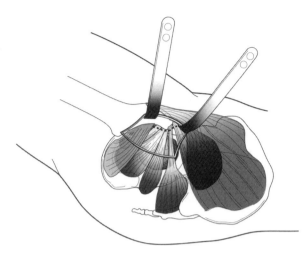

◘ **Fig. 7.36.** The incision through the capsule and small external rotators is shown by the dotted line. The quadratus femoris is not incised. This flap is closed at the completion of the operation (see Fig. 7.41)

be predictable. Following removal of the femoral head, the acetabulum is able to be visualized and retractor #4 is then placed on the posterior superior acetabulum between the bone and the posterior superior capsule and external rotators. This allows excellent visualization of the superior acetabular labrum and the anterior superior capsule which overhangs the acetabulum with the femur in this position. The number #2 retractor is moved to a position behind this anterior superior capsule for ease of removal of this corner of capsule. This is the only capsule that is removed in this operation. This tissue excision relaxes the anterior capsule and the iliofemoral ligament and allows the snake retractor (#5) to be positioned on the ilium. The only other capsular incision is through the posterior medial capsule (which includes the ischiofemoral ligament). This capsular incision relaxes this contracted tissue which further allows the femur to be retracted anteriorly, as well as allowing the femur to be internally rotated and flexed. It also makes easier the placement of retractor #7 against the cortical bone of the cotyloid notch.

Computer Registration of the Acetabulum

When the acetabulum is exposed, it is registered in the computer so that subsequent reaming and component placement can be tracked. Registration is performed by touching the edge of the acetabular walls and the medial floor with the probe creating a cloud of points which outlines the geometry of the acetabulum (❏ Fig. 7.37). A separate set of 6 points on the rim of the acetabulum allows the computer to measure the anatomic inclination and anteversion of the native acetabulum (see ❏ Fig. 7.38). In arthritic arthritic acetabulae these values are so variable that it is not prudent for the surgeon to match the acetabulum of the patient when placing the cup. These steps for

registration of the acetabulum requires one minute of operative time.

Reaming

Reaming is more dangerous when using a small incision because an error of reaming through an acetabular wall can occur. Reaming is significantly enhanced with the intra-operative computer. With any reamer the path of the reaming must be known by the surgeon, and the computer verifies this for the surgeon. The reamers have a light guide attached to them so that through the optical camera the computer can show the surgeon the position of the reamer in the bony acetabulum (❏ Fig. 7.39). By approximating the reamer to the yellow dots, the surgeon knows that he/she has reamed through the acetabular ridge to the medial wall (and conversely is protected against reaming through the medial wall). Likewise, by keeping the reamer inside the red dots, the surgeon knows the reamer is inside the walls of the bony acetabulum.

Reaming is initiated by using a straight-handled reamer transversely into the acetabulum for the purpose of reaming the acetabular ridge to the level of the cortical bone of the cotyloid notch. Using "half reamers"

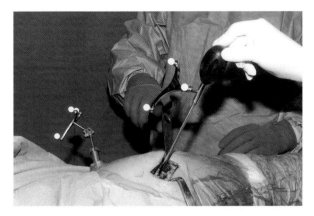

❏ **Fig. 7.37.** Probe is used to map out the bony acetabulum

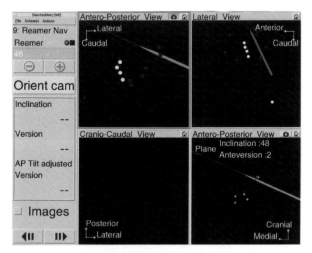

❏ **Fig. 7.38.** The *red dots* are the cloud of points made to outline the acetabular wall, and the *yellow dots* the medial wall in the anteroposterior and lateral views (*top two quadrants*). In the *lower right quadrant* the cloud of points has enabled the software to calculate the inclination and anteversion of the native acetabulum

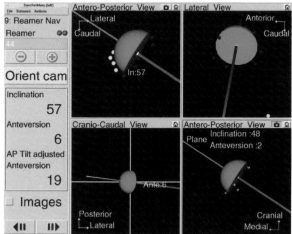

❏ **Fig. 7.39.** The computer allows navigation of the reamer by tracking its path within the *red dots* and to the *yellow dots* (medial wall). The lateral view shows this reamer is slightly eccentric and reaming into the anterior wall. The *lower left quadrant* shows the anteversion of the cup relative to the plane of the pelvis without tilt. The adjusted anteversion on the *left column* indicates the adjusted anteversion is 19°. The *lower right quadrant* shows the inclination of the reamer relative to that of the native acetabulum

(Zimmer, Warsaw, IN) gives much better visual confirmation of the reamer position in the bony acetabulum. The anterior wall of the acetabulum is at risk for being overreamed with this preparation. The reamer must be transverse, but also anteverted between the anterior and posterior walls of the bony acetabulum so that the reamer is not pointed at the anterior wall (see ◘ Fig. 7.39). When this preparation is complete, there will be cancellous bone exposed beneath the now absent ridge, and the cortical bone of the medial wall will form the floor of the acetabulum.

Reaming is completed with the curved reamer (◘ Fig. 7.40) used to prepare a hemisphere by shaping the iliac bone of the acetabulum. If a curved reamer is not used, the superior wall of the acetabulum is at risk because a straight reamer can be levered into an adverse superior position by the handle of the reamer abutting the distal wound edge. When the surgeon becomes experienced with this reaming technique, the acetabular preparation can usually be done with two reaming steps – the use of the straight reamer once and the curved reamer once. This preparation with a curved reamer can be more precise (less reaming time) for a press-fit of the cup than was the singular use of straight reamers when a long incision was employed.

Acetabular Component Placement

A curved holder is necessary for ease and accuracy of cup position (see ◘ Fig. 7.33). Just as with a straight reamer, a straight implant holder can abut on the distal wound edge and promote malposition of both the inclination and anteversion of the cup. The cup position is most precisely implanted with the computer. The cup holder has a light guide so that the computer can measure the position of the cup relative to the pelvis. Because pelvic tilt influences particularly the anteversion of the cup, the computer provides both the absolute anteversion and the adjusted anteversion (◘ Fig. 7.41). Adjusted anteversion is the most accurate measure of the true anatomic anteversion as has been confirmed from postoperative CT scans of the pelvis. For avoidance of impingement of the femoral component on the acetabulum, the cup position of choice is 40±5° inclination and 20±5° adjusted anteversion. Acetabular position with the computer adds one minute to the surgical time (but eliminates the indecision of the surgeon as to the cup position!)

A trial acetabular component should be used for greatest accuracy of fit. Reaming the bony acetabulum 1 mm smaller than the actual implants gives even

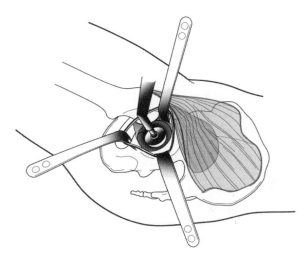

◘ **Fig. 7.40.** The curved reamer when used can correctly shape the acetabulum into a hemisphere with the anteversion desired without the reamer impinging on the distal wound

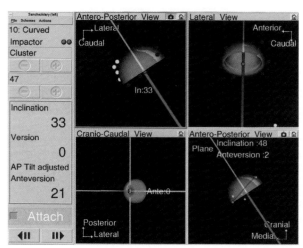

◘ **Fig. 7.41.** The *upper two quadrants* show the cup position within the acetabular walls and to the medial wall. This patient had 21° of posterior tilt so that the importance of the adjusted anteversion is apparent. The inclination at 33° relative to the native acetabulum is shown in the *lower right quadrant*. With 33° inclination, the risk of impingement with the metal femoral neck during flexion is increased

greater assurance that the fit will be secure without any adjunctive screws. A line-to-line fit with reaming is satisfactory if screws are to be used to fix the cup in every hip operation. To test the press-fit stability of the cup we try to lift the cup out of the bony acetabulum by pulling on the handle of the cup holder. If the cup moves, screws are required to provide immediate fixation stability. If manual evaluation of cup position is used, the medial edge of the cup should be level with the tear drop (the edge of the cortical bone of the cotyloid notch); the anterior edge should be about 5 mm below the pubic tubercle and preferably the metal edge of the cup is not proud above the anterior bony wall (so the iliopsoas tendon will not be irritated by the metal); superiorly, the metal edge of the cup should be below the anterior-superior acetabular bone to prevent impingement of the metal femoral neck against the metal edge of the cup in flexion; posterior superiorly there may be 5 mm of exposed metal which assures that the cup inclination does not exceed 45–50°.

Femoral Preparation and Implantation

Femoral preparation is performed with only the cut surface of the femoral neck as a bony reference. The quadratus femoris muscle obscures the femoral neck and lesser trochanter, although both can be felt. The use of a curved broach and implant holder will provide ease of broaching and implant placement. The computer can be used to verify the anteversion of the broach and the femoral component. The pointing probe is used to touch the surface of the metal neck and the light guides on the femoral registration device and the probe are aligned to measure the anteversion of the femoral component. This anteversion can be adjusted (or the cup position adjusted) to minimize any risk for impingement during range of motion of the hip.

The preparation of the femoral bone can be done using either reamers and/or broaches as necessary, followed by insertion of the implant. Insertion of the implant sometimes results in the metal femoral neck impinging on the jaws retractor so that the leg will need to be internally rotated to avoid this impingement (■ Fig. 7.42). The internal rotation of the leg for this maneuver must be done with the leg on the table (resting on the lower leg). Internal rotation of the leg, when it is hanging over the side of the table, can stretch the

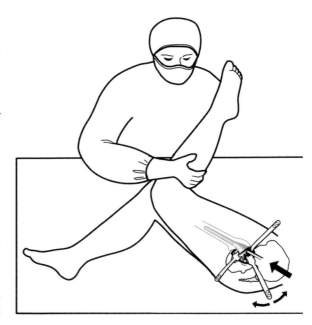

■ **Fig. 7.42.** The correct leg position for internal rotation of the hip. The operated leg is placed on the lower leg in the center of the table and then internally rotated. This does not cause a stretch of the sciatic nerve. This maneuver may be necessary to allow the metal femoral neck of the stem to clear the retractors of the hip

sciatic nerve. In the future, the use of modular necks with the femoral component will avoid this particular technical problem. Following implantation of the femur, the femoral head is placed onto the femoral neck using a tool that allows this to be accomplished inside the small incision.

Soft-Tissue Tension and Prevention of Impingement

The correct soft-tissue tension for the hip, which includes the correct leg length and offset, and prevention of impingement of the metal femoral neck against the cup or the femur against the pelvis, must be established with the trial implants in place. The leg length and offset of the femur are measured with the computer. The desired change from the pre-operative position can be measured on the pre-operative X-ray. Almost always an increase in the leg length up to 5 mm is needed to compensate for the lost cartilage. The greater the pre-operative deformity the greater change that will occur. By using the light guide in the distal femur, the leg can be placed in the same position as the initial measurement so that any change is exact. The use of modular heads allows adjustment of the leg length and off-set to the optimal desired position.

Previously, the leg lengths were manually confirmed by the position of the lesser trochanter to the ischium inside the hip and by overlaying the leg and measuring the position of the patella and the foot of the upper leg to the lower leg. Satisfactory off-set can be manually determined by taking the hip through an entire range of motion and using the index finger of the free hand to check that the femur clears the pelvis in the maximum flexed and internally rotated position; the maximally abducted and externally rotated position; and that the lesser trochanter clears the ischium in the maximally extended and externally rotated position. This clearance should be just by one fingerbreadth. Two fingerbreadth clearance means the off-set is increased, and impingement of the bone against the bone means that the off-set is too small. When checking the clearance of the femoral bone from the pelvis, the index finger can also be used to insure that the metal femoral neck is not impinging against the metal edge of the acetabular cup.

Closure is done with the capsule and external rotators sutured to the cut edge of the gluteus minimus (❑ Fig. 7.43). This closure helps improve the function of

the gluteus minimus muscle which is to contract against the femoral head and help hold it into position so that this closure gives further protection against dislocation. This closure also best eliminates any dead space between the closed capsule and external rotators and the metal femoral neck and head. A further help to reduce dead space in the closed hip is to use as large a femoral head as can be used in combination with the acetabular size. We have experienced that an additional benefit of the large femoral head will be improvement of the range of motion of the patient and further protection against impingement of either the metal femoral neck or the femoral bone.

Summary

Surgeons and patients must know that total hip replacement is predictable and reproducible with this posterior MIS operation or the mental and physical benefits for the patient are not of value. Studies have reported the same results with a posterior approach of 10 cm or less as have been reported with long incisions [3–5]. Our results have been summarized in two publications [2–6]. The publication of D'Gioia et al. [5] provides confirmation of the use of computer-assisted navigation for THR reconstruction. Their method used preoperative CT scans so that it is more expensive and time-consuming than our image-free method. Still, the principles remain the same.

Radiographic results showed that the average inclination angle of the acetabulum on X-ray was within 2° of that of the computer. While inclination remains the same, radiographic anteversion is, on average, 5° more than that of the computer and standing AP pelvis X-rays will measure, on average, 4 degrees more anteversion than the supine X-ray. These results demonstrate the influence of pelvic tilt in various body positions to the X-ray measurement of anteversion. The precision of the computer to provide an adjusted anteversion for the tilt of the pelvis on the operative table becomes very apparent. Our findings with these X-ray measurements compared to computer measurements are exactly the same as observed by Jaramaz et al. [7].

Since posterior MIS-THR surgery is reproducible and safe, surgeons must be aware of the desires of the patients and responsive to their needs. This is the art of medicine which heals many patients because patients

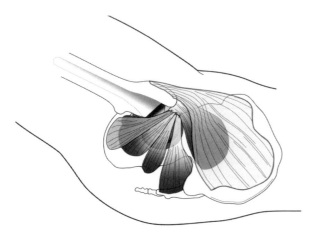

❑ Fig. 7.43. The external rotators and capsule are repaired together to the cut edge of the gluteus minimus. This provides a closure without any dead space of the hip joint and also allows the gluteus minimus to improve its function which is to contract against the femoral head

get better more quickly and more easily when they are mentally confident.

The human goals of the patient must be considered in treatment decisions, and it has been observed that as orthopedic surgeons we now must make not just professional decisions, but value judgments based on human goals [8]. Because orthopedic surgeons have done so well with scientific improvements of hip replacement, we must respond to the increased social expectations of the patients who now know their lives can be improved and want that improvement with as little violation of their body as possible. The use of computer navigation permits precise reconstruction of the hip in combination with a minimally invasive operation.

References

1. Madsen MS, Ritter MA, Morris HH: The effect of total hip arthroplasty surgical approach on gait. J Orthop Res 22: 44–50, 2004
2. Berry DJ, Berger RA, Callaghan JJ et al.: Minimally invasive total hip arthroplasty. Development, early results, and a critical analysis. J Bone Joint Surg 85A: 2235–2246, 2003
3. Wenz JF, Gurkan, I, Jibodh SR: Mini-incision total hip arthroplasty: A comparative assessment of perioperative outcomes. J Orthopedics 25: 1031–1043, 2002
4. Chimento G, Sculco TP: Minimally invasive total hip arthroplasty. Operative Techniques in Orthopedics 11: 270–273, 2001
5. DiGioa AM III, Plakseychuk A, Levison T et al.: Mini-incision technique for total hip arthroplasty with navigation. J Arthroplasty 18: 123–128, 2003
6. Dorr LD: Mini-incision for THR: Building a ship in a bottle: Orthopedics 27: 192–194, 2004
7. Jaramaz B, D'Gioio AM III, Blackwell M, Nikou C: Computer-assisted measurement of cup placement in total hip replacement. Clin Orthop 354: 70–80, 1998
8. Heck CV: The new style of medicine. J Bone Joint Surg 68A: 1–3, 1986

Posterior Approach with Minimal Invasive Surgery Utilizing Hip Navigation

R. Wixson

Introduction

The posterior approach to the hip for arthroplasty has been utilized extensively due to excellent exposure of the acetabulum and femur, its extensibility, and limited damage to the surrounding hip musculature [4, 11, 16, 23]. A major concern with the approach has been a high incidence of post-operative dislocation in the range of 1–5% [6, 10, 13, 18, 19, 21]. Modern techniques with retention of the anterior capsule and surgical repair of the posterior capsular structures and external rotators have reduced this problem while retaining the other advantages [5, 7, 12, 16, 24]. Pellicci [16] described a posterior capsular repair with a dislocation rate of less than 1% in a technique involving sewing the rotators and posterior capsule back through drill holes in the greater trochanter. Hedley [5] has described a similar technique, preserving the rotators and repairing the capsular structures to a tendinous cuff. This also reduced their dislocation rate to less than 1%.

To obtain the benefit of minimally invasive surgery, a number of surgeons have described utilizing a posterior approach that limits the proximal and distal extent of the incision and still allows adequate access to the joint [2, 3, 20, 23]. Chimento [2] described performing this through a 5–7 cm incision resulting in no change in post-operative complications or results. DiGoia's method was combined with CT-based computer-assisted techniques for implant placement [3].

Based on these descriptions and experiences, the author adapted the technique that he had been using for the posterior approach with a classic long incision to a minimally invasive method. Using the latter method, the posterior incision is limited to splitting the gluteus maximus tendon and not extending the incision into the ten-sor fascia overlying the greater trochanter. In both techniques, preservation of the anterior capsule and repair of the posterior capsule and external rotators was felt important to maintain joint stability. The goal of the smaller incision was to reduce the peri-operative morbidity and pain, reduce blood loss, and achieve more rapid patient mobilization while maintaining accurate component position, restoration of correct leg length and offset.

Particularly with reduced length of the incision and concerns about acetabular positioning, the use of navigation helps ensure that the acetabular component can be placed in the "safe zone" as described by Lewinnek and others [1, 9, 14]. It also provides an additional method of ensuring correct leg length and offset. DiGioia [3], using a CT-based system, has described the use of computer-assisted navigation methods in total hip replacement. Leenders [8] has shown more accurate acetabular cup placement with this method. The use of navigation based on anatomic landmarks without CT imaging has been described by Zheng [25].

The computer-assisted navigation system used by the author is made by Stryker Leibinger (Stryker Navigation, Kalamazoo, Michigan, USA). The system is based on trackers that are placed on pins located in the anterior iliac crest and distal femur. Light emitting diodes (LEDs) on the trackers send signals to a camera array that converts the position and motion information through a computer-software system onto a display monitor. With other trackers attached to instruments such as reamers and insertion handles, the position of the implants can be determined relative to the bone anatomy. The system is "image-free" and relies on manual determination of the anterior frontal plane by palpating the anterior superior iliac spines and the pubic symphysis. The femoral head center is determined by motion analysis.

Based on the combination of improved surgical methods with a minimally invasive posterior approach and computer-assisted navigation, the author now utilizes both of these as the standard technique in his primary total hip replacements.

Methods

The goal of the surgery is to reduce the trauma to the deep tissues. The length of the skin incision, while the focus of many discussions of minimally invasive surgery and what the patient observes, is perhaps less important in terms of recovery than minimizing the muscle and tendon damage that occurs during the exposure. The goal of this approach is to split only the gluteus maximus muscle and avoid incision of the tensor fascia over the greater trochanter.

The patient is positioned in a lateral decubitus position with radiolucent posts with soft-foam pad bolsters supporting the sacrum from behind and both anterior iliac crests from the front. Prior to making the skin incision, percutaneous pins are placed in the anterior iliac crest and lateral distal femur for attachment of the navigation tracker devices. By releasing the posterior support, the patient can be tilted back to palpate the two anterior iliac crests and the center of the public symphysis to establish the anterior frontal plane of the pelvis. After this, the patient is brought back to a lateral decubitus position and the posterior support is tightened.

The skin incision begins at the posterior-superior edge of the greater trochanter and extends posteriorly at 45° (◘ Fig. 7.44). In a normal patient, the incision is 7–10 cm, depending on the patient's size and thickness of the subcutaneous tissue. Heavier patients may have an extension of the skin incision posteriorly over the buttock tissue to allow adequate access to the femur. The skin incision is then carried down to the fascia, splitting the gluteus maximus in line with the incision and not extending into the tensor fascia beyond the point where the muscular fibers of the gluteus maximus end. By splitting the muscle, the bursa over the edge of the trochanter can then be identified, picked up and incised. Then finger dissection is used to create an interval between the gluteus maximus inner surface and the back of the trochanter and overlying gluteus medius. The

bursa and retinacular tissues over the gluteus medius and posterior trochanter are then incised and a retractor is placed underneath the gluteus medius elevating and exposing the piriformis tendon. A self-retaining Charnley type retractor is used to hold the wound open.

The next step is detachment of the short external rotators and posterior capsule from their bony insertions underneath the overhanging posterior trochanter and medius tendon. By lifting up the tensor fascia with a Hibbs retractor and looking with a headlight, the proximal attachments of the quadratus are released with electrocautery from just above the lesser trochanter to the base of the neck. By using an angled Beaver knife blade on the inner surface of the trochanter, the insertions of the short external rotators are released from their bony insertions and their length preserved as much as possible (◘ Fig. 7.45). Hemostasis may be needed for the perforating vessels of the medial femoral circumflex artery, which crosses the obturator externus and perforates the capsule between it and the obturator internus insertion.

After the short external rotators have been released, the capsular reflection of the gluteus minimus is elevated off the superior capsule and held back with a narrow retractor. A superior capsular incision is also made with the angled Beaver blade in the mid axial line along the long axis of the neck (◘ Fig. 7.46). The capsule and rotators are then reflected back and a meniscal clamp is used to grasp the inferior capsule just above the ischium. This is divided down to its bony insertion overlying the ischium, staying deep to the obturator externus muscle,

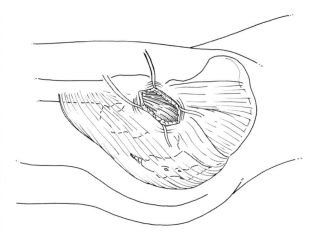

◘ **Fig. 7.44.** Location of skin incision overlying the fibers of the gluteus maximus and relationship to the underlying bony structures

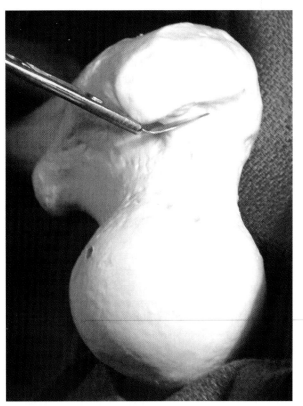

Fig. 7.45. Use of an angled knife blade to release the short external rotators from their attachments on the inner surface of the greater trochanter from a posterior approach

which lays on its surface. This creates a broad flap of tissue of capsule and the three short rotators. Hemostasis is then obtained and several sutures are placed through each of the short external rotator tendons (piriformis, obturator internus and externus) and three points on the reflected posterior capsule (■ Fig. 7.47).

At this point, manual determination of leg length is made from a mark on the trochanter up to the pin that has been placed in the anterior iliac crest for the navigation tracking system. Without navigation tracking, a mark can be made on the skin overlying the iliac crest and measurements made to that, or a pin placed in it for heavier patients with loose soft tissues.

The hip is then dislocated with a goal of disrupting the ligamentum teres and soft-tissue restraints after which it is relocated. A partial saw cut is made through the neck just below the head, the hip is dislocated, the cut completed and the head removed. This allows the remaining femoral neck to be positioned by internally rotating, adducting, and flexing the femur to make a second, definitive femoral neck cut.

The acetabulum is exposed by placing a Cobra retractor over the anterior and inferior aspect of the acetabulum and retracting the proximal femur anteriorly. Having released the inferior capsule near the ischium and the superior capsule at the top of the acetabulum, there is usually adequate exposure with no further releases being needed. The next steps are to debride the

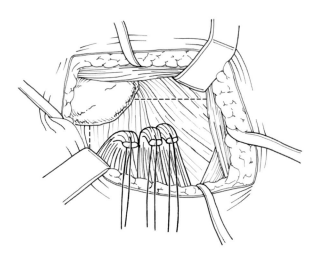

Fig. 7.46. Location of posterior hip capsular incisions after detaching the short external rotators with retraction of gluteus minimus and medius

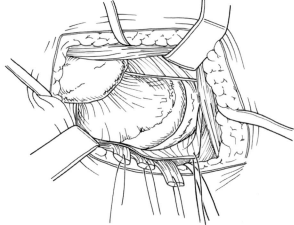

Fig. 7.47. Exposure of femoral neck and head after release of rotators and posterior capsular flap with sutures for later reattachment

acetabulum, remove the labrum and clear the acetabular fossa with control of any bleeding that may come through the artery at the ligamentum teres. After this, the computer-assisted surgery tool is used to register the acetabular fossa and articular surface of the acetabulum.

Following this, navigated reaming of the acetabulum can be performed, which allows simultaneous direct visualization of the reaming from the posterior approach and computer monitoring of the angle of the reamer's inclination as well as the depth of the reamer relative to the acetabular fossa. An offset, angled acetabular reamer may be utilized to get around the proximal femur and trochanteric area (◘ Fig. 7.48). Navigated reaming allows monitoring of the depth relative to the acetabular fossa as well as the inclination of the reamer. Following completion of reaming, debridement of the acetabulum and curettage of any large acetabular cysts with bone-grafting occurs as needed.

The acetabular cup, which is a press-fit bone ingrowth design, is inserted with an impactor that has a navigation tracker on its handle to guide it into the proper position of approximately 45° of abduction and 20° of flexion. By placing the cup in the opening of the acetabulum and removing all of the retractors, the soft tissues relax and allow the cup to be impacted in the proper position following the angles and depth of insertion on the computer monitor (◘ Fig. 7.49). In very heavy or obese patients, a secondary small incision can be made posterior to the femur and the cup impactor passed through it for cup placement and impaction with navigation. Following completion of the cup placement, the impactor can be removed through the incision, peripheral osteophytes removed, and the acetabular liner placed.

The incision that has been made is essentially the posterior arm of the classic posterior-lateral incision. With the femur internally rotated 90°, flexed and adducted, the proximal femoral osteotomy faces directly out of the wound. A small proximal femoral elevator can be placed underneath it along with the self-retaining retractor. A standard femoral preparation can be performed, opening the canal with a box osteotome, starter awls, and then reaming and broaching until the femoral trials can be placed for a trial reduction (◘ Fig. 7.50). The computer-assisted system aids in determining the appropriate amount of leg length and offset necessary to restore stability. Since the anterior capsule has been preserved, this is an additional aid in determining the proper soft-tissue tension. Once the appropriate prosthesis

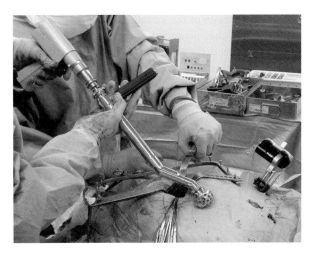

◘ **Fig. 7.48.** Angled acetabular reamer handle to improve access to acetabulum with proximal femur retracted anteriorly

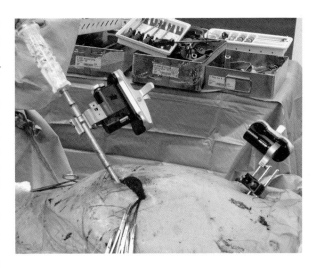

◘ **Fig. 7.49.** Acetabular cup impactor with hip navigation instrument tracker attached and pelvic tracker attached to the anterior iliac crest. Removal of retractors increases anterior positioning of the proximal femur by the impaction handle during navigated guidance of correct cup position

has been selected, it can be placed directly in the femur under direct observation to ensure correct rotation and avoidance of proximal calcar fractures. The technique also works well for cemented applications with preparation of the canal, irrigation, drying and pressure injection. Direct visualization of the canal ensures proper femoral rotation.

Following placement of the definitive prosthesis but before the head is impacted on, the trochanter is positioned in the center of the wound and four drill holes are made along the posterior border of the greater trochanter aimed toward the inside of the trochanter where the rotator tendons had been taken off. Pairs of sutures from adjacent tendons and capsule are then passed so that sutures may be tied over the bony bridges between them (◘ Fig. 7.51). The selected head is impact-ed on to the taper and the hip is reduced. After tying the sutures through the drill holes in the trochanter, the fascia over the gluteus maximus is repaired with absorbable sutures and followed by a standard closure.

Post-operatively, patients are managed in a standard fashion with an abduction splint, dislocation precautions, and mobilization with weight-bearing as tolerated on either the day of or day following surgery. Initial external support with crutches or a walker is advanced to a cane as patients recover strength and mobility.

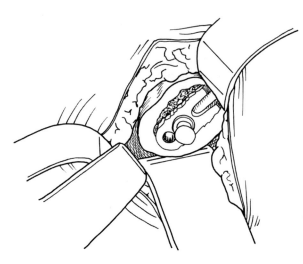

◘ **Fig. 7.50.** Exposure of proximal end of cut femoral neck through the posterior incision after placement of the trial broach

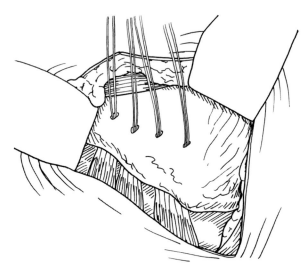

◘ **Fig. 7.51.** Location of drill holes for passing the sutures in the rotator tendons and posterior capsule. In order to have adequate access, the sutures are passed prior to placement of the femoral head and reduction of the hip. Once the hip is reduced, the sutures are tied over the bony bridges between the holes

Results

The MIS posterior approach has been used now in 250 cases with primary total hip replacements. The population is 43% female, 57% male with a mean age of 64 years (range 21–88). The diagnosis was osteoarthritis in 89.7%. The mean BMI was 30 (range 19–54). An uncemented, press-fit acetabulum was used in all cases. A proximal bone ingrowth tapered femoral stem was used in 88% of the cases with a cemented stem used in the remainder.

With minimally invasive surgical techniques, much of the emphasis has been on the length of the skin incision. The author has followed traditional surgical teaching to make an adequate exposure and minimize tension and damage that may occur to the skin. The benefit to the patient is the minimal disruption of the main muscle layer involved, the gluteus maximus, and avoidance of splitting the tensor fascia over the greater trochanter. Particularly in obese patients, there is a large amount of subcutaneous tissue in the buttock. Extending the skin incision posteriorly allows adequate access to the joint without undue tension on the skin. Since half the patients in this series are obese (BMI greater than 30), a larger skin incision was necessary to get down to the maximus fascia. All patients had a similar split in the gluteus maximus with the skin incision varying with the thickness of the subcutaneous tissue. While normal, thin patients can easily be done with incisions of 7–10 cm, the surgeon needs to decide how much tension is tolerable to the skin edges and corners to accomplish this. In this series, we avoided any excess pressure on the skin edges. The mean incision length for patients with a BMI under 30 was 11 cm, for a BMI between 30 and 40, it was 13 cm and for patients with a BMI over 40 and gross morbid obesity it was 18 cm.

While an increased dislocation rate has classically been associated with a posterior approach, the only dislocation occurred anteriorly in a non-computer-assisted hip where the cup position on radiographs was 55° of abduction and 22° of anteversion. This is a dislocation rate of 0.4%. Three non-displaced fractures, one of the greater trochanter and two in the proximal calcar, occurred at surgery that required fixation and extension of the wound distally. There were no late fractures or cases of distal migration. There were no cases with sciatic or peroneal nerve palsy after surgery. There was one superficial wound infection that was treated with no sequelae.

With the availability of computer-assisted hip navigation, almost all of the last 60 cases have been done with computer assistance using a MIS posterior incision. It is not used in patients with significant pelvic abnormalities such as previous acetabular and pelvic osteotomies. From analyzing the reports generated by the system after each case, the mean value for cup abduction was 42° (range 38–47°). The mean for cup flexion was 21° (range 15–29°). The surgical goal was to place the cup in 40–45° of abduction and 17–23° of flexion. This was achieved in 88% of the cases for abduction and 80% of the cases for flexion.

To determine the positions of the acetabular cup on digitized post-operative anterior-posterior radiographs, angular measurements were made using a computer-software program (SigmaScanPro, SPSS Science, Chicago, Illinois, USA). Abduction was determined from a line across the face of the cup and another across the bottom of the ischial tuberosities. Flexion was determined by the method of Pradhan [17], which is based on the elliptical appearance of the open face of the cup on a radiograph. Fifty-two radiographs of navigated cases were compared with 28 randomly selected radiographs of previously performed non-navigated cases. Both groups had similar means and ranges. For the navigated group the means were 43° abduction (range 34–54°) and 22° flexion (range 11–31°). For the non-navigated group the means were 45° abduction (range 37–53°) and 24° flexion (range 13–40°). Using an abduction goal of 40–45°, 65% of the navigated cases were in that range compared to 52% of the non-navigated cases. This was significant with a Pearson Chi-square test at $p=0.027$. With a cup flexion goal of 17–23°, 65% of the cases were in that range compared to 40% of the non-navigated cases. This was also signifi-cant with a Pearson Chi-square test at $p=0.044$. Since radiographic technique and positioning can affect the measured values, forthcoming studies comparing groups with CT scans would be expected to show more accurately any differences between the two groups.

Summary

The use of a limited posterior approach to the hip benefits patients by splitting only the muscular fibers of the gluteus maximus and avoiding disruption of the fascia lata tendon over the greater trochanter. The incision preserves the benefits of the posterior-lateral approach with extensibility and adequate access to the femur and acetabulum with direct vision. Combining the minimal posterior incision with computer-assisted hip navigation techniques allows the surgeon to place the total hip components accurately with minimal post-operative complications.

References

1. Barrack RL (2003) Dislocation after total hip arthroplasty: implant design and orientation. Journal of the American Academy of Orthopaedic Surgeons 11(2): 89–99
2. Chimento GF, Sculco TP (2001) Minimally Invasive Total Hip Replacement. Operative Techniques in Orthopaedics 11(4): 270–273
3. DiGioia AM, Plakseychuk AY, Levison TJ, Jaramaz B (2003) Mini-incision technique for total hip arthroplasty with navigation. Journal of Arthroplasty 18(2): 123–128
4. Gibson A (1953) The posterolateral approach to the hip joint. American Academy of Orthopaedic Surgeons, Instructional Course Lectures 10: 175–179
5. Hedley AK, Hendren DH, Mead LP (1990) A posterior approach to the hip joint with complete posterior capsular and muscular repair. Journal of Arthroplasty 5 Suppl: S57–66
6. Hedlundh U, Ahnfelt L, Hybbinette CH et al. (1996) Surgical experience related to dislocation after total hip arthroplasty. J Bone Joint Surg 78B: 206–209
7. Ko CK, Law SW, Chiu KH (2001) Enhanced soft tissue repair using locking loop stitch after posterior approach for hip hemiarthroplasty. Journal of Arthroplasty 16(2): 207–211
8. Leenders T, Vandevelde D, Mahieu G, Nuyts R (2002) Reduction in variability of acetabular cup abduction using computer assisted surgery: a prospective and randomized study. Computer Aided Surgery 7(2):99–106
9. Lewinnek GE, Lewis JL, Tarr R, Compere CL, Zimmerman JR (1990) Dislocations after total hip-replacement arthroplasties. J Bone Joint Surg 60A:217–220

10. Mallory TH, Lombardi AV, Fada RA et al (1999) Dislocation after total hip arthroplasty using the anterolateral abductor split approach. Clin Orthop 358:166–172

11. Marcy GH, Fletcher RS (1954) Modification of the posterolateral approach to the hip for insertion of femoral head prostheses. J Bone Joint Surg 36A:142

12. Martinez AA, Herrera A, Cuenca J, Panisello JJ, Tabuenca A (2002) Comparison of two different posterior approaches for hemiarthroplasty of the hip. Archives of Orthopaedic & Trauma Surgery 122(1): 51–52

13. Masonis JL, Bourne RB (2002) Surgical approach, abductor function, and total hip arthroplasty dislocation. Clinical Orthopaedics & Related Research (405): 46–53

14. McCollum DE, Gray WJ (1990) Dislocation after total hip arthroplasty: Causes and prevention. Clinical Orthopaedics & Related Research (261): 159–70

15. Moore AT (1959) A new low posterior approach. American Academy of Orthopaedic Surgeons, Instructional Course Lectures 16: 309–321

16. Pellicci PM, Bostrom M, Poss R (1998) Posterior approach to total hip replacement using enhanced posterior soft tissue repair. Clinical Orthopaedics & Related Research (355): 224–228

17. Pradhan R (1999) Planar anteversion of the acetabular cup as determined from plain anteroposterior radiographs. J Bone Joint Surg 81B(3): 431–435

18. Ritter MA, Harty LD, Keating ME, Faris PM, Meding JB (2001) A clinical comparison of the anterolateral and posterolateral approaches to the hip. Clinical Orthopaedics & Related Research 385: 95–99

19. Roberts JM, Fu FH, McClain EJ et al (1984) A comparison of the posterolateral and anterolateral approaches to total hip arthroplasty. Clin Orthop 187: 205–210

20. Sherry E, Egan M, Warnke PH, Henderson A, Eslick GD (2003) Minimal invasive surgery for hip replacement: a new technique using the NILNAV hip system. ANZ Journal of Surgery 73(3): 157–161

21. Vicar AJ, Coleman CR (1984) A comparison of the anterolateral, transtrochanteric, and posterior surgical approaches in primary total hip arthroplasty. Clin Orthip 188: 152–169

22. von Langenbeck B, Kocher D (1874) Ueber die Schussverletzungen der Huftgelenks. Arch Clin Chir 16: 236

23. Wenz JF, Gurkan I, Jibodh SR (2002) Mini-incision total hip arthroplasty: a comparative assessment of perioperative outcomes. Orthopedics 25(10): 1031–1043

24. Williams CR, Kernohan JG, Sherry PG (1997) A more stable posterior approach for hemiarthroplasty of the hip. Injury 28(4): 279–281

25. Zheng G, Marx A, Langlotz U, Widmer KH, Buttaro M, Nolte LP (2002) A hybrid CT-free navigation system for total hip arthroplasty. Computer Aided Surgery 7(3): 129–145

7.6

Posterior Minimally Invasive Total Hip Arthroplasty Using the Stryker HipNav Navigation System

J.B. Sledge

For the last 4 years, my standard technique for total hip arthroplasty (THA) has been to utilize a mini-posterior single incision and this has been augmented with the use of the Stryker Hip Navigation system for the past 18 months. I think that these are complimentary techniques, each maximizing the potential of the other. In our office once a patient is scheduled for a THA, they follow a standardized pre-operative protocol. Along with medical clearance this includes a SF-12v2, a Harris Hip Score, an X-ray with a calibration marker, and leg length by X-ray and by block test. The navigation system does not require a pre-operative CT scan or any other imaging intra-operatively. All outcome data is entered into a web-based database for multi-center collection and evaluation.

Prior to starting the case, all the patient demographic data and templating data are loaded into the computer. While we position the patient, the scrub nurse initializes all of the trackers and the circulator positions the optical camera. We have found that the optimum camera position for us is just above the arm board about 30 degrees off from parallel to the patient. We usually position the camera three times during the procedure: the initial position for registration and acetabular work, a second position for femoral broaching and stem insertion, and a final position for obtaining the kinematic range of motion data.

The patient is positioned in the lateral position with anterior and posterior bolsters. Initially the posterior bolster is not pushed in firmly against the sacrum, this allows the patient to role posterior into the "sloppy lateral" position which allows us access to the down anterior superior iliac spine (ASIS) and pubis. I use an 8–10 cm facial incision that is centered vertically over the tip of the greater trochanter and the length of the skin incision is determined by the thickness of the overlying fat. The

leg is placed in the position for preparation of the femur and the skin incision is placed over the junction of the anterior two-thirds and posterior third of the greater trochanter (◘ Fig. 7.52). The slightly posterior placement is to assist with access for the broach handle and for the neck on the stem.

With the incision drawn on the drape but not made, the pelvic tracker is placed, the pelvis is referenced, the femoral tracker is placed and the femur reference plane is established. For the placement of the trackers, two 4 mm pins from the external fixation set are placed through a clamp into the iliac crest. The tracker is placed far enough posteriorly so that when the patient is placed back into the true lateral position the tracker will be pointing at the camera. A bar-to-bar clamp then attaches the tracker pin to the clamp. Since the pointer is an active instrument, as are all of the trackers, we can

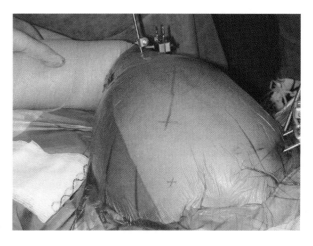

◘ **Fig. 7.52.** Left hip showing the location of the trackers and size and location of the incision

use any of them to advance the system as we step through the different functions so as not to interfere with the flow of the case. This also alleviates the need for an additional person to work the computer.

The user can select a three- or four-point pelvic referencing system. We have used both and prefer the three-point technique as we have found it to be more accurate. The ASIS are marked through the drapes on both sides with the pointer. We have not had difficulty locating the ASIS even in our heaviest patients as on the down side there is a fold that can be followed and there is little subcutaneous fat over the bone at this location. We have found the best way to find symphysis pubis is to "follow the foley", this brings one to the inferior pubis below to the pubic fat pad. From this point, one must slide proximally pushing the fat pad out of the way until the anterior lip of the symphysis pubis is felt. By following this technique, and by using the computer which calculates in real time the distance to the mid line, we have found excellent intra- and inter-observer reliability.

The femoral tracker is then placed in the femur far enough distally so that it does not impair the procedure or the retractors. Once again two 4 mm pins are placed through a clamp and the tracker is attached to the clamp. This tracker is aimed posteriorly and proximally at about 45°. This is done so that the tracker is visible with the leg in extension and external rotation, and also in flexion and internal rotation. We place it in this fashion so that it will be optimal for the kinematic range of motion test and accept that we will have to move the camera during femoral broaching and stem insertion. Both trackers are now removed, leaving only the stable low profile clamp in place, thus minimizing the chances that a tracker will get bumped.

The skin incision is made with the hip flexed and a standard Kocher–Langenback approach to the hip is performed. The fascia is split distally far enough to palpate the lesser trochanter and great care is taken to split the gluteus maximus along its fibers. The skin, the subcutaneous tissue and the muscle are all infiltrated during the approach with 20–30 cc of Lidocaine HCL 1% with 1:100 000 Epinephrine and Bupivacaine 0.5% with 1:200 000 Epinephrine as a 50/50 mix. With the hip in extension, the piriformis is tagged and reflected posteriorly. This exposes the gluteus minimus which is elevated off of the superior capsule and reflected with a hip cobra retractor. The capsule is incised parallel to the neck at the junction of the inferior two thirds and the superior

one third. The capsule and muscle are taken off the bone and tagged to enhance later repair. A superior capsulotomy is performed as is an inferior capsulotomy, the latter being done without injury to the transacetabular ligament. The femoral head is dislocated posteriorly and the distances from the lesser trochanter to the center of rotation and from the medial border of greater trochanter to the center of rotation are measured. The femoral tracker is placed back on the femur so the piriformis fossa, the popliteal fossa and the achillies tendon can be marked so as to be able to calculate the version of the femoral component.

During preparation of the acetabulum, I use special retractors that are now available from most implant manufactures and from several instrument companies. I place a sharp Hohmann at the inferior margin of the insertion of the indirect head of the rectus outside the labrum but inside the capsule. A two-pronged retractor straddles the ischium just outside of the labrum (this retractor is placed first and is done with the leg in extension). A third retractor is placed superiorly to control the superior capsule if needed. Using the HipNav pointer the Fovea is scribed to find its deepest point; the articular surface is scribed to determine the acetabular size and location; the acetabular rim is scribed to determine its orientation. I rarely try to medialize the acetabular component so I start with a reamer 2 mm smaller then the computer's calculated size so that I have to only pass two or three reamers through the soft tissues. Due to the accuracy of the computer, I no longer use an acetabular trial so I am able to place the real liner immediately after the shell.

As attention is now directed towards the femur, the camera is repositioned, the pelvic tracker is removed and the femoral tracker is applied. I use special retractors on the femoral side as well. I place a hip skid under the femoral neck that has two prongs to elevate the femur away from the retractor to allow access for the calcar reamer. A curved two-pronged retractor straddles the iliopsoas tendor under the inferior skin edge (this retractor is placed before the femur is maximally internally rotated). A third retractor is placed deep to the minimus along the anterior insertion of the medius to protect the muscles from the reamers and the broaches. Since the computer gives us real time data on the version and the change in leg length and offset as we broach, we can minimize internal femoral rotation and proceed quickly to the correct broach and depth (◘ Fig. 7.53).

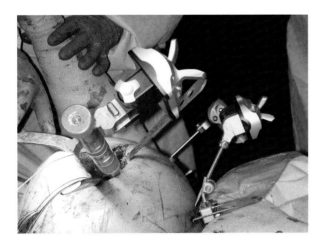

Fig. 7.53. Inserting the femoral prosthesis using the instrument tracker

We confirm the final head position by comparing the computer calculations to the pre-operative and intra-operative measurements. We perform a trial reduction to check stability and compare the computer's calculated leg length and offset to that measured by the computer during the reduction. The real femoral component is then inserted and the hip is placed through a range of motion. The kinematic data includes range of motion and when subluxation occurs. Posterior capsular repair is followed by routine multilayer closure, a subcuticular skin closure and then full length half inch steri-strips.

I think that the patient's post-operative recovery rate during the first several weeks is more closely related with the patient's comorbid factors and personality then the specifics of the procedure performed. The surgical factors that have the greatest impact on initial outcomes are not the length of the skin incision or the surgical time, but are the stability of the implants, the amount of damage to the soft tissues and the avoidance of peri-operative complications. The advent of an imageless active tracker navigation system has allowed us to incorporate navigation with little change to our previous surgical technique. The navigation allows more consistent placement of the components irrespective of the exposure and allows us to minimize the surrounding soft-tissue damage by requiring fewer passes of instruments through the soft tissues, fewer trial reductions and fewer fiddles. The above technique has been very successful for us and our patients in maximizing their short-term recovery while optimizing the long-term success of their implants.

Single, Posterolateral, Mini-Incision Approach to the Hip

A.J. Timperley, J.R. Howell, M.J.W. Hubble

Introduction

It is widely reported that the growth in minimally invasive surgery (MIS) of the hip has been driven by patient demand. Whilst there is certainly now truth in this assertion, a fundamental question is: how did the public become aware that this type of surgery is possible and how have they been convinced that MIS surgery is desirable? MIS surgery has been marketed by implant companies directly to patients for commercial advantage before there is yet scientific evidence that it confers any clinical advantage. MIS surgery has not yet been conclusively shown by randomized prospective studies to confer any of the clinical benefits reported in the marketing brochures and on commercial Web sites. Multi-center randomized, prospective studies are ongoing and initial results are expected soon. It will then become clearer which of the surgical approaches confer any type of short-term benefit; conversely it may be shown that some of the MIS techniques adopted are associated with unacceptably high complication rates. Only in the longer term will it become clear if any short-term benefit to the patient (if proven) is to become overshadowed by compromised function of the joint in later years.

Orthopedic surgeons should not lose sight of the fact that the indication for re-operation in over 70% of patients requiring further surgery after their index arthroplasty is mechanical loosening of the prosthesis [1]. It will therefore take much longer to show that the long-term result for patients is not compromised by the use of some of the new techniques. RSA studies [2] could be used to prove or disprove the thesis that some MIS approaches may compromise initial mechanical stability of implants, but studies of this type were not carried out before these techniques were popularized by their advocates and no information of this sort is available.

We should, therefore, conclusively and scientifically prove the benefits of each approach to MIS surgery before employing them on a large numbers of patients. This proof should ideally be sought through randomized prospective studies. A step-wise approach to the introduction of techniques of this sort, akin to that advocated for new implants, would have been desirable [3].

An advantage of carrying out small-incision surgery through a reduced posterolateral approach in contradistinction to, for instance, the two-incision approach, is that the surgical modifications necessary may be practiced to the surgeon's satisfaction without threatening the end result of surgery for the patient. The size of the incision can then be sequentially reduced as expertise is gained. At any point in a procedure the exposure may be enlarged should circumstances dictate to ensure the best surgical result.

Advantages of the Mini-Posterolateral Approach

Advantages inherent in the minimal posterolateral approach over other mini approaches therefore include:
- It is easily extendable if, at any point, it is felt that the operative procedure is being compromised by lack of exposure.
- The incision length can be progressively reduced as the surgeon gains experience with the technique.
- It is based on an approach with which many surgeons are already familiar, and fluoroscopy is not required.

— It requires disruption of only the small external rotators of the hip and preserves the hip abductors. There is no fear of damage to the superior gluteal nerve.

— The acetabulum and femur are exposed through a single incision.

— It is suitable for the insertion of both cemented and uncemented components in the acetabulum and the femur.

Pre-Operative Planning

Pre-operative planning is an essential part of performing total hip replacement through a mini-incision. Particular attention should be paid to the following areas:

— **Patient selection:** We would advise that surgeons should gain initial experience with patients whose build, diagnosis and bony anatomy are conducive to total hip replacement through a less extensive approach. As confidence is gained with the technique more patients will be deemed suitable for the use of a smaller incision.

— **Patient examination:** The patient should be carefully assessed for leg-length discrepancy, pelvic obliquity and fixed deformities to guide patient positioning on the operating table (vid. inf.) and the subsequent surgery.

— **Templating of radiographs:** Pre-operative radiographs should be analyzed using the manufacturers templates or digital templates to determine the correct leg length, center of rotation of the hip joint, femoral offset and the size of prostheses.

Equipment

Although the operation can be performed with difficulty using non-customized instruments, there are definite advantages to using equipment that has been specifically developed to allow exposure of the hip through a smaller incision (■ Fig. 7.54). These instruments include a range of narrower, longer retractors and a longer gluteus medius retractor that can retract both muscle and skin edge (■ Fig. 7.55). Most importantly a range of femoral elevators are desirable that not only allow direct access to the cut section of the femoral neck but also create sufficient space on the anterior aspect of

the femur in order that the implant may be inserted in the correct amount of anteversion (■ Fig. 7.56).

Modified cement accessories are deemed to be essential in order to prevent compromise of the cementing technique. For acetabular cementing, an aspirator-retractor, used in the proximal end of the wound, enhances exposure and helps to promote adequate intru-

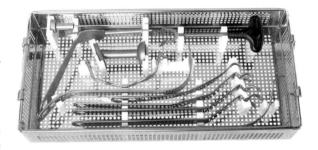

■ **Fig. 7.54.** Tray containing instruments for Limited Incision cemented Exeter hip replacement

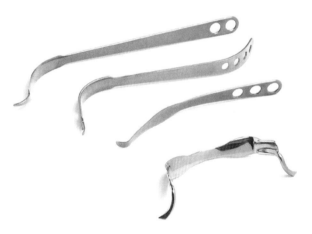

■ **Fig. 7.55.** Acetabular retractors: from above down: inferior, anterior, Homan and gluteus medius retractors

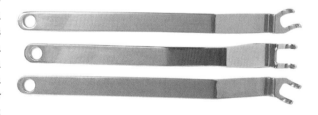

■ **Fig. 7.56.** Angled and non-angled femoral elevators

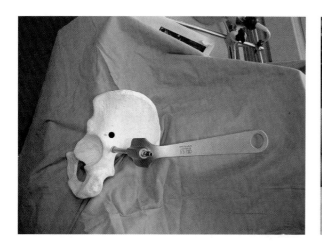

Fig. 7.57. Acetabular retractor – aspirator

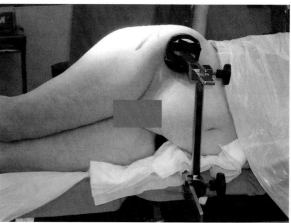

Fig. 7.58. Patient held in position by sacral pad and supports on both anterior spines

sion of cement into trabecular bone whilst minimizing accumulation of blood at the interface (■ Fig. 7.57). For femoral cementing, smaller sorbothane accessories are required with an extended metal backing plate over the gun nozzle and proximal femoral seal and a handled femoral seal-pusher for use around the femoral neck once the implant has been seated to the correct depth.

Patient Positioning

Place the patient on the operating table in the lateral decubitus position. It is helpful to position the patient towards the far side of the operating table since this reduces the chance of impingement of the operated leg on the table, facilitating maximal adduction for subsequent femoral exposure. Ensure also that the opposite leg can be extended so that it does not oppose later adduction of the operated leg.

We advocate the use of supports on both anterior superior iliac spines in combination with a sacral prop for secure and accurate stabilization of the patient on the table (■ Fig. 7.58). The props should be applied so that the anterior iliac spines are over each other in both vertical and horizontal planes and the degree of pelvic flexion is assessed by palpating the position of the pubis. It should be borne in mind that flexion of the contralateral hip may flex the pelvis, as will obliteration of the normal lumbar lordosis [4]. Additionally, the anterior spine may adduct by 10–15 degrees in the coronal plane.

With strong retraction, sometimes necessary when a mini-incision is used, movement of the pelvis within the soft tissue envelope may lead to malpositioning of the acetabular component unless this movement is identified and corrected for by the orientation of the acetabular introducer. Navigation will reduce the incidence of malpositioning from this cause.

Operative Technique

Skin Incision

The routine skin incision for a mini-posterolateral approach is sited more posteriorly and obliquely than a standard incision (■ Fig. 7.59) although it is possible to carry out the procedure through a variety of different orientations of skin incision. The routine incision starts distally over the femur and runs obliquely, passing 2 cm posterior to the tip of the greater trochanter, and continuing proximally a further 5 cm. By convention, the incision should be less then 10 cm in length to be called a "mini-approach" [5].

Deep Dissection

The fascia lata is divided in line with the skin incision, extending the fascial incision 1–2 cm proximally and distally to the skin incision splitting the gluteus maximus muscle in the line of its fibers. This reveals the posterior aspect of the greater trochanter and the trochanteric bursa. The latter is incised posterior to the trochanter and swept back by digital pressure to expose the short external rotators. The sciatic nerve, which lies posterior to these tendons can be easily palpated and need not be exposed. It must be protected at all times during the procedure. Internal rotation of the hip at this point will lengthen the short external rotators and the view is further enhanced by retracting the posterior border of the gluteus medius in an anterior direction. This exposes the underlying gluteus minimus tendon and piriformis, which lies immediately posterior to it. These

two tendons may be separated and a retractor passed over the femoral neck in the interval between the rotators and gluteus minimus (◘ Fig. 7.60). Then, keeping the hip internally rotated, piriformis and obturator internus with associated gemelli are tagged with stay sutures and then divided along the posterior aspect of the greater trochanter thus leaving as long a length of tendon as possible for later repair. The piriformis tendon may be preserved in many cases; it is then retracted with the medius and minimus tendon. The external rotators may be raised with the posterior capsule as a composite flap or the two layers may be raised separately, but in either case these layers should be firmly repaired at the end of the procedure. The capsule is further split proximally in line with the original direction of the piriformis tendon and then distally as near to the trochanteric attachment as possible, and then along the posterior border of the femoral neck and inferiorly towards the transverse ligament.

Dislocation and Neck Resection

In most cases the femoral head is now easily dislocated and the neck sectioned after placement of retractors around it (◘ Fig. 7.61). If the head is very large or the hip is ankylosed then the neck may be sectioned at the correct level prior to dislocation, a further section of proximal neck removed, to enhance exposure and then the head removed piecemeal.

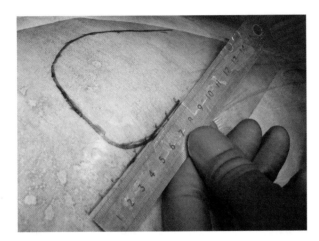

◘ **Fig. 7.59.** Position and orientation of skin incision

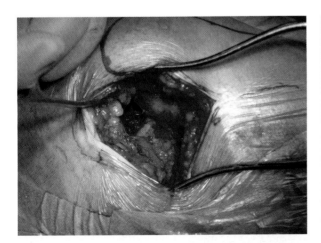

◘ **Fig. 7.60.** Superior retractor beneath gluteus minimus and medius exposing piriformis and other external rotators

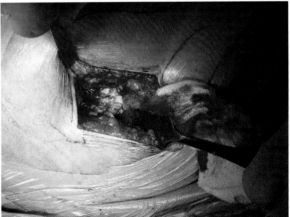

◘ **Fig. 7.61.** Retractors placed above and below femoral neck prior to osteotomy

Acetabular Exposure

Exposure of the acetabulum may be achieved by placing the anterior retractor (■ Fig. 7.62) over the anterior column and retracting the femoral metaphysis anteriorly. This retractor can either be stabilised by an assistant, or secured with a weight and chain. Release of the iliofemoral ligament and the reflected head of rectus femoris by running a knife from anterior to posterior on the ilium just above the superior acetabular rim can dramatically improve access (■ Fig. 7.63). Incising the inferior capsule further down to the transverse acetabular ligament improves anterior mobilisation of the femur and assists in acetabular exposure. The inferior retractor is placed immediately distal to the transverse acetabular ligament, underneath the cotyloid notch with its tip in the obturator foramen and a weight may be used to hold this retractor in position. At the proximal end of the wound the aspirator-retractor may be hammered in to the wing of the ilium. After defining the plane between the posterior capsule and acetabular labrum, one blade of a self retaining retractor (such as a Norfolk and Norwich retractor) is placed in this interval and the other jaw under the gluteus minimus muscle anteriorly (■ Fig. 7.64). The acetabulum can now be prepared for either a cemented or uncemented component in a standard fashion. Access to the acetabulum is not usually a problem. However, if it proves difficult to correctly orientate the acetabular reamer then positioning of the aspirator-retractor may be left until the stage of lavaging and

cementing the acetabular component. For a cemented implant a trabecular bone bed is prepared wherever possible and multiple drill holes made in the dome and around the rim. The surface is thoroughly lavaged using a powered system and the aspirator-retractor attached to a vacuum. Care is taken with this device not to remove an excessive amount of host blood. Bone graft is routinely placed on the cortical surface of the true medial wall prior to introduction of the cement and prolonged pressurization with a proprietary pressurizer (■ Fig. 7.65). Using simplex cement at 21 °C the pressurizer is usually applied at 3 min after the beginning of

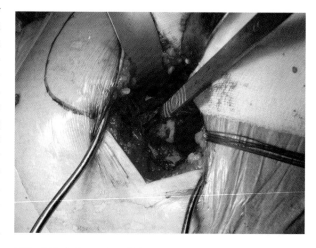

■ **Fig. 7.63.** Release of the iliofemoral ligament and the reflected head of rectus femoris by running knife over superior aspect of acetabular rim

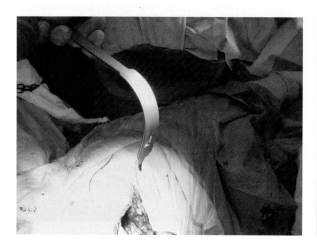

■ **Fig. 7.62.** Anterior acetabular retractor

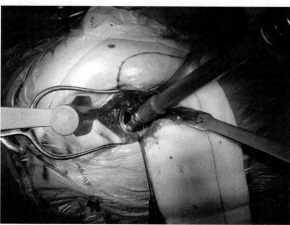

■ **Fig. 7.64.** Full acetabular exposure

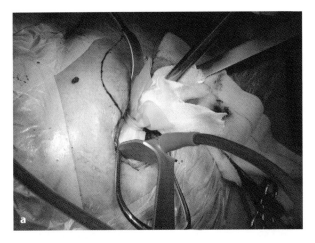

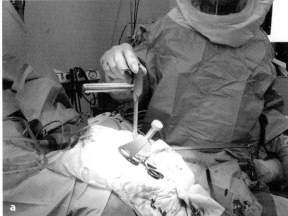

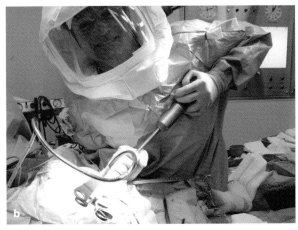

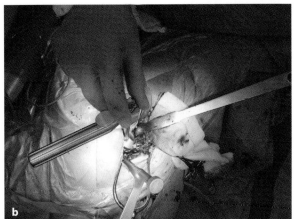

☐ **Fig. 7.65a,b.** Acetabular pressurization using exeter pressurizer

☐ **Fig. 7.66a,b.** "Charnley style" Acetabular introducer

mixing and used until 6–7 min have elapsed after mixing until the viscosity of the cement is rising. A flanged polyethylene socket with its flange accurately trimmed to fit concentrically within the acetabulum is then firmly pushed into place. The lateral "Charnley style" acetabular introducer is ideal to position the acetabular implant since it does not impinge on the femoral neck (☐ Fig. 7.66).

Femoral Exposure

To expose the femur, the acetabular retractors are removed and then the non-operated leg is moved into full extension. This allows the operated leg to be placed in maximum adduction, thus helping deliver the proximal femur into the wound. A range of 3 elevators (straight, right- and left-angled) are available, and use of two elevators will often improve exposure (see ☐ Fig. 7.56). The leg is internally rotated and one or more femoral elevators placed under the femoral neck. The forks of the elevator can be placed on either side of the iliopsoas tendon as it inserts into the lesser trochanter, or more proximally. The gluteus medius retractor (☐ Fig. 7.67) is then introduced with the spike rotated around minimus and through the fleshy anterior fibers of medius, to allow direct access to the femoral canal (☐ Fig. 7.68).

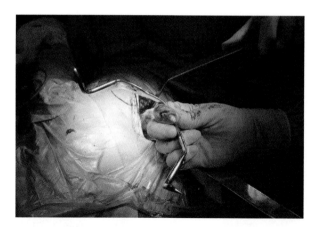

■ **Fig. 7.67.** Gluteus medius retractor

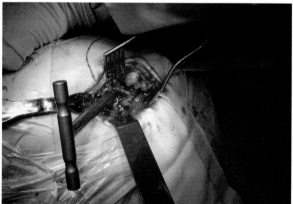

■ **Fig. 7.69.** Taperpin reamer pointing to middle of popliteal fossa

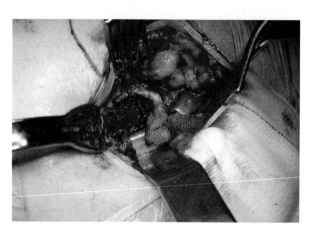

■ **Fig. 7.68.** Gluteus medius retractor and two femoral elevators in position

Femoral Preparation for a Cemented Stem

The posterolateral corner of the cut femoral neck is opened with a box chisel to allow in-line access to the femoral canal. Taper pin reamers are then used to open the femoral canal. To prevent varus stem placement the canal should be opened posteriorly and laterally into the base of the trochanter if necessary so that the taper pin reamer points to the middle of the popliteal fossa when viewed down its axis (■ Fig. 7.69).

The femoral canal is then prepared with the rasps. Modular rasp are available and are easier to insert at this stage than the routine monobloc rasps with necks. However, it should be remembered that there must be sufficient space anteriorly for the stem to be inserted in the correct degree of anteversion without impingement of the device on the retractor or soft tissues. Further internal rotation of the leg may help to prevent such impingement. It is important to rehearse this step to make certain that the stem can be accurately inserted into the cement mantle without impingement and consequent movement of the stem inside the polymerizing cement.

After final seating of the definitive rasp a trial reduction is performed to confirm appropriate leg length, stability and choice of offset. When satisfied, the femur is marked with diathermy or methylene blue dye at a level opposite one of the leg-length markers on the rasp. These marks correspond to marks on the definitive implant.

Femoral Cementing

The canal diameter is measured and an appropriate cement plug inserted. The femoral canal is then thoroughly washed to remove bone fragments and fat from the endosteal surface. A suction catheter is inserted to aspirate any accumulating blood from the distal canal and a peroxide soaked ribbon gauze is packed into the femur. These are removed immediately prior to retrograde injection of cement, using a cement gun about 3 min after mixing. The new reduced-size femoral seal and extended backing plate (■ Fig. 7.70) are designed for optimum cement pressurization through a mini-incision and these are used until approximately 6 min after mixing. The stem is inserted down the axis of the femur to the pre-rehearsed position. Following stem insertion, cement pressurization is maintained until polymeriza-

7.7

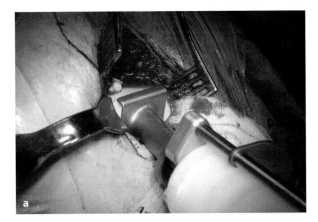

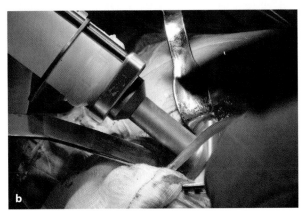

Fig. 7.70a,b. Femoral cement pressurisation using gun, extended metal backing plate and sorbothane proximal femoral seal

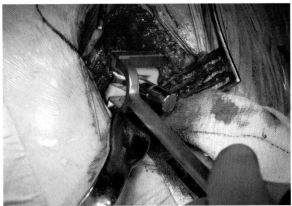

Fig. 7.71. Mini horse-collar and angled stem seal pusher to maintain pressure in femoral canal after stem insertion

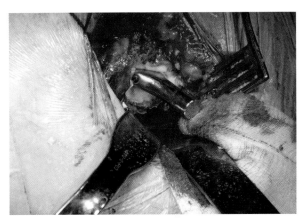

Fig. 7.72. Ideal position of stem towards posterior aspect of femoral neck

tion using the mini-horse-collar and angled stem seal pusher (**Fig. 7.71**). It is essential that the femoral component is not allowed to move inside the cement mantle once it is fully seated. The correct position of the stem is towards the posterior aspect of the cut surface of the femoral neck in order to ensure a complete mantle of cement just below the lesser trochanter (**Fig. 7.72**).

Reduction and Closure

A further trial reduction may now be performed and the appropriate neck length chosen to establish exact leg length as well as optimal soft-tissue balance and stability of the hip. After the selected head has been engaged on the Morse taper, the hip is reduced and the posterior structures repaired through drill holes in the greater trochanter (**Fig. 7.73**). Repair of these structures is

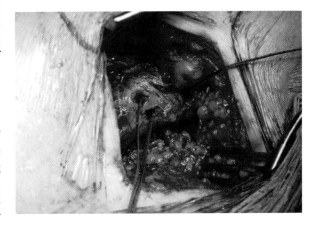

Fig. 7.73. Posterior capsule and external rotators re-attached through drill holes in greater trochanter

important in minimizing the risk of post-operative dislocation of the hip [6–8].

Conclusions

If practiced in the manner advocated above, we believe it is possible to carry out a cemented hip arthroplasty through a mini-posterior incision without compromising the end result for the patient. There is no doubt that patients like the cosmetic result of a smaller wound, and with increasing experience of the technique it has become evident that the traditional length of wound is rarely required, even in larger patients. Whether the smaller MIS incision, less than 10 cm, confers any other clinical advantage is yet to be conclusively demonstrated.

References

1. Malchau H, Herberts P, Soderman P, Oden A. Prognosis of total hip replacements. Update and validation of results from the Swedish National Hip Arthroplasty Registry 1979–1998. Scientific exhibit at the 67th Annual Meeting of the American Academy of Orthopaedic Surgeons, Orlando, USA, 2000
2. Karrholm J, Herberts P, Hultmark P, Malchau H, Nivbrant B, Thanner J. Radiostereometry of hip prostheses. Review of methodology and clinical results. Clin Orthop 344: 94–110, 1997
3. Malchau H. On the importance of stepwise introduction of new hip implant technology. Goteborg, 1995
4. McCollum DE, Gray WJ. Dislocation after total hip arthroplasty. Causes and prevention. Clin Orthop 261: 159–170, 1990
5. Howell J, Garbuz D, Duncan C. Minimally invasive hip replacement: Rationale, applied anatomy and instrumentation. Orthop Clin North Am 35(2): 107–118, 2004
6. Pellicci PM, Bostrom M, Poss R. Posterior approach to total hip replacement using enhanced posterior soft tissue repair. Clin Orthop 335: 224–228, 1998
7. Chiu FY, Chen CM, Chung TY, Lo WH, Chen TH. The effect of posterior capsulorrhaphy in primary total hip arthroplasty: a prospective randomized study. J Arthroplasty 15: 194–199, 2000
8. Robinson RP, Robinson HJJ, Salvati EA. Comparison of the transtrochanteric and posterior approaches for total hip replacement. Clin Orthop 147: 143–147, 1980

7.7

Tissue-Preserving, Minimally Invasive Total Hip Arthroplasty Using a Superior Capsulotomy

S.B. Murphy

Introduction

Conventional total hip arthroplasty in its many forms has been well established as a reliable procedure with predictable recovery. The high volume of procedures has allowed the incidences of the most common post-operative complications to be determined. Early complications vary widely by surgical approach and method of fixation, but generally include infection, dislocation, abductor morbidity, intra-operative fracture, and, rarely, nerve palsy. Preliminary reports of total hip arthroplasty using minimally invasive techniques have shown a tendency towards higher, rather than lower, complication rates [1, 6, 17, 19, 20]. Reasonable goals for evolving total hip arthroplasty include reducing the incidence of these peri-operative complications while simultaneously accelerating recovery.

The incidences of complications following conventional total hip arthroplasty depend largely on the surgical approach used to perform the procedure.

- THA performed using a posterior exposure may be complicated by post-operative dislocation [10, 18].
- THA performed using a direct lateral exposure may be complicated by incomplete abductor muscle recovery [5, 15].
- THA performed using a trans-trochanteric exposure may be complicated by trochanteric non-union and dislocation [16].
- THA performed using an anterior exposure may be complicated by abductor muscle injury and difficulty instrumenting the femur [6, 8, 9].

The current chapter reviews the rationale, technique, and results of tissue-preserving minimally invasive THA using a single incision through a superior capsulotomy.

Rationale and Design of the Surgical Technique

While at first glance, less invasive techniques might be anticipated to offer only short-term, but no long-term benefits. In fact, the principle of preserving all of the important structures around the hip joint is well founded. The principle of tissue preservation may facilitate early recovery because these methods are also minimally invasive, but the greatest benefit may be in the long term for hip-joint stability, muscle strength, and the more normal state of the soft tissues surrounding the joint at the time of any revision procedure. Further, since dissection of the surrounding soft tissues is minimized, the hip joint remains extremely stable, allowing unrestricted motion post-operatively, with minimal risk of dislocation.

Design of any minimally invasive total hip technique requires decisions regarding patient position, dependence on or independence from imaging and or traction, the ability to perform a trial reduction, and the tissue intervals to be used to avoid releasing important structures.

Patient Position

The lateral position was chosen for this procedure for several reasons. In the lateral position, gravity facilitates separation of the subcutaneous tissue layers and the posterior borders of the gluteus medius and medius are easily visualized. Since the lateral position is the most common position used to perform THA in the United States, the position is familiar to many surgeons, affording an opportunity to transition from familiar, conventional techniques to a more tissue-preserving technique. This also allows the rapid transition from a minimally invasive technique to a conventional technique if any aspect of the surgery cannot be adequately managed through a more limited tissue interval.

Tissue Intervals

Minimizing abductor morbidity is essential for rapid recovery of muscle strength following surgery. Similarly, avoiding release of the posterior capsule and short external rotators is essential to allow full, unrestricted motion following surgery. Any successful minimally invasive technique must be performed without disturbing these structures. Minimizing abductor morbidity requires that components be inserted either posterior or anterior/inferior to the gluteus medius and minimus. Splitting of the abductors for insertion of the femoral component cannot be performed because of the adverse affect on abductor recovery. Similarly, allowing unrestricted motion after surgery dictates that the posterior capsulotomy and short rotators cannot be incised [18, 21]. Further, posterior displacement of the femoral head out of the acetabulum requires partial disruption of the posterior capsule and short external rotators, even if they are not incised surgically. This means that the femoral head must be excised without dislocation or dislocated anteriorly to prevent injury to the posterior structures.

Anterior exposures such as the Watson–Jones and the Smith–Petersen exposures provide excellent visualization of the acetabulum but poor exposure of the femur. Performing the entire procedure, including femoral component insertion, through one of these exposures requires either some release of the anterior gluteus medius and minimus or skeletal traction. The use of skeletal traction during surgery has the great disadvantage that the performance of a trial reduction is either extremely difficult or not possible at all. Assessment of the reconstructed hip for stability, soft-tissue tension, and prosthetic impingement is a critical aspect of performing total hip arthroplasty, especially when hard bearings are used. As a result, this procedure was designed to be performed without the use of skeletal traction and to allow trial reduction for proper assessment of the joint.

Technique

The patient is placed in a lateral position. Most of the procedure is performed with the leg placed in the position of sleep (60 ° of flexion, 15 ° of internal rotation, and maximum adduction). A 6–8 cm incision is made starting at the tip of the greater trochanter and extending proximally (● Fig. 7.74). The skin incision can be longer in heavier patients as necessary. The gluteus maximus fibers are bluntly separated in line with their course to reveal the thin bursa tissue overlying the gluteus medius. The posterior border of the gluteus medius

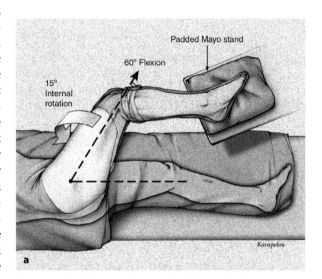

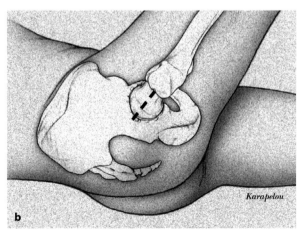

● **Fig. 7.74.** The patient is placed in a lateral position. Most of the procedure is performed with the leg in the position of sleep (60° of flexion, 15° of anteversion)

is mobilized anteriorly to reveal the piriformis tendon. The anterior border of the piriformis tendon is developed to reflect the piriformis posteriorly. The insertion of the piriformis can be released and repaired as necessary since most uncemented femoral components require removal of the bone that the piriformis tendon inserts upon. A blunt Hohmann retractor is placed in between the short external rotators and posterior capsule. The posterior border of the gluteus minimus muscle is developed and the minimus is mobilized anteriorly, taking care to fully develop the interval between the minimus tendon insertion and the anterior capsule. A blunt Hohmann retractor is placed around the anterior femoral neck in between the minimus and capsule. A spiked Hohmann retractor is placed into the anterior ilium to protect the medius and minimus. A second spiked Hohmann retractor is placed into the posterior/superior ilium. These four retractors allow complete exposure of the superior capsule and are levered to form four corners of a rectangle to maintain exposure throughout the procedure (◻ Fig. 7.75).

A vertical capsulotomy is performed from the trochanteric fossa to the acetabular rim along the previous course of the retracted piriformis tendon. An anterior capsular flap by creating two incisions in the anterior capsule; one along the acetabular rim, and one along the anterior femoral neck, deep to the minimus tendon insertion. The two blunt Hohmann retractors are then switched from being extracapsular to intracapsular, around the femoral neck anteriorly and posteriorly (◻ Fig. 7.76).

With the trochanteric fossa fully exposed and the surrounding tissues protected, a reamer is placed through the superior part of the femoral neck into the medullary canal. A tapered metaphyseal miller is used to expand the proximal opening, ensuring that subsequent reamers pass in line with the femoral shaft axis. After the diaphysis is reamed to size, the superior portion of the head and neck are removed with an osteotome to allow the femur to be prepared with broaches. The femoral head and neck are left in situ during this part of the procedure because the head provides stability to the femur during broaching, the neck provides a fulcrum for leverage retractors, and it also provides reinforcement to the calcar region to reduce the likelihood of femoral fractures during femoral preparation (◻ Fig. 7.77). The femoral broach is left in place.

Once the femur is fully prepared, a pelvic reference frame is percutaneously affixed to the pelvis if surgical navigation of the pelvis is to be performed [2–4, 7, 11–14]. A pre-reconstruction leg-length measurement is made. If fluoroscopic navigation is to be used for acetabular component insertion, fluoroscopic images may be

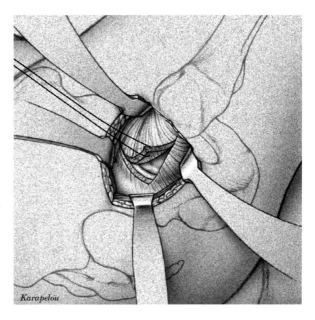

◻ **Fig. 7.75.** The superior capsulotomy, leaving the posterior capsule intact

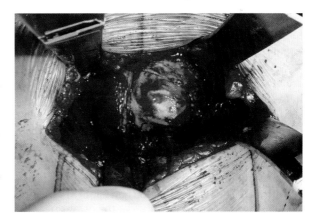

◻ **Fig. 7.76.** Exposure of a right hip through a superior capsulotomy. The femoral head and labrum are seen in the center of the photograph. The blunt Hohmann in the upper left is inside the anterior capsule, around the femoral neck. The spiked Hohmann in the upper right is in the ilium, underneath the minimus and medius. The spiked Hohmann in the lower right is inside the ilium above the posterior-superior portion of the acetabulum. The blunt Hohmann in the lower left is inside the posterior capsule, around the femoral neck. The entire THA procedure can be performed through this exposure

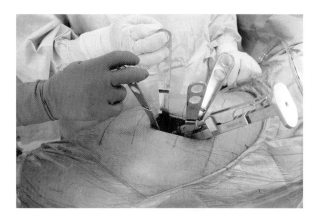

◘ **Fig. 7.77.** Femoral broach fully inserted through the exposure. The femur is fully prepared through the top of the femoral neck, prior to removal of the femoral head so long as the hip adducts sufficiently to allow this. The femoral head is left in place to stabilize the femur during preparation and to allow leverage retractors (blunt Hohmanns) to facilitate exposure

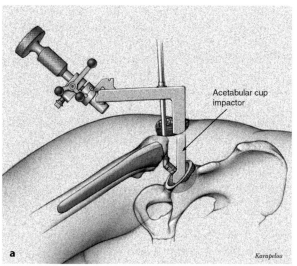

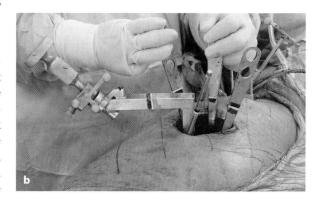

◘ **Fig. 7.78. a** Acetabular insertion device with a reference frame for surgical navigation. The impactor turns 45° from the cup plane to allow the instrument to exit the incision. Adding a 90°- and a second 45° angle allows the cup-insertion handle to be oriented in line with the cup. **b** Navigated acetabular impactor during cup insertion. The cup impactor is designed with two 45°- and one 90° angle to allow the cup impactor to exit the incision above the greater trochanter while still allowing impaction of the cup in line with the cup axis. (Acetabular cup impactor courtesy of Wright Medical Technology, Memphis, TN)

acquired at this point. The femoral neck is then transected, using the blunt Hohmann retractors to protect the surrounding soft tissues from the saw blade. The femoral head can also be split longitudinally to facilitated excision. Schanz screws are placed into the head/neck segments to control the bone fragments as they are excised. If CT-based navigation is being used, data points on the pelvis and acetabulum are now acquired, to achieve pelvic registration, after excision of the femoral head and prior to acetabular reaming.

The blunt Hohmann retractors are now placed around the acetabulum anteriorly and also posteriorly in the lesser sciatic notch. The entire acetabulum can be seen and remnants of the labrum are excised. A very low profile, 45-degree-angled reamer is then used to prepare the acetabulum. A z-shaped acetabular impactor is used to insert the acetabular component (◘ Fig. 7.78). If surgical navigation is employed, the cup is generally inserted with a goal of 41° of abduction and 25° of anteversion (◘ Fig. 7.79). While acetabular screws are rarely used for fixation, they may be inserted by passing the instruments from posterior, just above the edge of the retracted posterior capsule. Alternatively, screws may be inserted percutaneously through the Watson–Jones interval, using standard hip-arthroscopy cannulas and straight screw-insertion instruments.

After the cup is inserted, potentially impinging bone is trimmed, the trial or real acetabular liner is inserted,

a trial femoral head is inserted, a trial neck is affixed to the broach and reduced into the trial head in situ using a bone hook for traction and maximal muscle relaxation. The head and neck are not generally assembled before reduction because the surrounding soft tissues are so stable that even displacement to allow reduction of a 32 mm head may be difficult or cause disruption of surrounding tissues. An intra-operative radiograph

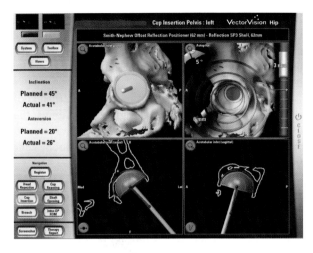

Fig. 7.79. Display of CT-based cup navigation during insertion of the acetabular component

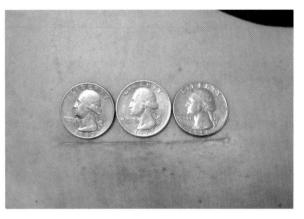

Fig. 7.80. 7.5 cm incision at the completion of the procedure. The procedure has been performed leaving the abductors and posterior capsule fully intact

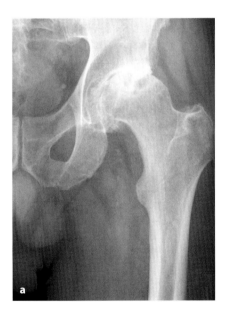

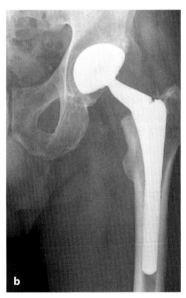

Fig. 7.81a,b. Pre- and post-operative radiographs of an uncemented alumina ceramic-ceramic total hip arthroplasty performed surgical navigation using the tissue-preserving, minimally-invasive technique described

may be taken to confirm proper component size and position as necessary. Trial reduction should produce a hip that cannot be dislocated in any direction without traction.

After satisfactory trial reduction, the trial components are removed, the real acetabular liner and femoral head are inserted, the real femoral component is inserted, and the femoral neck is again reduced into the femoral head *in situ* as before. The hip-joint capsule is closed. The piriformis tendon may be repaired with transosseous suture. The gluteus minimus and medius return to their native positions when the retractors are removed. The fascia overlying the gluteus maximus is closed prior to subcutaneous and skin closure (■ Fig. 7.80). Post-operatively, the patient may progress motion and weight-bearing without restriction (■ Fig. 7.81).

Clinical Experience and Results

This technique of tissue-preserving total hip arthroplasty can be performed in approximately 95% of primary procedures [14]. Modestly obese patients can often be managed just as effectively as thinner patients although with a slightly longer cutaneous and fascial incision may facilitate exposure. Clinical circumstances that may preclude use of the technique include hips with existing femoral hardware, severe deformities of the femur, and morbid obesity. Clinical assessment of patients postoperatively has shown a dramatic acceleration in return to walking without support as compared to patients treated by the direct lateral exposure by the same surgeon using the same implants. In the first 85 procedures, the two surgical complications were a greater trochanteric fracture repaired intraoperatively and an unrecognized displacement of an acetabular cup during stem insertion requiring prompt cup revision. These complications occurred in procedures #12 and 18 respectively, with no surgical complications in procedures #49 to 85. 48 of the last 50 primary hips performed were performed using this exposure. Of the two that were performed with conventional techniques, on patient had Paget's disease and the other had protrusio. None of the hips have dislocated, despite being allowed to regain motion without restriction. There have been no calcar or femoral shaft fractures.

Risks, Benefits and Conversion to a Conventional Exposure

Total hip arthroplasty through a superior capsulotomy is an approach that is nearly the opposite of anteriorly based exposures. Using a superior capsulotomy, the femoral instruments can be straight, while the acetabular instruments must be angled. This makes fixing an acetabular component with screws and direct visualization of superolateral screw holes more difficult. Also, since the femur is prepared with the femoral head in place, this technique is more difficult in patients whose hips cannot adduct into the position of sleep. More deformed and contracted hips can be managed by performing an osteotomy of the femoral neck early in the procedure and levering the leg into proper position. Alternatively, the femoral head can be excised prior to femoral preparation.

Reduction of the trail and real components can also be challenging since the tissues surrounding the hip are largely intact and limit displacement of the femur. Complete muscle relaxation at the time of implant assembly is very helpful.

With the patient in a lateral position and the exposure performed posterior to the gluteus minimus, the mini-posterior exposure is the most logical exposure to expand the procedure into if any factors cannot be controlled with the more limited exposure.

There are many benefits to the technique over conventional exposures and anteriorly based minimally invasive techniques. First, anteriorly based exposures must adversely affect the abductors whether the femoral component is placed anterior and inferior to the medius and minimus, or if a second exposure is used to blindly insert the femoral component through or behind the abductors. Second, the entire procedure can be performed through a single, short incision while preserving the abductors, posterior capsule, and short rotators. Since the femur is prepared prior to femoral head excision, the neck and head reinforce the calcar region, reducing the risk of femur fracture, a common complication of minimally invasive techniques. Finally, since the hip is so stable, the risk of hip dislocation appears to be minimized, even without placing any restriction on hip motion post-operatively.

In summary, experience with total hip arthroplasty through a superior capsulotomy demonstrates that the technique combines the rapid abductor recovery of posterior exposures, the hip-joint stability of the direct lateral exposure, and leaves the patient in position for more extensile exposures as necessary.

Acknowledgements. The author wishes to acknowledge Marc Mosier, M.D. and Korena Larsen, P.A.

References

1. Berry DJ, Berger RA, Callaghan JJ, Dorr LD, Duwelius PJ, Hartzband MA, Lieberman JR, Mears DC. Minimally invasive total hip arthroplasty. Development, early results, and a critical analysis. Presented at the Annual Meeting of the American Orthopaedic Association, Charleston, South Carolina, USA, June 14, 2003. J Bone Joint Surg Am 2003, 85-A(11): 2235–2246
2. DiGioia AM, Plakseychuk AY, Levisoin TJ, Jaramaz B. Mini-incision technique for total hip arthroplasty with navigation. J Arthroplasty 2003, 18(2): 123–128
3. DiGioia AM, Jaramaz B. Plakseychuk A et al. Comparison of a mechani cal acetabular alignment guide with computer placement of the socket. J Arthroplasty 2002, 17: 359

4. DiGioia AM, Jaramaz B, Blackwell M et al. Image guided navigation system to measure intraoperative acetabular implant alignment. Clin Orthop 1998, 355: 8

5. Gore D, Murray P, Sepic S, Gardner G. Anterlateral compared to posterior approach in total hip arthroplasty: difference in component positioning, hip strength, and hip motion. Clin Orthop 1982, 165: 180

6. Hartzband M. MIS meets CAOS. Pittsburgh, April 2003

7. Jaramaz B, DiGioia AM, Blackwell M, Nikou C. Computer assisted measurement of cup placement in total hip replacement. Clin Orthop 1998, 354: 70

8. Kennon RE, Keggi JM, Wetmore RS, Zatorski LE, Huo MH, and Keggi KJ. Total hip arthroplasty through a minimally invasive anterior surgical approach. J Bone Joint Surg 85-A [Suppl 49: 39–48

9. Light TR, Keggi KJ. Anterior approach to hip arthroplasty. Clin Orthop 1980, 152: 255–260

10. Morrey BF. Instability after total hip arthroplasty. Orthop Clin North Am 1992, 23: 237

11. Murphy SB, Deshmukh R. Clinical results of computer-assisted total hip arthroplasty. In: Langlotz F, Davies B, and Bauer A (eds) Computer-assisted orthopedic surgery. Steinkopff-Verlag, Darmstadt. 2003, pp 250–251

12. Murphy SB, Deshmukh R. Minimally invasive computer-assisted total hip arthroplasty. In: Langlotz F, Davies B, and Bauer A (eds) Computer-assisted orthopedic surgery. Steinkopff-Verlag, Darmstadt. 2003, pp 254–255

13. Murphy SB. Minimally-invasive THR using image-guided surgical navigation. The Hip Society, Washington, D.C., 2003

14. Murphy SB. Alumina Ceramic-Ceramic Total Hip Arthroplasty using computer-assisted surgical navigation and a new minimally invasive techniuque. In: Bioceramics in joint arthroplasty. Steinkopff, Darmstadt, 2004

15. Roberts JM, Fu FH, McCain EJ, Ferguson AB. A comparison of posterolateral and anterolateral approaches to total hip arthroplasty. Clin Orthop 1983, 187: 205

16. Schinsky MF, Nercessian OA, Arons RR, Macaulay W. Comparison of complications after transtrochanteric and posterolateral approaches for primary total hip arthroplasty. J Arthroplasty 2003, 18(4): 430–434

17. Waldman BJ. Minimally invasive total hip replacement and perioperative management: early experience. J South Orthop Assoc 2002, 11: 213–217

18. Weeden SH, Paprosky WG, Bowling JW. The early dislocation rate in primary total hip arthroplasty following the posterior approach with posterior soft-tissue repair. J Arthroplasty 2003, 18(6): 709–713

19. Wenz JF, Gurkan I, Jibodh SR. Mini-incision total hip arthroplasty: a comparative assessment of perioperative outcomes. Orthopedics 2002, 25: 1031–1043

20. Woolson ST. Primary total hip arthroplasty using an incision <12 cm in length. The Hip Society. Washington, D.C., September 11th, 2003

21. Wright J, Crockett H, Sculco T. Mini-incision for total hip arthroplasty. Orthopedic Special Edition 2001, 7: 18

Minimally Invasive Total Hip Arthroplasty Using the Two-Incision Approach

R. Berger

Introduction

Minimally invasive surgery has the potential for minimizing surgical trauma, pain and recovery. These minimally invasive techniques in total hip replacement include single-incision and two-incision techniques. This chapter describes a minimally invasive hip-replacement procedure performed with two incisions: one incision for acetabular preparation and placement, the other for the femoral preparation and placement. This new minimally invasive technique avoids transecting any muscle or tendon, thereby minimizing morbidity and recovery. Unique instruments have been developed to facilitate this technique. Fluoroscopy aids in many steps in this process to ensure the proper starting points for the incisions and accurate component position and alignment. Standard implants are used to maintain the present expectation for implant durability.

Surgical Technique

A radiolucent operating-room table is used. The patient is placed in the supine position with a small bolster under the ischium on the effected side. The leg and hip are prepped and draped. The fluoroscope is used to define the femoral neck. A metal marker is used to mark the midline of the femoral neck from the junction of the head distally 1.5 inches (■ Fig. 7.82). An incision is made directly over the femoral neck from the base of the femoral head distally 1.5 inches. The fascia of sartorius is present in the proximal-medial incision whereas the tensor fascia lata lies at the distal-lateral portion of the incision. The sartorius muscle and tensor fascia lata can be seen beneath the fascia. Just medial to the tensor fascia lata, the fascia is incised longitudinally, parallel to the

sartorius muscle and tensor fascia lata. This lateral fascial incision avoids the lateral femoral cutaneous nerve, which is located superficial to the sartorius muscle. Sartorius is retracted medially, and tensor fascia lata is retracted laterally, exposing the lateral border of rectus femoris. The medial retractor is repositioned to retract the rectus muscle medially (■ Fig. 7.83). This exposes the lateral circumflex vessels, which are coagulated with an electrocautery. The fat pad then is retracted medially and laterally exposing the capsule over the femoral neck.

Two curved lit Hohmann retractors (part of the minimally invasive two-incision instruments [Zimmer, Warsaw, IN]) are placed extra-capsularly around the femoral neck, illuminating the capsule. The capsule is incised in line with the femoral neck. This incision is made from

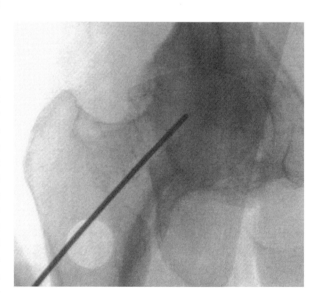

■ Fig. 7.82

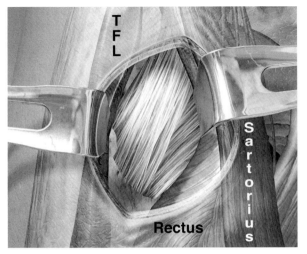

Fig. 7.83

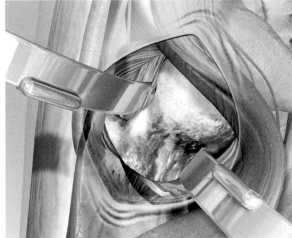

Fig. 7.84

the edge of the acetabulum distally to the inter-trochanteric line. The capsule can be elevated approximately 1 cm medially and laterally along the inter-trochanteric line if additional exposure of the femoral neck and head is needed. The two-curved lit Hohmann retractors are repositioned intra-capsularly to expose the femoral head and neck from the acetabulum to the inter-trochanteric line (**Fig. 7.84**).

The head is removed in two pieces. The first neck cut is made at the equator of the femoral head with an oscillating saw and a second cut is made 1 cm distal to this (**Fig. 7.85**). The small 1 cm wafer of bone is removed using a threaded Steinmann pin. Next, a threaded Steinmann pin is placed into the femoral head and the head is removed. If the ligamentum teres is intact, a curved osteotome is used to transect the ligamentum teres. Based upon pre-operative templating, the final femoral neck osteotomy is completed. Appropriate femoral neck resection is confirmed with fluoroscopy or by flexing and externally rotating the hip in a figure-of-four, which exposes the lesser trochanter.

Three curved lit Hohmann retractors are placed around the acetabulum, one anteriorly around acetabulum, a second posteriorly around the acetabulum, and the third directly superiorly over the brim of the acetabulum. This retracts the capsule and allows excellent visualization of the acetabulum (**Fig. 7.86**). The labrum is excised, exposing the entire peripheral bony rim of the acetabulum.

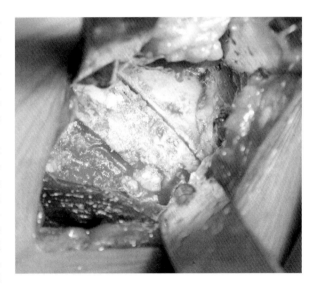

Fig. 7.85

The superior retractor is removed while the anterior and posterior retractors are left in place. Specially designed, low-profile reamers (part of the minimally invasive two-incision instruments), which are cutout on the sides, are used to ream the acetabulum. These reamers are aggressive with square cutting teeth; therefore, it is possible to start with a reamer that is close in size to the intended final reamer to avoid inserting and extracting many reamers. Furthermore, the open design of these reamers

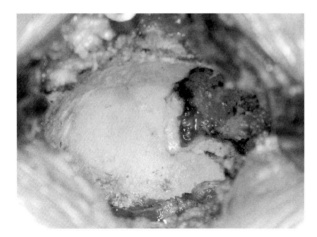

◻ Fig. 7.86

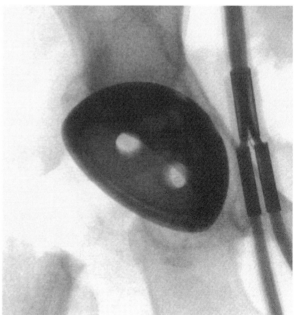

◻ Fig. 7.88

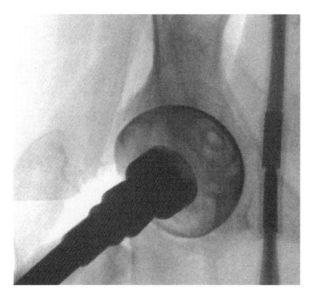

◻ Fig. 7.87

allows visualization of the acetabulum during reaming. With gentle traction on the leg, the reamer is inserted in line with the femoral neck, with the cutouts of the reamer aligned with the two retractors. The acetabulum is reamed at 45° of abduction and 20° of anteversion. The fluoroscope is used for visualization as the acetabulum is reamed (◻ Fig. 7.87). The acetabulum is sequentially reamed until a healthy bleeding bed of cancellous bone is present throughout.

A specialized dog-leg acetabular inserter (part of the minimally invasive two-incision instruments) with the supine positioner is used to place the chosen acetabulum shell. The anterior and posterior retractors are left in place, as gentle traction is placed on the leg. The bolster beneath the ischium is removed so that the patient is completely supine. The acetabular component is inserted as the retractors keep the capsule from invaginating. The acetabulum is viewed with the fluoroscope as the cup is positioned in 45° of abduction and 20° of anteversion, following the native acetabulum. The cup is then impacted in place and the inserter is removed (◻ Fig. 7.88). With the curved lit acetabular retractor in place around the acetabulum, the stability of the shell is assessed. Two supplemental screws are placed in the posterosuperior quadrant of the shell. Finally, a small-curved osteotome is used to remove any osteophytes around the rim of the acetabulum and the polyethylene liner is impacted into the shell. All retractors are removed from the acetabulum and attention is turned to the femur.

The leg is adducted fully and placed in neutral rotation. A 1- to 1.5-inch incision is made in the posterior lateral buttocks, co-linear with the piriformis fossa allowing access to the femoral canal. A Charnley awl is guided through the posterior incision, posterior to the abductors and anterior to the piriformis fossa down the femoral canal. Fluoroscopy can aid this starting point and can be used to visualize the leg in a frog lateral position to ensure this is well centralized anteriorly and posteriorly. Specially designed lateralization side-cutting reamers (part of the minimally invasive two-incision instruments) are used to enlarge this starting hole and position the starting point laterally against the trochanteric bed. These lateralization reamers are used sequentially through the posterior incision within the same track as the Charnley awl (⬛ Fig. 7.89). Flexible reamers are used to ream the canal until cortical chatter is obtained. Straight reamers with a tissue-protecting sleeve then are used to ream the femoral diaphysis until good cortical chatter is obtained.

After reaming to the appropriate size, broaching is done. With visualization though the anterior wound, the rasp is rotationally aligned to the calcar. The rasp is fully seated. Rasps then are sequentially introduced and seated, finishing with appropriate size (⬛ Fig. 7.90). When the final rasp is seated, care must be taken to visualize the rotation of the rasp in the anterior wound to ensure alignment with the metaphysis.

A trial reduction may be performed. The trial neck and head are placed on the broach from the anterior wound. The hip is then put through a range of motion to assess stability. The hip should be stable in full extension with 90° of external rotation and 90° of flexion with 20° of adduction and at least 50° of internal rotation. The fluoroscope can be used to assess leg lengths by comparing the level of the lesser trochanters with the obturator foramen. In addition, with the patient in the supine position, the medial malleoli may be checked to assess leg length. When the trial reduction is complete, the head and neck are removed through the anterior incision and the broach is removed through the posterior incision.

Two Hohmann retractors are placed into the posterior wound, one anterior to the femoral neck and one posterior to the femoral neck. These retract the soft tissue as the stem is placed into the femoral canal. The stem then is introduced into the femoral canal from the posterior incision and impacted into place (⬛ Fig. 7.91). Visualization through the anterior incision ensures no soft-tissue entrapment between the calcar and the collar and assures correct stem version.

With the actual component in place, repeat trial reduction is performed, placing the head from the anterior incision. The hip should be stable and leg lengths equal. With the hip in external rotation and the bone hook around the neck, the real head is then placed on

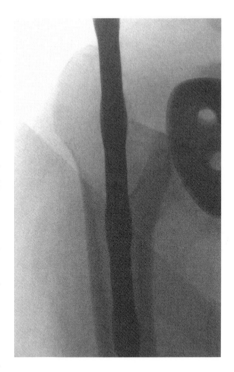

⬛ Fig. 7.89

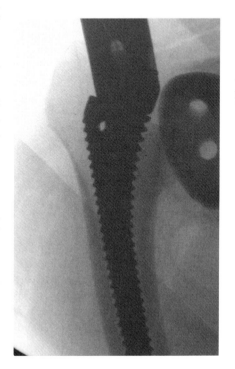

⬛ Fig. 7.90

7.8

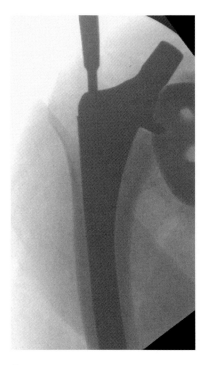

◘ Fig. 7.91

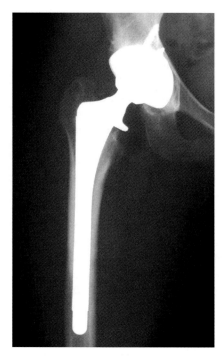

◘ Fig. 7.93

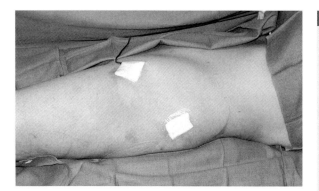

◘ Fig. 7.92

Conclusions

Minimally invasive surgery has the potential to minimize surgical trauma and pain while improving functional recovery in patients having total hip replacement. The minimally invasive two-incision total hip
technique described here, where no muscle or tendon is cut, shows substantial short-term pain and
functional improvement over traditional hip replacement. In fact, in the last 100 patients done at Rush
Hospital with this procedure, all surgeries have been
performed as an outpatient. Furthermore, unique
instruments and fluoroscopic assistance enabled
accurate component position and alignment.
While this minimally invasive two-incision technique
shows great promise, this technique requires meticulous surgical technique, specialized instrumentation,
and special instruction. As such, preclinical exercises,
anatomy laboratories, cadaver training, and proctor-
ing programs are strongly recommended for surgeons interested in this new technique to minimize
complications and ensure the success of this new
procedure.

the neck and gently impacted in place. The hip is located with gentle traction and internal rotation. The capsule is then closured. The fascia between the sartorius
and the tensor fascia lata is closed, followed by closure of
the anterior and posterior incisions. Two 2×2 inch bandages are used to cover the incisions (◘ Fig. 7.92). Figure
◘ 7.93 demonstrates the pre-operative and post-operative radiographs of this case example.

Anterior Double Incision

G.F. Heynen

Introduction

The concept of two separate incisions in total hip arthroplasty was originally introduced and popularized by Dana Meers, though Kristaps Keggi has extensive long-term experience with multiple incision surgery. The idea being each implant, i.e. cup and stem, are introduced through separate portals, thereby allowing for smaller incisions and less muscle release and disruption. The theoretical benefit of this so called "muscle sparing" approach is less pain, faster return of function and therefore earlier discharge from hospital and overall quicker recovery. It appears from preliminary data that these are viable goals, but safety in terms of complications and longer term questions of implant positioning and fixation have yet to be answered.

Anatomical Considerations

The double-incision approach as described by Meers incorporated an anterior incision centered over the neck of the femur in the interval between sartorius and tensor fascia muscles and a second incision above the trochanter. The anterior incision approaches the acetabulum via an internervous plane, the Smith–Peterson interval (■ Table 7.1).

From experience with pelvic osteotomy and anterior approaches to the hip, there are numerous problems with this incision. Unless the incision is oriented in the line of the groin crease, the anterior incision tends to heal with a certain degree of spreading and puckering, which in a situation where one of the indications for the technique is cosmesis, the ugly nature of the resultant scar is a concern.

The lateral cutaneous nerve of the thigh, which supplies a large area of sensation over the antero-lateral thigh is at risk in this interval, and damage either by traction or directly can cause permanent aggravating numbness or paresthesia.

For most orthopedic surgeons in the world, except our European colleagues, an anterior approach to the hip is unfamiliar and this contributes to the learning curve especially in relation to acetabular reaming and implant placement. To this end the surgical technique recommends the use of 32 mm heads and offset liners, where the offset is placed anteriorly, to reduce the risk of anterior dislocation. There is a tendency to increased anteversion of the acetabular component.

If problems arise during the procedure, the anterior approach is not extensile and therefore a separate third incision is required, positioned more laterally and allowing more conventional exposure of the proximal femur and the hip.

Based upon these concerns I embarked upon an anatomical study and cadaveric dissection to see whether these problems could be overcome. The only way to reliably do this was to shift the anterior incision laterally, and use the interval between gluteus medius and tensor facia, i.e. the Watson–Jones interval.

The incision is lateral over the anterior border of the trochanter, in line with the femur, and cosmetically heals more acceptably. The nerve supply to tensor fascia passes high on the interval and is not at risk, and concerns over the lateral cutaneous nerve are removed.

The patient can be placed supine or in the lateral decubitus position, and the interval provides a much straighter access to the acetabulum, both for reaming and implant placement. The incision is easily extensile into a modified Hardinge approach, and it is recom-

□ Table 7.1

	Advantages	Disadvantages
Smith–Peterson	1. True internervous plane 2. Easy access to femoral neck 3. Easier access for trial necks and heads	1. Lateral cutaneous nerve at risk 2. Cosmesis of scar 3. Increased risk of eccentric reaming 4. Increased difficulty in accurate cup placement, i.e. anteversion 5. Not extensile
Watson–Jones	1. Relatively internervous plane 2. Patient supine or lateral decubitus 3. Scar cosmesis better 4. Straighter access for acetabulum reaming and up insertion 5. Easily extensile	1. More difficult access to femoral neck for trial neck and head insertion

mended that surgeons new to the procedure can familiarize themselves with it by using a single longer skin incision, then placing the cup with full exposure of the trochanter and gluteus medius, going anterior to that muscle. The femoral preparation can then be performed by the standard gluteal split as for the anterior two-incision approach.

The difficulty with moving the incision laterally is access to the top of the femur for neck trial and head placement as the femoral neck is directed medially away from the incision. This difficulty has been overcome with specialized instruments for manipulating the neck trials and the femoral heads.

Implant Selection

Selection of implants has played an important role in the development of the minimally invasive two-incision surgery. Whereas virtually any type, size or shape of implant can be placed with single mini-incision techniques, there are specific restrictions, especially on the femoral side, at present with two-incision surgery, using existing implant systems.

Mini-incision surgery allows better visualization of the proximal femur and hence cemented stems and proximal fit/fit style cementless stems can be utilized. For two-incision surgery this access is restricted and hence more certainty is achieved with cementless fixation using fully porous coated stems, or in my hands the Taperloc design of the Accolade System.

Surgical Technique

Patient Positioning

The patient is placed supine with a bolster under the involved sacro-iliac joint, elevating the buttock and hip off the bed (□ Fig. 7.94). This position is favored as leg-length determination can be more accurately assessed compared to the lateral decubitus position and allows easier access to pelvic landmarks for computer navigation. The patient's arm is elevated and adducted across the chest out of the way. The whole leg is painted up to the costal margin, across to the midline, groin and buttock, and the leg is free draped.

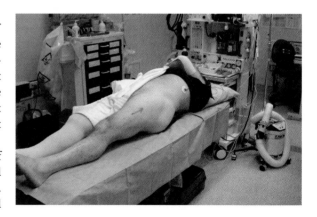

□ Fig. 7.94. Patient supine with bolster under buttock. Should be positioned appropriately on radiolucent table if image intensification required, also allows easy registration for Computer Navigation

Acetabular Placement

The skin incision is placed along the anterior border of the trochanter, starting approximately 1 cm distal to the tip, and is usually 5–6 cm in length. The size of the skin incision is determined by the pre-operative template size of the acetabular component, and the size of the patient (■ Fig. 7.95, 7.96). A 68 mm acetabular component will not fit in a 40 mm skin incision no matter how hard you try!

On exposure of fascia lata, tensor can usually be seen coming down obliquely to its insertion into fascia, and a longitudinal incision is made through fascia where the muscle inserts, and extends proximally in line with the skin incision. The interval between the muscles is easily defined and an index finger can be passed through the interval onto the anterior capsule. This is partially covered by fat, the origin of vastus intermedius fibers and more medially rectus muscle.

The hip is flexed and a curved pointed Hohmann style retractor is placed under rectus over the antero-superior rim of the acetabulum. Rectus can be released if necessary. A specially developed light-source retractor greatly aids visualization at this point through the small incision.

Fat and vastus are stripped from the capsule and narrow curved Hohmann retractors placed superiorly and inferiorly fully exposing the anterior capsule. An anterior capsulectomy is then performed (■ Fig. 7.97).

A superior capsulotomy both on the acetabulum and femoral side at this point will help with femoral preparation. The narrow retractors are then placed around the neck inside the capsule to protect the soft tissues and a femoral neck osteotomy is performed (■ Fig. 7.98).

A segment of neck can be removed, as this allows easier extraction of the femoral head from the acetabulum using a corkscrew. I have not found this always necessary, as long as the neck osteotomy is complete and mobilized (■ Fig. 7.99).

The complete circumference of the acetabulum cannot be visualized, but with sequential placement of retractors the whole margin can be exposed in a stepwise fashion from anterior, superior to posterior to allow debridement of labrum and osteophytes.

The acetabulum is reamed in the usual fashion with a straight reamer. Traction on the femur certainly aids in seating the reamers and removal of acetabular retractors. Reaming should not be performed until palpation

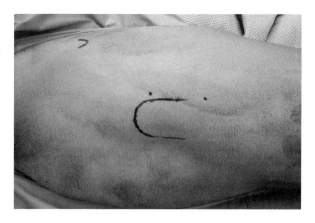

■ **Fig. 7.95.** Incision along anterior border of trochanter, the length of which is determined by the size of the acetabular component

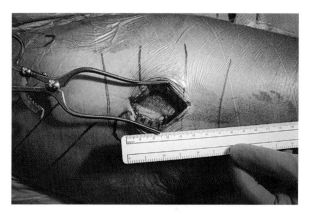

■ **Fig. 7.96.** Tensor Fascia Lata insertion identified, and incision through fascia is parallel to the skin incision, along this insertion

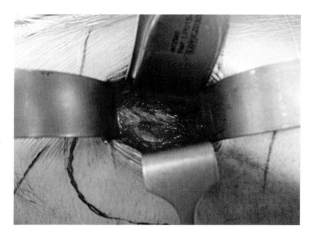

■ **Fig. 7.97.** Retractors placed with low profile light source to expose the anterior capsule, all the way medially to the acetabular margin

7.9

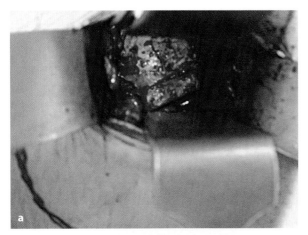

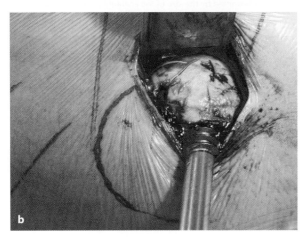

Fig. 7.98. a Segment of neck removal aids in easy extraction of the femoral head. **b** Femoral head easily removed with a thredded extractor

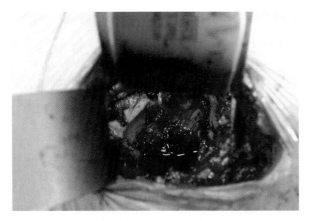

Fig. 7.99. Good views are obtained of the acetabulum, though sequential positioning of the retractors is required to perform a circumferential debridement

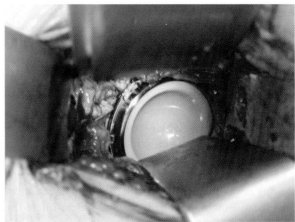

Fig. 7.100. Component positioning is easier with more direct visualisation than with the more anterior window

has confirmed that the reamer is centered in the acetabulum.

Acetabular placement can be performed with a straight inserter, but a curved inserter allows easier positioning, using the curvature to help clear the femur and the inferior aspect of the wound. Seating of the component can be inspected by replacement of the light-source retractor and viewing the polar hole.

I use a standard 28-mm articulation with an offset acetabular insert placed superiorly. Using a ceramic articulation sometimes requires the use of larger heads, determined by the size of the acetabular component in the Trident acetabular system. Ceramic liners are neutral without offset available (**Fig. 7.100**).

Femoral Preparation

The preparation of the femur is far more familiar in concept for most surgeons, as it equates fairly closely to closed rodding of a femoral fracture.

The superior neck is palpated and a curved scissor is then pushed through gluteus medius, out towards the skin as close to the tip of the trochanter as possible. During the maneuver the leg is flexed and adducted across the other leg. The tip of the scissors are advanced until easily palpated under the skin, then a 3 cm incision is made onto the tips, with the alignment of the skin incision according to the estimated version of the component to facilitate insertion of the stem (**Fig. 7.101**).

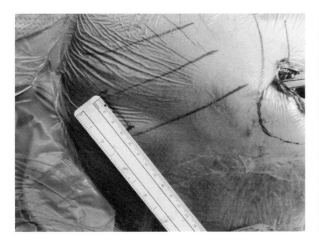

Fig. 7.101. Orientation of the second skin incision is according to the version of the femoral component

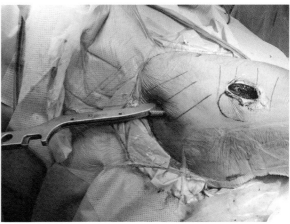

Fig. 7.102. Minimise the number of passes through the skin and abductors with instruments to reduce the potential for skin contamination and muscle damage. A finger in the inferior incision can be used to help direct instruments, and to check their position

From cadaveric dissection, the split in gluteus medius tends to be at the junction of middle and posterior third, and the importance of keeping the split as close to the tip of the trochanter is emphasized, as the anterior branch of the superior gluteal nerve is at risk with insertion of the stem. Rasping does not pose the same risk as these do not usually have a neck segment.

An important part of the femoral preparation is to ensure that the bone of the superior femoral neck is removed. This can be performed through the lateral incision or with a box chisel from above. The straight awl should be introduced with control coming from the first incision, and as it is advanced, the handle should be pulled laterally to ensure straight placement and not varus. A similar technique is adopted for broach seating.

During femoral preparation the leg is kept in its adducted flexed position, and orientation of the broaches judged using the position of the femur and knee. If the final broach size differs greatly from the templated size then this usually indicates the broach is in varus. This can be checked using image intensifier if necessary, and certainly with initial experience, an image intensifier adds confidence (**Fig. 7.102**).

A specially designed reverse-offset broach handle for the Accolade system is required for femoral preparation, as the standard and straight rasp handles tend to impinge on the skin and soft tissues, and not enough clearance makes it difficult to impact onto them with a hammer.

Trial Reduction

After seating of the final broach, the handle is disengaged and removed through the superior incision. The femoral neck trial appropriate along with the trial head is grasped in the special reduction forceps. A bone hook is placed either into the trochanter or around the medial femoral neck and the proximal femur is distracted away from the side of the pelvis and the reduction forceps and the head/neck trial is introduced onto the spigot of the trial broach. External rotation and traction by the assistant on the leg can facilitate this maneuver. The lighted retractor can be re-introduced for this part of the procedure. Leg lengths and stability are checked, the hip is re-dislocated and the reduction forceps re-introduced to remove the head/neck trial.

It is occasionally necessary to place the head/neck trial into the acetabulum, and then reduce the femur onto it, once again using the reduction forceps to manipulate the head/neck trial.

Femoral Stem Insertion and Final Reduction

The broach handle is then re-inserted through the superior incision and engaged, and the broach is removed.

The most difficult and taxing part of the procedure is the femoral component insertion. Soft-tissue impinge-

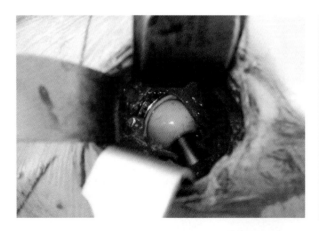

Fig. 7.103. Final position, tissue tension and stability can all be checked by direct visualisation via the inferior incision

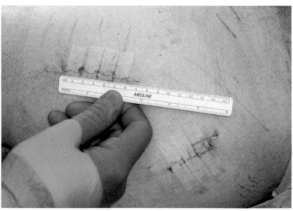

Fig. 7.104. The size of the skin incisions are determined by the size of the implants, but on average are 5cm for the lateral incision and 3cm for the buttock incision

ment on the neck and morse taper tends to push the implant into anteversion, especially the superior capsule and acetabular rim. Care must be taken using palpation and visualization that the stem is not catching as it is being impacted. The penalty for not taking care with this step is seating in increased anteversion and risking a proximal femoral fracture. To assist with this, it is a good idea to pull the neck segment through into the hip before final seating of the implant. This is achieved by traction on the leg, using a finger through the lateral incision, palpating the trunion and ensuring it is moving through the gluteal split and not catching on the superior capsule and acetabular margin (Fig. 7.103).

Once the stem is seated, a further trial reduction can be performed, externally rotating the leg and slipping the trial head onto the trunion.

The final head is introduced via the lateral incision using the specially designed head impactor.

Closure

As the anterior capsule is excised, there is no tissue available for deep or capsule closure, therefore only deep fascia, fat and skin require closure (Fig. 7.104).

Discussion

There is a considerable amount of skepticism surrounding the need for or advisability of minimally inva-

sive techniques in hip replacement considering the success of conventional exposures and techniques. Skeptics view it as a cosmetic procedure with no clinical benefit and certainly from the standpoint of someone with considerable experience, it does make the procedure slightly more complex, but only because it is currently based upon the use of existing implant and instrument designs.

Cosmesis is certainly a valid reason and should not be discounted. The average age of patients presenting for joint replacement is decreasing and body image is playing a far more important role in today's society. If a patient is offered the same procedure, with a choice between an 8 cm incision or a 15–20 cm incision, 9 patients out of 10 would choose the smaller incision. As surgeons we have already seen this trend in our practices due to the popularizing and marketing of minimally invasive surgery via the internet and popular press.

The clinical expectation of patients in terms of recovery is also affected by the size of their incision, and our study (see chapter 4) has shown that discharge times and early recovery can be improved with both two-incision and mini-incision surgery.

From a technical perspective, there is a significant learning curve for two-incision surgery, as the emphasis moves away from full exposure and visualization to a combination of exposure and tactile feedback and, in the future, computer navigation. To this end, the technique needs to have strong educational backup provided by the companies, preferably with a mentoring system available.

Clinical Results

In my own series, there has been a significant improvement in operating times and complications, though interestingly my average in-patient time has not reduced as my experience improves (□ Table 7.2). In-patient stay over my consecutive series from day 1 using two-incision surgery is 2.4 days, compared to 4.2 days for my first 200 cases using a mini-posterior approach.

Complications

There have been many valid concerns raised about the popularization of two-incision hip-replacement surgery. The principle flies in the face of basic surgical tenet "Exposure, Exposure, Exposure" and therefore must be scrutinized with careful scientific study to ensure safety.

Of the complications that have occurred in my consecutive series, one calcar fracture became significant when the patient stumbled and fell landing heavily on the hip 3 weeks after surgery. The fracture propagated to become a periprosthetic fracture with implant subsidence and required a second procedure to cable the proximal femur.

The infection rate is of concern. Currently the technique entails insertion of instruments and implants past the skin edges and hence the theoretical risk of contamination. The one infection in the series presented 6 months after the index procedure with ongoing pain, an elevated C-reactive protein and sedimentation rate. The infecting organism was coagulase negative *Staphylococcus* and the patient required a two-stage revision.

As instruments and implants evolve for the procedure, I am sure, safety will improve, and computer navigation will certainly improve feedback and confidence with the technique.

Conclusions

Minimally invasive two-incision surgery is in its infancy, but the technique offers advantages over conventional exposures by improving the early post-operative recovery.

Two-incision surgery using the more laterally based Watson–Jones interval for acetabular insertion offers significant advantages over the more anteriorly positioned Smith–Peterson interval:

1. more cosmetic skin healing,
2. avoiding lateral cutaneous nerve of the thigh,
3. straighter access to the acetabulum, improving orientation of reamers and cup insertion,
4. fully extensile to direct lateral approach,
5. allows use of single larger lateral skin incision with two incision deep dissection as part of the early learning of the procedure.

The technique will evolve, assisted by more sophisticated instrument design and soft-tissue protection, the integration of computer navigation, and the development of specific implants to overcome some of the technical challenges currently encountered with the technique.

□ **Table 7.2.** Case number

	0–20	21–40	41–60	61–80
Operative-time average	117	112	84	76
Blood-loss average	890	860	640	520
Hospital stay	2.4	2.2	2.4	2.0
Complications	2 fractures	1 fracture, 1 infection	Nil	1 fracture

Anterior Double-Incision Lateral Decubitus Approach

J.P. Nessler, G. Nelson

Introduction

Total hip arthroplasty has become a commonplace and highly successful surgical procedure. Improvements in prosthetic design and bearing surfaces have led to expanded indications for hip replacement in younger, active patients. The demands of younger patients and increased expectations for earlier return to activity in older patients has led to a growing interest in less invasive methods of total hip arthroplasty. Mini-incision anterior, posterior, and multiple incision approaches have been described [1, 3, 4, 6–8]. So-called muscle-sparing procedures utilizing a modified anterior Smith–Petersen approach have been promoted as the least disruptive approach to the soft tissues in hip arthroplasty. There has been some hesitancy amongst surgeons to adopt these newer techniques that employ different surgical approaches to the hip when combined with a different patient positioning. The majority of North American surgeons have traditionally performed total hip arthroplasty with the patient in the lateral decubitus position. Muscle sparing anterior and multiple incision approaches have typically been described with the patient in the supine position [1, 7]. In an attempt to minimize changes in surgical routine a procedure and instrumentation were adapted to allow a two-incision muscle-sparing surgical approach with the patient in the lateral decubitus position. It is the authors' firm belief that by maintaining standard patient positioning the surgeon is already familiar with, component placement errors can be minimized, and the requisite learning curve shortened.

Surgical Technique

Positioning and Acetabular Exposure

The patient is placed in the lateral decubitus position with the affected side up. Low profile pelvic positioners may be placed at the pubic symphysis level and at the sacrum to stabilize the pelvis. Care should be taken such that any positioning devices do not interfere with hip range of motion. The lower extremity is prepped and draped free. Anatomic landmarks are identified as follows: the anterior superior iliac spine (ASIS), the greater trochanter (GT), and the lateral border of the patella. The anterior skin incision is made just lateral and parallel to the line extending from the lateral border of the patella to the ASIS. The incision starts proximally at the level of the proximal tip of the GT, and extends distally 4–10 cm based on patient size and muscle mass (◘ Fig. 7.105). The lateral femoral cutaneous nerve lies in proximity to the incision, if identified efforts should be made to protect it, often retracting it medially with the underlying sartorius [2, 5]. The underlying tensor fasciae latae muscle (TFL) is identified. The muscle fasciae is incised along the medial border of the muscle (in large heavily muscled individuals the dissection may proceed 1–3 cm lateral to the medial border of the TFL muscle) and blunt finger dissection is carried out to the hip-joint capsule overlying the femoral neck (◘ Figs. 7.106, 7.107). Retractors are placed inferior and superior to the hip-joint capsule. The anterior capsule is tightened, and exposure enhanced by placing the leg in an abducted and externally rotated position. The reflected head of the rectus femoris muscle may be resected or bluntly elevated of the capsule. Frequently, the ascending branch of the lateral femoral circumflex artery is in the operative field and may need to be ligated [5]. A complete resection of the pathologic anterior and superior capsule is performed. Osteotomy of the femoral neck is performed at the level determined by pre-operative templating. A second osteotomy is made proximal to this to remove a wedge of bone and facilitate femoral head removal. Acetabular retractors are placed to expose the socket. Lighted retractors may be used, alternatively, the author's preference is to use a headlight for visualization. Acetabular reaming is carried out in the usual fash-

ion. Special angled acetabular reamer shafts are helpful with smaller incisions (○ Fig. 7.108). Excision of osteophytes, labrum, and capsular releases are carried out as necessary. Implantation of the acetabular component is carried out in the usual fashion, curved acetabular insertion handles are utilized. Through the anterior incision, the GT is visualized and a ronguer is used to make a notch along the medial aspect of the GT. This notch will serve as a palpable landmark for the starting point of the femoral reamers and broaches to avoid varus positioning of the component.

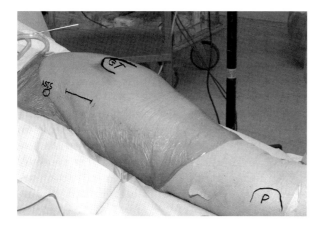

○ **Fig. 7.105.** Patient in the lateral decubitus position with landmarks identified and proposed skin incision marked. *GT* Greater trochanter, *ASIS* anterior superior iliac spine, *P* patella

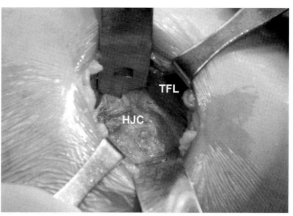

○ **Fig. 7.107.** Retractors are placed superior and inferior to the hip joint capsule (*HJC*), the tensor fasciae latae is seen in the lateral aspect of the wound

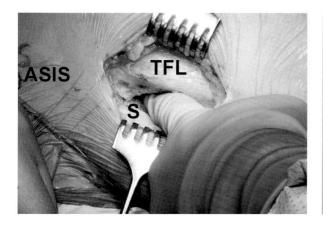

○ **Fig. 7.106.** After making the skin incision the medial edge of the tensor fasciae latae muscle (*TFL*) is identified, the sartorious (*S*) lies medial to it. Blunt finger dissection is performed at this interval down to the hip joint capsule

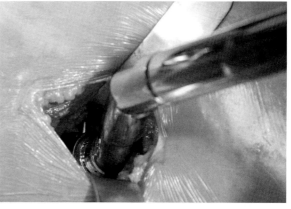

○ **Fig. 7.108.** Angled reamer shaft allows acetabular preparation through smaller skin incision

7.10

Femoral Preparation

The surgeon moves to the opposite side of the operating table, behind the patient. The limb is placed in the figure-4 position over the table. This allows consistent positioning of the femur to control anteversion during preparation of the femur. A smooth Steinmann pin is placed percutaneously through the skin to enter the femur near the notch created in the GT. Palpation and direct visualization of the proximal femur through the anterior incision confirms appropriate positioning of the pin. Once satisfactory pin placement is obtained it is used as a reference for the skin incision. A 2–5 cm skin incision is made in line with the proposed anteversion of the femoral component. Preparation of the femur is carried out specific to the implant design. The author's preference is for a proximally fixed wedge-taper design stem. The femoral canal is opened with a starter reamer followed by a trochanteric lateralizing reamer to prevent varus and flexion, a self retaining retractor with deep 60–70 mm feet protects the soft tissues (❑ Fig. 7.109). Sequential femoral broaching is performed, based on pre-operative templates. Correct broach placement is confirmed by inspection through the anterior incision. Through the anterior incision, the calcar can be inspected for cracks and to ensure complete seating of broaches/implants. The femoral implant is then inserted (❑ Fig. 7.110) and trial reduction performed to determine head length. The femoral head is placed on the trunion through the anterior incision.

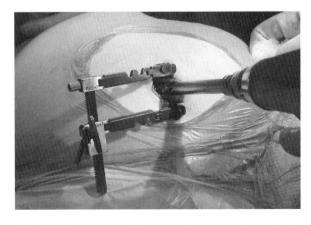

❑ **Fig. 7.109.** Assistant maintains leg in figure-4 position while the surgeon prepares the femur. 70 mm deep retractors protect the soft tissues

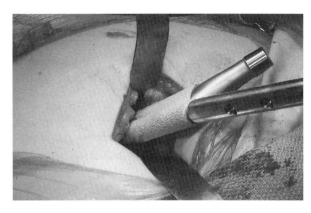

❑ **Fig. 7.110.** Femoral component being inserted percutaneously from the posterior incision

Stability and Range of Motion Check

With the lateral decubitus position, no special operating tables are necessary and hip range of motion can be checked in all directions including hyperextension. The hip is brought into full or slight hyperextension, adducted and externally rotated to check anterior stability. Anterior stability is further tested in varying degrees of flexion (to 110° or more), external rotation and adduction. Posterior stability is tested in external rotation throughout the flexion–extension arc. Wound closure is a simple layered closure utilizing a subcuticular absorbable suture. Drains are not routinely used. All wounds are infiltrated with 0.25% bupivicaine with 1:200 000 epinephrine, 30–90 cc, based on body weight. Antibiotic ointment, non-adherent dressings and a clear occlusive dressing cover the wounds.

Post-Operative Care

Passive range of motion is started immediately in the recovery room. The patient is allowed out of bed, full weight-bearing the day of surgery. Patients are allowed to advance to a single cane when tolerated, usually within the first 10 days post-operatively. Many patients leave the hospital utilizing a single cane for support. Most patients do not regularly use any assistive devices after 2–3 weeks post-operatively. Dressings are changed on day 2 post-operatively, then daily. Showers are allowed anytime after the initial dressing is removed. No specific hip precautions are observed after 3–4 weeks after surgery.

Results and Complications

In the first 150 patients utilizing this technique no dislocations have occurred. Calcar cracks, recognized intra-operatively and cabled prophylactically occurred in 3/150 patients. One patient without an intra-operatively recognized calcar crack sustained a post-operative fracture upon arising from a chair and twisting. This was successfully treated by femoral revision and cabling. If an intra-operative calcar fracture is identified, it can be easily treated with cerclage wires or cables through the anterior incision (■ Fig. 7.111). All calcar cracks occurred early in the learning curve, no cracks occurred in the last 112 surgical procedures. In extremely osteoporotic bone, prophylactic cerclage wires may be placed. If more extensive exposure is required, the anterior approach is extensile and can be extended distally to expose the entire femoral shaft and proximally to expose the lateral aspect of the ilium [4]. Post-operative radiographs demonstrate the ability to consistently place the components in the appropriate position. Neutral femoral alignment was obtained and average acetabular abduction on post-operative radiographs measured 46° (■ Fig. 7.112). Five percent of patients required homologous blood transfusion.

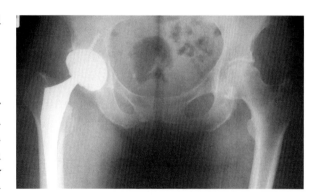

■ **Fig. 7.112.** Post-operative radiograph showing ability to obtain excellent alignment of components through the muscle-sparing approach

Conclusions

A muscle-sparing two-incision surgical approach with the patient in the lateral decubitus position affords the surgeon the ability to maintain landmarks and orientation he is already accustomed to. The technique described appears to be safe and allows for an extensile approach should untoward intra-operative complications arise. Subjective patient satisfaction is high and demand for this procedure continues to grow. Long-term studies of this and other muscle-sparing approaches will be necessary to determine if overall outcomes are similar to or superior to conventional approaches.

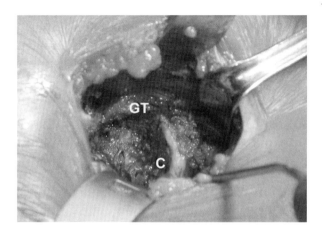

■ **Fig. 7.111.** Excellent exposure of the proximal femur can be obtained and cerclage cabling carried out if necessary. *C* calcar, *GT* greater trochanter

References

1. Berger R et al (2003) Minimally-invasive total hip arthroplasty. J Bone Joint Surg 85-A 11: 2235–2246
2. Clemente C (1981) Anatomy, a regional atlas of the human body. Urban & Schwarzenberg, Munich
3. DiGioia A et al (2003) mini-incision technique for total hip arthroplasty with navigation. J Arthroplasty 18: 123–128
4. Goldstein W et al (2003) Minimal-incision total hip arthroplasty. J Bone Joint Surg 85-A [Supp 4]: 33–38
5. Hoppenfeld S, deBoer P (2003) Surgical exposures in orthopedics. Lippincott Williams & Wilkins, Philadelphia
6. Kelmanovich D et al (2003) Surgical approaches to total hip arthroplasty. J South Orthop Assoc 12: 90–94
7. Kennon R, Keggi J et al (2003) Total hip arthroplasty through a minimally invasive anterior surgical approach. J Bone Joint Surg 85-A [Supp 4]: 39–48
8. Waldman B (2003) Advancements in minimally invasive total hip arthroplasty. Orthopedics 26(8) [Suppl]: 833–836
9. Wenz J et al (2002) Mini-incision total hip arthroplasty: A comparative assessment of peri-operative outcomes. Orthopedics 25(10): 1031–1043

Minimally Invasive Approach to Metal-on-Metal Resurfacing Hip Arthroplasty

C.M. Thomas, M.A. Mont, H.P. Bezwada, P.S. Ragland

Introduction

Resurfacing is a type of hip replacement that conserves bone of the proximal femur and involves preparing the femoral head with special tools that allows for putting a cap on the remaining head. Presently, this femoral head will typically articulate with a metal acetabular component. The use of resurfacing is not a new concept as these prostheses predated the use of stemmed femoral components. They were used commonly in the 1970s with metal-on-polyethylene articulations, but fell out of favor due to high rates of bone resorption and loosening within 5 years [2]. Presently, there has been a resurgence in the use of this technology because of the advent of new metallurgical techniques which have allowed for better metal-on-metal articulations in general. Recently, there have been excellent mid-term results reported with a number of these devices [1, 4, 5]. This review will focus on our use of a minimally invasive approach for resurfacing with a device called the Conserve Plus™ (Wright Medical, Arlington, Tennessee). However, most resurfacings are very similar in design and the techniques that are described in this report can be applied generically to almost all resurfacing devices.

Resurfacing is not a new concept as it has been used as a general standard in total knee replacement. Simply resurfacing the worn joint surfaces has uncommonly been used as a means of a total hip replacement. There are a number of theoretical advantages of resurfacing. An obvious advantage is that it saves bone on the femoral side. This allows the patient to avoid the use of an intra-medullary device that is used in standard total hip replacements. Unfortunately, this necessitates a more difficult surgical dislocation and exposure required to prepare the acetabulum because the femoral head is not being sized and can be in the way. In addition, for a truly conservative procedure one would like to take less bone from the acetabulum. Until recently, with newer designs in shells, this has not typically been the case as more acetabular bone stock has been resurfaced.

Other advantages of the resurfacing include possibly better stress transfer to the proximal femur and because of the large femoral head (typically sizes range from 36–54 mm), there has been more range of motion with these replacements than conventional total hips and there has typically been a lower dislocation rate. In one study, the gait mechanics more closely resemble a normal hip than conventional hip replacements [4].

A final advantage is that, when necessary, the revision of the femoral component should be much easier than revising a standard intra-medullary femoral component in a conventional total hip replacement. The contemporary components have an acetabular bearing that removes very little acetabular bone stock and in the event of a revision, there is less inflammatory bone loss of metal-on-metal bearings. In the event of a femoral side failure, the acetabular component can be left in place and mated to a standard femoral component with a large diameter femoral head (◘ Fig. 7.113) [3].

In summary, there are various possible advantages of resurfacing over standard total hip replacements including the preservation of bone stock, the possibly better stress transfer with more range of motion, lower dislocation rates, and perhaps in many cases, an easier revision.

Indications for Resurfacing

The indications for resurfacing hip replacement include most of the indications that are used for any standard hip replacement for any arthritic condition. The indications have gradually been expanded from the use in all forms of primary osteoarthritis, as well as developmental dysplasia of the hip and post-traumatic arthritis, to patients with osteonecrosis and rheumatoid arthritis when there is an adequate bone stock. If any patient, including patients with inflammatory arthritis, have the appearance on X-rays of inadequate bone stock of the femoral head and neck, they would not be candidates for this procedure. Patients have generally been under 55 years of age, but it should be emphasized once again that good bone stock is imperative and that there are certainly patients over this age who have been indicated. Another assessment of bone-stock adequacy can be made through pre-operative DEXA scans.

Although these are no contra-indications, the worst results have been reported in patients who are tall, of female gender, and who have had femoral head cysts greater than 1 cm, which may lead to increased risk for later component failure [1].

Contraindications for resurfacing include patients who obviously have a lack of a femoral head- or neck-bone stock and would not be able to have a resurfacing femoral component. In addition, patients with bone-deficient acetabulae would not be candidates as most resurfacing components on the market do not have screws available for ancillary fixation. As these second generation devices are developed with ancillary fixation aids for

the acetabulum, more people with dysplasia or acetabular bone deficiency may be candidates.

Excellent indications for resurfacings include
- patients who have retained hardware of the proximal femur that would be difficult to remove for a standard stem replacement,
- patients with certain diagnoses that may have a high risk for failure or dislocation in standard total hip replacements (such as sickle-cell disease or chronic alcoholics),
- patients with a proximal femoral deformity which makes putting a standard-stem prosthesis difficult or impossible to place (Fig. 7.114, 7.115).

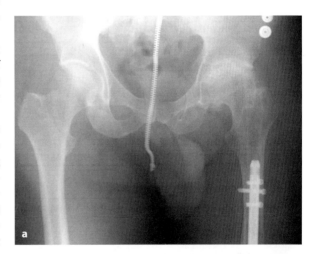

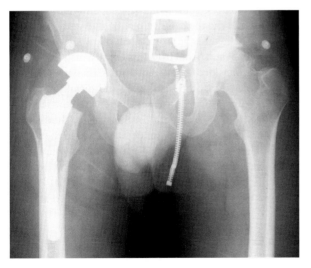

 Fig. 7.113. Post-operative radiograph showing standard femoral component with large diameter femoral head

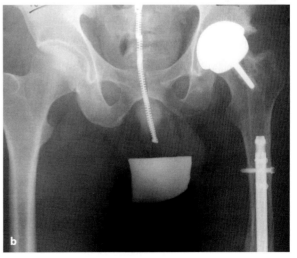

 Fig. 7.114a,b. Pre- and post-operative radiograph of femur with intra-meduallary rod

7.11

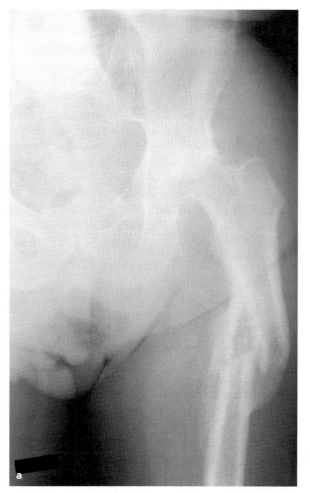

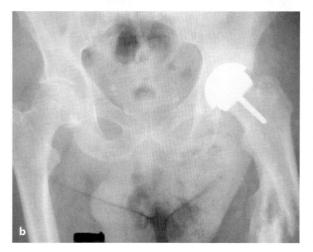

Fig. 7.115a,b. Pre- and post-operative radiograph of femur with proximal mal-union

Surgical Technique – Anterolateral Approach

Equipment

As the instrumentation to perform minimally invasive surgery for resurfacing is in an evolutionary stage and still being developed, minimally invasive metal-on-metal resurfacing hip arthroplasty may still be performed using current instrumentation without any substantial increase in the degree of difficulty. In addition to the standard metal-on-metal instruments provided by the vendor, only a few additional instruments are necessary to perform minimally invasive metal-on-metal resurfacing hip arthroplasty. Listed below are the instruments required to perform this procedure.

- Weitlander retractors for skin retraction
- Cobb elevator for tensor fascia latae exposure
- spike or Taylor retractor for acetabulum exposure.

Placement of Incision

The ability to perform minimally invasive metal-on-metal resurfacing hip arthroplasty without compromising appropriate placement of components, begins and ends with the important placement of the incision. First, outline the greater trochanter. Use the pre-operative radiographs to grossly determine the location of the center of the femoral head in relation to the greater trochanter. Remember that many of these patients will have deformed femoral necks, with variable neck-shaft angles. Often, different patient's landmarks for the incision will not be the same. Once the center of the head is approximated, mark a straight line 3 cm proximal and distal from this point, which will be the initial base incision. The surgeon should then mark an additional line 2 cm, both proximally and distally, if extension is required during the case. Thus, overall the incision can range from 6–10 cm total for most cases. The skin incision is deepened through subcutaneous fat to the tensor fascia latae. A single retainer is used for retraction, as well as to tamponade subcutaneous bleeding. One should avoid the use of electrocautery at this superficial level, if possible, to minimize the extent of fat necrosis created.

Deep Exposure

The tensor fascia latae is identified and a Cobb elevator is used to establish a plane approximately 5 cm in every

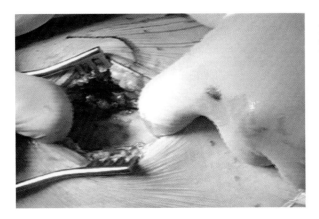

☐ **Fig. 7.116.** Exposure of the tensor fascia latae

direction (☐ Fig. 7.116). This step cannot be over-emphasized. It allows for mobilization of the skin incision, essentially converting a 6 cm skin incision into an 8–12 cm working incision.

The leg is held in slight abduction to relax the tensor and the fascia is incised in both a proximal and distal directions. Be careful not to extend the tensor fascia incision much beyond the boundaries of the mobile skin incision. If this is done later, closure can be difficult. Next, identify the anterior 20% of the gluteus medius muscle. With one finger under the gluteus medius and above the minimus, detach the anterior 20–30% of the medius from its insertion on the greater trochanter.

Next, continue dissection along the neck, until the plane between the gluteus minimus and the anterior capsule is identified. At this point, place a Hohmann retractor superiorly and inferior to the neck. Next, a Cobb elevator is placed between the gluteus minimus and anterior capsule. The tip of the Cobb is placed on the rim of the acetabulum. The anterior capsule is dissected free of any gluteus minimus fibers either with scissors or blunt dissection as the gluteus minimus is completely lifted off the capsule. Once the capsule is completely exposed, a standard capsulectomy is performed, and the remaining capsule is released from the neck, using a Smillie meniscal knife, in both a superior and inferior direction, being careful to stay adjacent to the femoral neck.

Next, all instruments are removed and the hip is dislocated. A bone hook should not necessarily be used, as the point of the hook can penetrate the femoral neck, leading to an unnecessary stress riser. The posterior limb of the tensor fascia latae will impede dislocation unless a greater trochanteric retractor or a blunt Hohmann is placed on the bone to keep the tensor posteriorly. With the head dislocated, the femoral neck is debrided free of any remaining capsule. A key step is that a neck measurement is made to adequately determine the matching acetabular shell size that will correspond with the femoral head size to avoid notching of the femoral neck. For example, a neck diameter approximately measured in two planes will be the minimum diameter of the reamer than can be used on the femur to avoid notching the femoral neck. This minimum diameter will then direct the minimum acetabular cup size that must be reached to insert a cup that will not lead to notching of the femoral neck. The presence of any neck osteophytes must be incorporated into the neck sizing. The leg is now brought back into extension, and the acetabulum is prepared for placement of the acetabular cup. When the head is dislocated through a small incision, it is tempting to lengthen the incision at this time. The surgeon should resist this tendency. The incision may often stretch 1–2 cm as a result of retraction for the acetabular preparation.

Exposing the Acetabulum

This is the hardest part of the case to master. The hip is placed in varying degrees of flexion depending on the neck deformity present. Usually, 30–40° are sufficient to allow for the head to be retracted posteriorly. First, an anterior retractor is placed anterior-inferiorly (approximately 4:30 position). Next, a curved Hohmann is positioned on the posterior-inferior acetabular rim (approximately 7:30 position). Placement of this retractor may be difficult, secondary to neck deformity and remaining posterior capsule. A Cobb elevator may be used to release posterior capsule from the posterior femoral neck. Many patients will have a deficient anterior and posterior wall and it is important not to lever the retractors on the acetabular walls to avoid fracture. At this point, only 20% of the acetabulum may be visualized. A spike or tailor retractor is then placed superiorly. The psoas tendon is identified to avoid cutting it. The remaining medial capsule is then excised in an elliptical fashion. In the majority of cases, this will be sufficient to provide adequate exposure for acetabular reaming. In some cases, the femoral head deformity will not allow adequate exposure. In these cases a skim cut of the femoral head in line with the femoral neck may be utilized. It is important not to notch the femoral neck, as this may increase the chance of a femoral neck fracture. With adequate visualization, reaming of the acetabulum is initiated.

Currently there are no acetabular cups with screws available; therefore, concentric reaming is a must, and intra-operative radiographs should often be utilized to confirm that the cup has bottomed out. After the cup is properly inserted, all osteophytes should be removed either with an osteotome or a burr. This is yet another critical step in achieving a good outcome by maximizing range of motion and avoiding impingement. Often, young patients may have deformed femoral necks and will often impinge on the osteophytes. If osteophytes are not removed at this time, it becomes a formidable task after the femoral head is resurfaced.

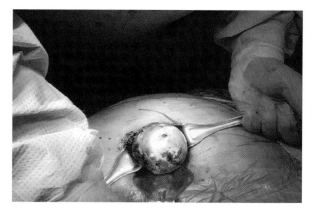

Fig. 7.117. Dislocated head with variety of retractors used to protect overlying skin

Femoral Resurfacing

The hip is now externally rotated into view, holding the leg in a figure-of-4 position. The skin may be protected with a variety of retractors (Fig. 7.117). We prefer to use a combination of smooth Bennett retractors and Richardson retractors to protect the tissue. A smooth 32-mm pin is aligned at an angle between 135–140° with the use of a goniometer. The pin is appropriately placed, using the "spin-around" guide to avoid neck impingement. After the pin is inserted, the epicondylar axis of the knee is placed horizontal to the floor and the angle is checked (Fig. 7.118). Next, the femoral head is reamed with a reamer 6 cm above the final size, determined by the size of the acetabular cup (Fig. 7.119). The "spin around" is used to confirm that the neck, including osteophytes, will not be notched. If the potential for notching exists, the pin is translated in the appropriate direction, making sure not to change the angle of the pin. If there is any doubt, one should re-check the angle with the goniometer. With the pin positioned appropriately, the final femoral head reaming is performed. Next, the "donut" is placed on the cut head and positioned to resect approximately 5–10 mm of proximal femoral head. The central hole is then drilled through the "donut tower" to the appropriate depth to provide for the short stem. Next, the chamfer cuts are made, with care not to torque the femoral neck. The chamfer reamer must be started with the reamer off the bone (Fig. 7.120). A trial head, which is not reduced, is placed to ensure that the central hole is large enough to allow the head to seat flush with the proximal femoral

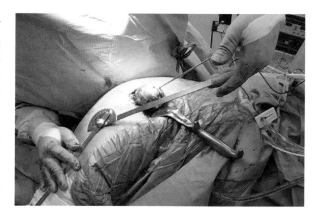

Fig. 7.118. Use of goniometer to confirm neck shaft angle

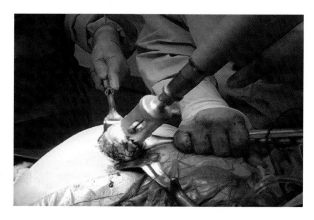

Fig. 7.119. Cylindrical reaming of femoral head

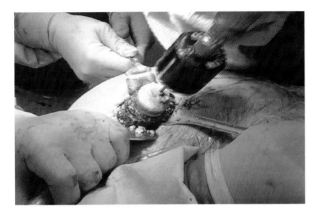

◘ **Fig. 7.120.** Chamfer preparation, with reamer started off bone

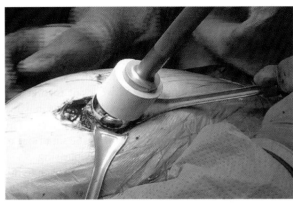

◘ **Fig. 7.122.** Impaction of femoral component

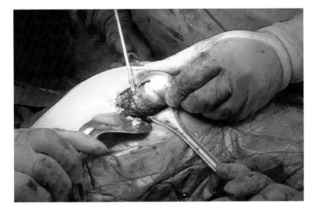

◘ **Fig. 7.121.** Trial femoral head placed, ensuring proper seating. The inferior edge of the trial is marked to ensure accurate placement

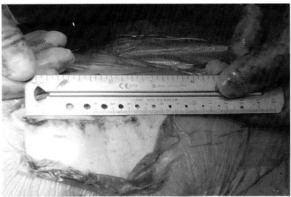

◘ **Fig. 7.123.** Closure of wound showing a 6-cm incision

head cut (◘ Fig. 7.121). If not, one can simply enlarge the central hole. The next step involves cementing the femoral head in place, and reducing after cure (◘ Fig. 7.122). The hip should be then taken through a range of motion. One should be assured that there is no neck impingement. These patients may have a large shuck, but this is usually of no clinical significance, secondary to the large femoral head. The rest of the closure is performed in a standard manner (◘ Fig. 7.123).

Post-Operative Care

The patient should be kept at 20–50% weight-bearing for 6 weeks, and then advanced to full weight-bearing from weeks 6–12. No restrictions are placed after 12 weeks.

Discussion

Many of the techniques using this approach have evolved from the standard approaches for an anterolateral approach to the hip. This procedure here has specifically focused on the anterolateral approach, but many of the concepts mentioned here can be applied to the posterior approach. Surgeons should start with a large incision first (over 10 cm long) and move down to a small incision. This should certainly be an evolutionary process, because the most important feature of doing these resurfacings is adequate exposure of the acetabulum while keeping the femoral head in place.

Patients with this minimally invasive approach have so far had superior short-term results when compared to patients with a standard, long-incision technique. The patients have reported less pain, have been able to use less narcotic analgesics, and are able to leave the hospital almost a full day earlier than patients with standard techniques. The authors are at the present time looking at various modalities, such as gait analyses, to see the true effects of this approach and we await further follow-up to see if these short-term apparent gains in using this approach will be beneficial in the long term. The patients themselves are very happy with the small size of their incision as it has been cosmetically pleasing.

In summary, this minimally invasive approach to hip resurfacing has a tremendous advantage over standard hip-arthroplasty approaches. It should be an evolutionary process that most surgeons, familiar with the techniques of resurfacing, should be able to learn. Further refinements of this approach will allow its general use for any surgeon.

References

1. Amstutz HC, Beaule PE, Dorey FJ, LeDuff MJ, Campbell PA, Gruen T. Metal-on-metal hybrid surface arthroplasty: Two to six-year follow-up study. J Bone Joint Surg Am 2004; 86: 28–39
2. Amstutz HC, Grigoris P, Dorey FJ. Evolution and future of surface replacement of the hip. J Orthop Sci 1998; 3: 169–186
3. Etienne GE, Ragland PS, Mont MA. Use of modular large femoral heads without liners in hip arthroplasty: A case report. Am J Orthop 2004 (submitted)
4. Mont MA, Bhave A, Etienne G, Ragland PS, Starr R, Erhart J. Gait analysis of resurfacing hip arthroplasty compared to hip osteoarthritis and standard total hip arthroplasty. Present at Hip Society 2003. Clin Orthop 2004 (submitted)
5. Mont MA, Etienne G, Schmalzried TP. Hip resurfacing arthroplasty: Past, present, and future. J Am Acad Orthop Surg 2004 (submitted)

The Standard Anterior Medial Parapatellar Approach to TKA

W. Frueh, P. Sharkey

Introduction

The standard surgical approach used in total knee arthroplasty (anterior medial parapatellar) was first described in 1945 by Abbott and Carpenter. It has since been modified to become the standard approach for total knee arthroplasty (TKA). Simple and extremely utilitarian, the standard approach offers excellent visualization, extensibility, and reproducibility. As is the origin of many surgical exposures in orthopedics, the anterior medial parapatellar approach was first utilized in treating infection, namely septic arthritis. The advent and success of TKA, however, brought its effectiveness to the forefront of adult reconstructive knee surgery.

The manner in which the approach is prepared for and carried out at our institution reflects our goals of patient safety, surgical precision and speed; maximizing surgical exposure while minimizing surgical time.

Positioning and Preparation

The patient is placed supine on the operating room table. If a Foley catheter is used (as is done at our institution after induction of spinal/epidural anesthesia), care is taken to route the catheter posterior to the non-operative leg in order to reduce the risk of catheter kinking and obstruction during surgery. A non-sterile tourniquet is placed as proximally as possible on the thigh to maximize area for surgical exposure if needed. The tourniquet is set at between 250 and 350 mmHg as is necessary given the patient's mean blood pressure and body habitus. A non-sterile clear plastic drape is placed just distal to the cuff to prevent betadine prep from saturating and soiling the tourniquet. The foot is wrapped in a non-sterile clear

drape to define the surgical field and area to be prepped. A foot-stop bump is attached to the table maintaining approximately 90–100° of knee flexion when the foot is resting on it. After standard prep and draping has been performed, landmarks are outlined on the skin. The superior, inferior, medial and lateral borders of the patella are marked, as well as the tibial tubercle. With the knee flexed to 90°, a 13–17 cm line is marked for incision centered over the femoral shaft, patella, and medial aspect of the tibial tubercle (◨ Fig. 8.1). A betadine impregnated

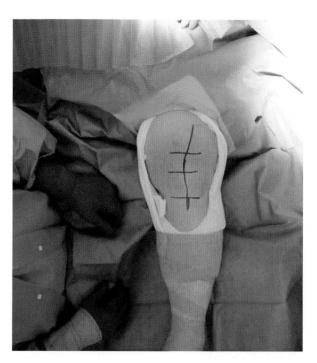

◨ **Fig. 8.1.** A 13–17 cm incision is marked out over the femoral shaft, patella and medial aspect of the tibial tubercle

plastic drape is then placed over all exposed skin. The leg is exsanguinated with the use of an esmarche, and the tourniquet is inflated.

Superficial Dissection

The skin incision is carried out using a scalpel through skin and subcutaneous tissues down to the level of the patellar retinaculum (◘ Fig. 8.2). Using bovie electrocautery and tissue forceps, meticulous hemostasis is maintained so as to prevent post-operative deep or superficial hematoma formation. The medial skin and subcutaneous tissues are dissected sharply away from the underlying fascia in order to expose the medial edge of the patella and its adjoining retinaculum. If the patient is obese, a lateral flap is created by subcutaneous dissection. This facilitates patellar eversion by creating a "pocket" under the skin where the patella can be stably placed.

Deep Dissection

A large Richardson-type retractor is placed proximally exposing the proximal edge of the quadriceps tendon (◘ Fig. 8.3). Taking care to maintain a 3 mm medial cuff of tendon, the medial parapatellar arthrotomy is carried out from proximal to distal, beginning with the quadriceps tendon (◘ Fig. 8.4). The arthrotomy is done with the entire depth of the scalpel blade, in line with the tendon fibers in order to prevent the creation of multiple tissue planes that would hamper good repair at closure. As the arthrotomy approaches the patella, it is curved sharply medially along its border, again taking care to maintain a 3 mm cuff of patellar retinaculum laterally for repair. The arthrotomy is continued distally along the medial edge of the patellar tendon and tibial tubercle (◘ Fig. 8.5). The knee is then extended, and the patella gently everted 180°, exposing the anterior aspect of the knee-joint surface. The knee is then returned to 90° of flexion with the patella everted, taking care to protect the patellar tendon insertion into the tibial tubercle (◘ Fig. 8.6). The surgeon resects the patellar fat pad using scalpel dissection, leaving a thin layer of adipose tissue on the undersurface of the tendon to minimize scarring and tendon contracture (◘ Fig. 8.7).

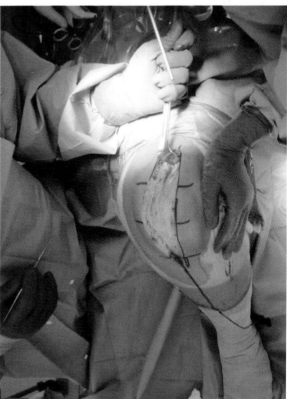

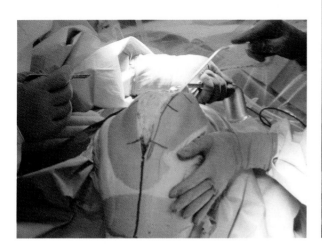

◘ **Fig. 8.2.** The skin incision is carried out with a scalpel down to the depth of the patellar retinaculum

◘ **Fig. 8.3.** A Richardson-type retractor is placed proximally to facilitate exposure of the quadriceps tendon

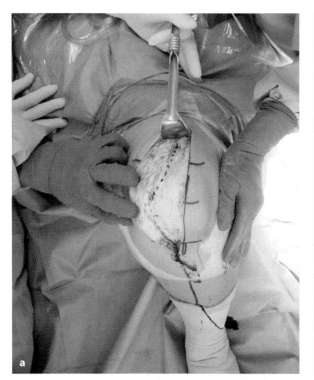 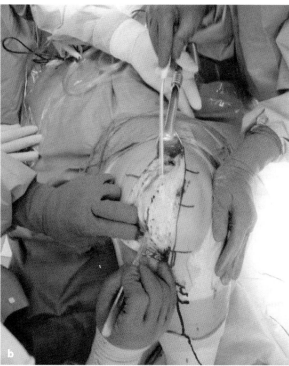

Fig. 8.4a,b. The medial arthrotomy is carried out from proximal to distal taking care to maintain a 3 mm cuff of tendon for later repair

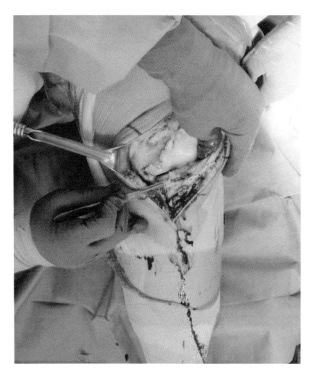

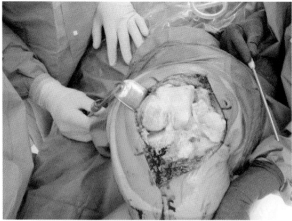

Fig. 8.6. The knee is flexed, patella everted laterally, and the knee returned to 90 degrees of flexion taking care to protect the patellar tendon insertion into the tibial tubercle

◄

Fig. 8.5. The arthrotomy is completed distally along the medial edge of the tibial tubercle

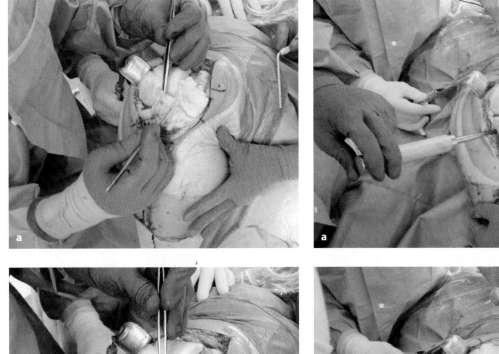

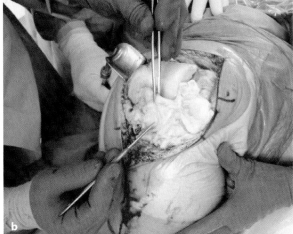

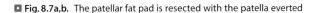

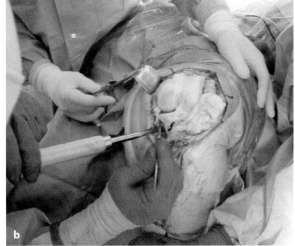

◘ Fig. 8.7a,b. The patellar fat pad is resected with the patella everted

◘ Fig. 8.8a,b. The medial release is performed with a scalpel, using a large Cobb elevator to protect the MCL

Medial Release, Cruciate Resection and Knee Dislocation

In order to allow surgical dislocation of the knee without the risk of tearing the medial collateral ligament, a medial release is performed. Using a Cobb periosteal elevator and scalpel, sub-periosteal dissection is performed. A medial release is carried out at a 45° angle to the shaft of the tibia to the level of the meniscal rim. A

Cobb elevator is then used to continue this dissection around the medial side of the tibial plateau, elevating and protecting the MCL (◘ Fig. 8.8). The release is carried posteriorly back to the insertion of semimembranosus and distally about 1–1.5 cm (the approximate width of a large Cobb periosteal elevator). Minimal medial release is performed if the patient has a preoperative valgus deformity. The anterior and posterior cruciate ligaments are then resected using a scalpel or

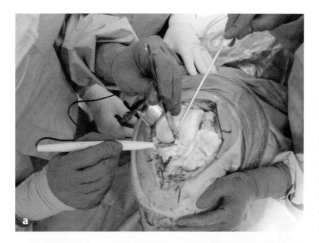

bovie (assuming a posterior stabilized knee system is to be used as is the case for all TKAs at our institution) (◘ Fig. 8.9). Using a large posterior reverse (Hohmann) retractor, the knee is gently dislocated anteriorly with applied external rotation to the tibia (◘ Fig. 8.10). The menisci are resected (medial first, then lateral) using a large Leahy and scalpel (◘ Fig. 8.11). The lateral patellofemoral ligament is incised with a scalpel or bovie (◘ Fig. 8.12). The superior lateral geniculate artery is cauterized after it is exposed during resection of the lateral meniscus (◘ Fig. 8.13). Any cruciate remnants are resected from the posterior tibia. Care is taken to completely expose the tibial plateau to help facilitate the tibial cut (◘ Fig. 8.14).

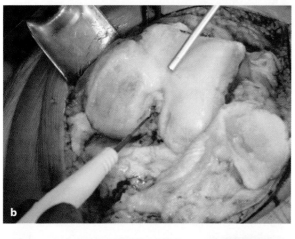

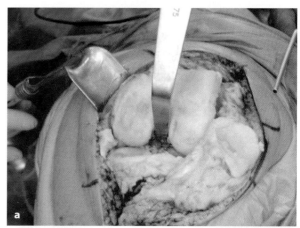

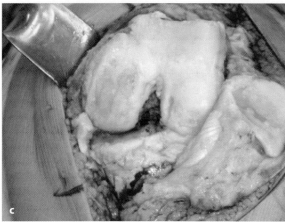

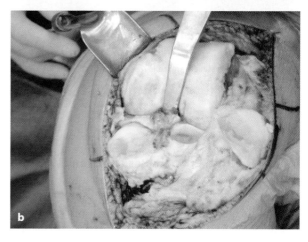

◘ **Fig. 8.9a–c.** The cruciate ligaments (ACL, then PCL) are resected using bovie electrocautery dissection

◘ **Fig. 8.10a,b.** Using a large reverse (Hohmann) retractor and anterior translation with external rotation, the knee is dislocated

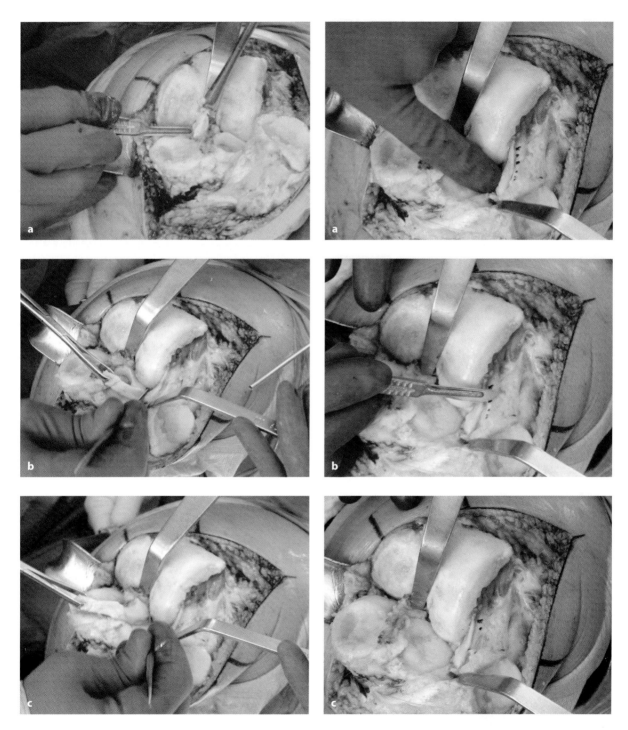

◨ **Fig. 8.11a–c.** The menisci are resected at the menisco-synovial junction (medial meniscus, then lateral) using a scalpel

◨ **Fig. 8.12a–c.** The lateral patellofemoral ligament is incised taking care to protect the underlying LCL

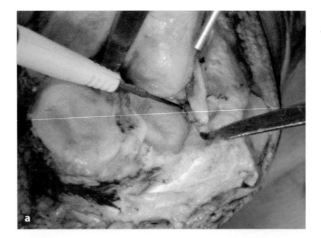

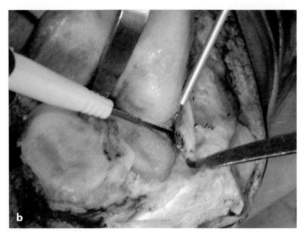

◩ **Fig. 8.13a,b.** The superior lateral geniculate artery is cauterized

References

1. Abbott LC, Carpenter WF: Surgical approaches to the knee joint. J Bone Joint Surg 27: 277, 1945
2. Guyton JL: Arthoplasty of the ankle and knee. In: Canale ST (ed) Campbell's Operative Orthopaedics (9th edn). Mosby, St. Louis, pp 232–295, 1998
3. Hoppenfeld S et al.: The knee. In: Hoppenfeld S, deBoer P (eds) Surgical exposures in orthopaedics: The Anatomic Approach (2nd edn). Lippincott-Raven. Philadelphia, pp. 429–482, 1994
4. Insall JN: A midline approach to the knee. J Bone Joint Surg Am 53: 1584–1586, 1971
5. Insall JN: Surgical techniques and instrumentation in total knee arthroplasty. In: Insall JN (ed): Surgery of the knee. Churchill-Livingstone, New York, 1993
6. Johnson DP et al.: Anterior midline or medial parapatellar incision for arthroplasty of the knee. J Bone Joint Surg Br 68: 812–814, 1986
7. Johnson DP: Midline or parapatellar incision for knee arthroplasty. J Bone Joint Surg Br 70: 656–658, 1988
8. Parker DA et al.: Surgical exposure for primary total knee arthroplasty. In Callaghan JJ (ed) The adult knee. Lippincott Williams & Wilkins, Philadelphia, pp. 1095–1109, 2003
9. Whiteside LA et al.: Exposure options in the difficult knee. Orthopedics 24(9): 895–896, 2001

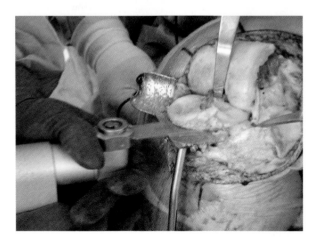

◩ **Fig. 8.14.** The entire tibial plateau is completely exposed prior to proceeding with the tibial bone cut

Minimally Invasive Approaches to the Knee

Minimally Invasive Total Knee Arthroplasty – Midvastus Approach

P.M. Bonutti

Introduction

Despite the intra-operative trauma inflicted to the knee joint, patients receiving traditional total knee arthroplasty (TKA) have demonstrated long-term success with regard to mobility and return to some activity – walking and stairs [2, 4, 8, 9, 14, 16, 17]. In addition to a large surgical incision of 8–12 inches, TKA also results in joint dislocation, patella eversion, quadriceps mechanism disturbance, tibiofemoral capsular dislocation, as well as extensive soft tissue disruption. Patient demand for a less invasive surgical approach reducing the trauma induced to the joint has resulted in the development of minimally invasive surgery (MIS).

Unfortunately, the clinical definition and criteria for MIS have not been firmly established. Various parameters can be used to define MIS, including length of incision, location of incisions, muscle-sparing approaches, reduced in-patient hospital stay, and rapid muscle recovery. However, the most definitive characteristics of MIS, which include reduced soft-tissue trauma and enhanced postoperative functional recovery, are often overlooked. Recent studies conducted with the MIS approach indicated that a VMO snip, a variation of the midvastus approach, may be the most universal MIS approach to TKA as it allows for adequate exposure of the joint cavity and improved postoperative recovery and pain relief [1–3, 13].

TKA performed through a reduced incision and with limited exposure is more difficult than the standard surgical approach to TKA. A successful MIS knee replacement requires that the surgeon possess a thorough comprehension and comfort level with the implants, instrumentation, and surgical techniques employed in this procedure. A graduated "evolutionary" approach, with regard to reducing the length of the incision, should be performed once the surgeon becomes comfortable with the MIS specific instrumentation. The objective of the paper is to provide an overview of various MIS TKA approaches and to describe the current approach utilized by the author with preliminary results.

Alternate MIS TKA Approaches

Several approaches have been described for MIS TKA. Vaughan et al. described the mini-TKA as a reduced incision with a standard median parapatellar approach with patellar eversion [19]. They performed this procedure in a group of selected patients with good pre-operative range of motion (ROM), and weight of less than 250 lbs. Post-surgical results observed in his patients identified a reduction in the number of post-surgical in-patient hospital days.

Tria performed a "quad sparing approach" (i.e. the subvastus approach) on a group of selected patients with good pre-operative ROM, low BMI, and minimal joint deformity [18]. Patients were discharged from the hospital at 2 days, however, they were required to spend an additional 5 days in an acute rehabilitation facility for in-patient therapy prior to final discharge.

Data collected from a study conducted by Scheibel et al., demonstrated that the subvastus approach in TKA increased a patient's risk of injury to musculoarticular branch of the femoral artery, and the saphenous nerve [15]. Scheibel et al. also found that further mobilization of the surrounding tissues increased the risk of damage to the femoral artery and vein in patients when the subvastus approach was used.

In contrast to these MIS TKA approaches, a VMO snip is an excellent alternative and may serve as a universal approach to MIS TKA. This new approach, which does not evert the patella, allows for adequate exposure of the joint and improved post-operative recovery and pain relief. Trauma to the quadriceps muscle is reduced as only VMO is split along its fibers during this procedure. MIS-specific instruments were utilized to facilitate joint-cavity exposure.

Five articles have been published on midvastus with everted patella [6, 7, 11, 20, 21], albeit not solely for MIS techniques. Results from studies conducted by Maestro, White, Dalury, and Engh indicated that patients who received the VMO split had less post-operative pain, a faster return of the quadriceps mechanism, improved ROM, and reduced rate of lateral release. However, Keating reported on data, which detected no significant differences between a modified median parapatellar and midvastus approaches in his TKA patients [10]. Keating did not violate the quad tendon with his modified parapatellar approach explaining the similarity of results [10]. Cooper found that VMO muscle can be split up to 8.8 cm safely [5].

The Bonutti MIS TKA Surgical Technique

The MIS TKA surgical procedure requires cooperation between the patient, anesthesiologist, surgeon, and surgical assistants. An experienced surgical team is recommended as the MIS procedure produces challenging conditions, such as reduced visualization and increased operating-room time, for the surgeon.

To begin, the patient should be positioned either supine or with a suspended leg technique [1]. The suspended leg technique is similar to arthroscopic procedures and may have several distinct advantages including posterior joint and ligament balancing. Appropriate anesthesia should be administered to the patient to ensure optimal muscle relaxations. A spinal epidural or epidural was utilized in almost all of our patients.

Once the patient is properly positioned, place the affected leg in flexion and demarcate the tibial tubercle and patella. An adjustable leg holder to vary flexion and extension is recommended. A skin incision should be made slightly medial to the patella (approximately 1–2 cm), and proximal to the tibial tubercle. The length of the incision may be extended during the procedure as needed ◘ (Fig. 9.1).

After an incision is made, the knee should be placed in 70–90° of flexion to allow full exposure of the VMO

fibers and capsule. A complete medial arthrotomy to the knee should be performed. A sharp VMO split of 1.5–2 cm is performed along the muscle fibers. Blunt dissection can split the VMO further – up to 8.8 cm safely [5] (◘ Fig. 9,2).

A Hohmann retractor should be placed underneath the patella with the leg in full extension. Inferior capsular releases should be performed to remove a portion of the fat pad and additional attachments to the anterolateral tibia. Following this release, a proximal capsular release, underneath the quadriceps mechanism, should be done to release a portion of the proximal capsule. This combination of proximal and distal releases should mobilize the patella and allow it to slide laterally over the lateral condyle to expose the anterior femur and tibia (◘ Fig. 9.3).

The knee should be placed into flexion again between 60° and 90° of flexion to avoid additional stress to the quadriceps mechanisms that result from everting the patella. Retracting the patella laterally should reduce the degree of stress to the entire quadriceps mechanism.

Tibial releases should be performed, followed by a tibial osteotomy using an extramedullary system and a downsized cutting jig (◘ Fig. 9.4). The tibia should be cut from anteromedial to posterolateral in situ, without dislocating the tibiofemoral joint. The proximal tibial cut should be removed in a piecemeal fashion to expose the PCL. At this point, the PCL should either be maintained or resected.

It is the author's preference to use anterior referencing instruments. However, posterior referencing guides

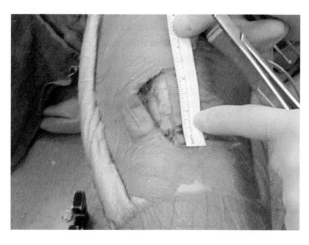

◘ **Fig. 9.1.** Initial surgical incision – 1 finger breath above tibial tubercle to superior pole of patella

could be used as well. The quadriceps is elevated to expose the anterior femur (◘ Fig. 9.5). Because the establishment of rotational alignment of the femur in MIS TKA can be difficult, the following guides are recommended to attain appropriate rotational alignment:

1. custom L-shaped guide (position on medial epicondyle and intercondylar notch – indirectly pointing to the lateral epicondyle);
2. intercondylar axis;
3. tibial cut at 90° flexion;
4. posterior condyles;
5. anterior femur.

These rotational landmarks can be utilized to set appropriate rotation once the correct cuts have been made. The rotational orientation can then be evaluated against the "Grand Piano Sign" to ensure that the anterior femoral resection removes more anterolateral than anteromedial and does not notch the femur.

After completing the anterior cut to establish the rotational plane the distal femoral cut is made with intramedullary reference guide. The distal femoral cut should be made in approximately 50–70° of flexion to allow the quadriceps muscles to relax (◘ Fig. 9.6) After sizing the medial condyle the femoral cuts are complet-

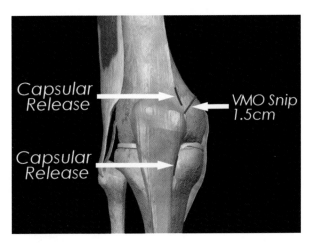

◘ **Fig. 9.2.** Initial surgical approach – VMO Snip with superior and inferior releases to mobilize the patella laterally

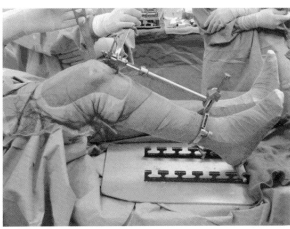

◘ **Fig. 9.4.** Lateral view of extramedullary tibial instrumentation and adjustable leg holder

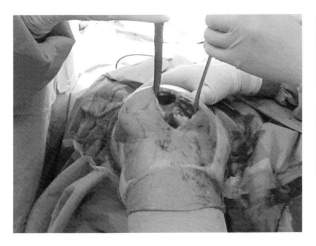

◘ **Fig. 9.3.** Initial exposure with patella retracted laterally

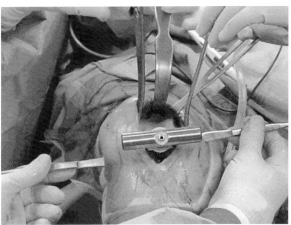

◘ **Fig. 9.5.** Exposure of femur with quadriceps mechanism elevated and intramedullary alignment. Landmarks for femoral rotation

9.1

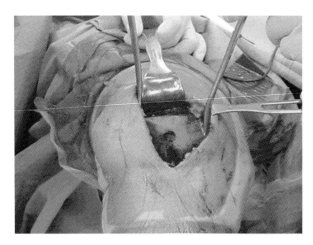

Fig. 9.6. Exposure of anterior femur after distal and anterior femoral cuts

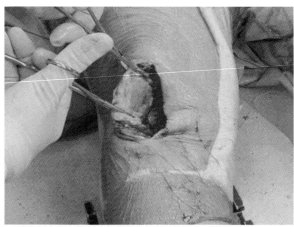

Fig. 9.8. Patella exposure and osteotomy in full extension

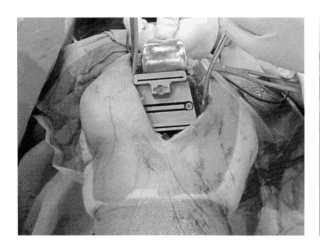

Fig. 9.7. Down-sized femoral 4-in-1 cutting block

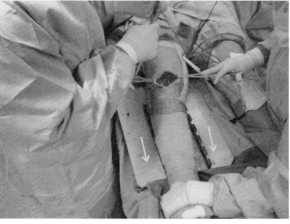

Fig. 9.9. Distraction of an extremity in full extension to expose anterolateral tibia and femur

ed with a downsized 4-in-1 cutting block (Fig. 9.7) The patellar osteotomy can be done earlier should the surgeon experience difficulty positioning the femoral cutting block. With our approach, the surgeon has the option of resurfaced or unresurfaced patella. The patella osteotomy is done in full extension without everting it (Fig. 9.8).

Evaluation of the bone cuts, osteophytes, and loose bodies should be performed, both visually and manually through finger manipulations, when placing the leg through a range of motion. Additional evaluations should be executed by distracting the leg in full exten-sion to allow better visualization and access to the lateral tibia and femur. Distracting the joint in full extension will allow not only the removal of laterally based osteophytes but also the surgeon to examine the lateral femur and tibia for complete tibial and femoral osteotomies (Fig. 9.9).

Before the prosthesis is implanted into the joint cavity, trialing and ligament balancing should be performed in flexion and extension. Implanting a cemented MIS TKA may be challenging. Appropriate cement techniques with direct anterior exposure, variable degrees of knee flexion allow enhanced visualization of

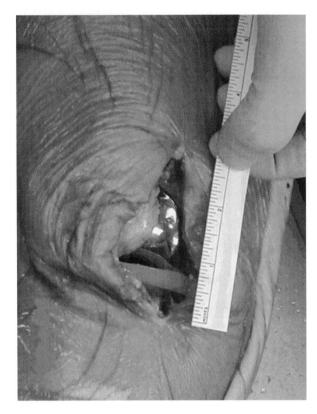

Fig. 9.10. Incision after all components cemented in position

ative day. Patients were discharged from the hospital, on average, in 3 days post-operatively with 95° of flexion, independent transferring, and the ability to climb stairs [2]. Functional recovery appeared to be significantly more rapid. Over 75% of patients were ambulating with the occasional use of a cane 2 weeks post-operatively and almost all patients with unilateral TKA were ambulating independently 4 weeks post-operatively. In addition, most patients were able to perform an unassisted chair rise test by 4 weeks post-operatively. Other studies have not demonstrated similar successful results, with only 64% of patients capable of rising from a chair unassisted at 3 months [12]. Higher demand functional activities such as kneeling, squatting and quadriceps strength are currently under evaluation. MIS TKA patients with a minimum 2-year follow-up also scored an average Knee Society Score of 96 [3]. Case reports with patients undergoing standard TKA on one knee and MIS TKA on the opposite knee show recovery 2 months faster on MIS group.

Pitfalls and Complications

Clearly, MIS TKA is a more challenging procedure than the standard TKA. There is an increase in operating-room time with a greater risk for complications. Complications may be reduced with early radiographic reviews performed by an objective independent reviewer. Some general surgical risks to avoid include:
— excessive traction to the skin with skin breakdown;
— quadriceps trauma (stretching against the quadriceps mechanism which can cause intrinsic damage to the muscle or shredding of the muscle);
— inappropriate bone/osteophyte/cement removal due to decreased visualization;
— femoral malrotation;
— injury to the patella due to excess retraction;
— difficult tibial keel implantation (risk of damaging the lateral femoral condyle);
— flexion of the femoral component; and
— inadequate cement pressurization and implantation.

the joint space and adequate cement pressurization, both in the tibia and femur. The tibial keel may also prove difficult to implant and caution should be exercised to avoid injuring the lateral femoral condyle. Impaction of the femoral component will require increased flexion and retraction of the patella laterally. Proper cement removal especially when excising lateral cement prior to implanting the patella is essential and deserves particular attention and detail. The "Scorpio" TKA is implanted (☐ Fig. 9.10, note incision size). ROM and stability are evaluated and the wound is closed in flexion, one stitch in the VMO.

Post-operatively, patients start rehabilitation in the recovery room with a CPM to 100° of flexion. Physical therapy is initiated two times a day, with weight-bearing as tolerated on the first day post-operation.

Our research demonstrated that straight leg raises occurred in majority of patients by the first post-operative day, and unassisted transfer by 48 h. Many patients were also ambulating with a cane by the third post-oper-

Re-operations in our first 500 MIS TKA included: 10 manipulations, 10 arthroscopies, and 8 open re-operations including 1 traumatic PCL, 2 infection/sepsis post colonoscopy, 1 patellar instability, 1 traumatic quad tear, 2 poly-exchange, 2 tibial component revisions. The number

■ **Fig. 9.11.** Immediate post-operative AP and lateral X-ray with arrows denoting staple line – incision length

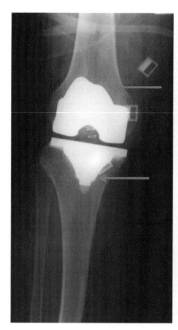
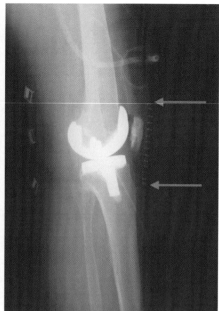

of re-operations performed since 1999 indicates that a strong learning component exists when mastering this technique and should be recognized by all surgeons operating with this procedure for the first time.

Conclusions

MIS TKA continues to evolve and be redefined. After 500 consecutive TKAs, the non-patellar everting, muscle splitting VMO snip with downsized soft-tissue instruments, and in situ bone cuts may be performed on all patients regardless of age, weight, and joint deformities. An evolutionary and cautionary approach of gradually downsizing the incision should be taken to reduce the risk of trauma to the knee joint and surrounding muscles. Moreover, careful attention to detail during surgery and analysis of post-operative techniques and X-rays is imperative to successful patient outcomes. A MIS TKA with as little as a 2-inch (5.5 cm) incision – 9.1 cm average – can be performed (■ Fig. 9.11).

The VMO muscle splitting technique appears to be universally accepted as a safe and effective approach to MIS TKA. Our progressive technique to TKA has been described at the (OCNA) Orthopedic Clinics of North America 2004 conference and presented with 2 year

▼

minimum follow-up [3] in addition to a Suspended Leg Technique Manual [1]. The suspended leg technique is similar to arthroscopic procedures and may have several distinct advantages including posterior joint and ligament balancing. Study results of up to 4-year follow-ups, suggest the MIS TKA technique merits further evaluation to confirm that the midvastus approach (VMO snip – non everted patella, in situ cuts, and downsized instruments) is a universal technique for MIS [3].

References

1. Bonutti P, Neal D, Kester M (2003) Minimal incision total knee arthroplasty using the suspended leg technique. Orthopedics 26: 899–903
2. Bonutti P, Mont M, Kester M (2004) Minimally invasive total knee arthroplasty: a 10-feature evolutionary approach. Orthop Clin North Am 35(2): 217–226
3. Bonutti P, Mont M (2004) Minimum 2 year follow-up of MIS TKA. Podium Presentation AAOS 2004. San Francisco, CA
4. Buechel F (2002) Long-term follow-up after mobile-bearing total knee replacement. Clin Orthop 404: 40–50
5. Cooper RE, Trinidad G, Buck WR (1999) Midvastus approach in total knee arthroplasty: a description and cadaveric study determining the distance of the popliteal artery from the patellar margin of the incision. J Arthroplasty 14(4): 505–508

9.1

6. Dalury DF, Jiranek WA (1999) A comparison of the midvastus and paramedian approaches for total knee arthroplasty. J Arthroplasty 14(1): 33–37

7. Engh GA, Parks NL (1998) Surgical technique of the midvastus arthrotomy. Clinical Orthopedics 351: 270–274

8. Font-Rodriguez DE, Scuderi GR, Insall JN (1997) Survivorship of cemented total knee arthroplasty. Clin Orthop 345: 79–86

9. Hanssen A, Rand J (1988) A comparison of primary and revision total knee arthroplasty using the kinematic stabilizer prosthesis. J Bone Joint Surg Am 70: 491

10. Keating E.M. et al (1999) Comparison of the midvastus muscle-splitting approach with the median parapatellar approach in total knee arthroplasty. J Arthroplasty 14(1): 29–32

11. Maestro et al. (2000) The midvastus surgical approach in total knee arthroplasty. Int. Orthopedics, pages 104–7.

12. Mahoney OM, McClung CD, dela Rosa MA, Schmalzried TP (2002) The effect of total knee arthroplasty design on extensor mechanism function. J Arthroplasty 17: 416–421

13. Mont MA, Stuchin SA, Bonutti PM et al. (2004) Different surgical options for monocompartmental osteonecrosis of the knee high tibial osteotomy versus unicompartmental knee arthroplasty versus t. Course Lectures 53: 265–283.

14. Rand JA, Ilstrup DM (1991) Survivorship analysis of total knee arthroplasty: Cumulative rates of survival of 9200 total knee arthroplasties. J Bone Joint Surg Am 73: 397–409

15. Scheibel MT et al. (2002) A detailed anatomical description of the subvastus region and its clinical relevance for the subvastus approach in total knee arthroplasty. Surg Radiol Anat 24: 6–12

16. Scott W, Rubinstein M, Scuderi G (1988) Results after knee replacement with a posterior cruciate-substituting prosthesis. J Bone Joint Surg Am 70: 1163

17. Stern S, Insall J (1992) Posterior stabilized prosthesis: Results after follow-up of nine to twelve years. J Bone Joint Surg Am 74: 980

18. Tria AJ Jr (2003) Advancements in minimally invasive total knee arthroplasty. Orthopedics 26: 859–863

19. Vaughan L (2003) Presented at the 17th Annual Vail Orthopaedic Symposium. Hospital Stays Shortened in Study of Minimally Invasive Total Knee Replacement. Zimmer Press Release

20. White et al. (1999) Clinical comparison of the midvastus and medial parapatellar surgical approaches. Clin Orthop 117–122

21. White RE Jr, Allman JK, Trauger JA, Dales BH (1999) Clinical comparison of the midvastus and medial parapatellar surgical approaches. Clin Orthop 367: 117–22

The Subvastus Approach in Total Knee Arthroplasty

O.M. Mahoney

Introduction

The concept of minimizing soft-tissue invasion during the surgical approach to the knee is not new. In fact, the subvastus muscle-sparing approach was originally described in 1929 by Erkes [6]. The proposed advantages of this approach were the reduction of post-operative pain and a more rapid recovery of motion. Over the next 40 years, there were few references to this technique in the American literature [1, 9]. Interest in the subvastus approach has been rekindled over the past decade as surgeons and patients have begun to focus their interests on improving the rate of recovery after knee arthroplasty. An internet search of the literature in 2004 (PubMed medline query) yielded 17 citations concerning the effect of the approach on total knee recovery published since 1991, and 11 of those have been written in the past 4 years.

Several short-term advantages of the muscle-sparing approach have been well documented in peer-reviewed journals. Studies have confirmed that the need for a lateral release is reduced using this technique. Bindeglass and Vince noted a lower release rate in a review of 83 cases using a posterior stabilized total knee [2]. This finding has been confirmed by two other retrospective studies [13, 15]. In an in vivo strain study, Ogata et al. demonstrated a reduction in post-implantation retinacular strain in subvastus cases, as well as a reduction in the lateral release rate [14]. In 1993, Faure et al. published a prospective randomized series confirming better patellar tracking with the extensor-sparing approach [7]. The study by Faure also revealed a more rapid recovery of strength in subvastus patients when compared to the conventional median parapatellar approach

patients. Several retrospective studies have also demonstrated improved muscle strength in cases where the muscle-sparing approach is used [3, 4]. In a more recent randomized prospective study Roysam and Oakley also reported a more rapid recovery of strength, significant reductions in blood loss and narcotic requirements, and improved range of motion with the subvastus approach [18, 19].

The muscle-sparing approach also offers the theoretic advantage of preserving blood flow to the patella by preserving the medial retinacular artery [12]. This preservation of patellar blood supply, even in the presence of a lateral release, along with the well-documented findings of reduced pain, more rapid recovery of strength, quicker recovery of motion, and improved patellar tracking make the subvastus approach an obvious choice for minimally invasive knee replacement.

Anatomy

The subvastus region provides a muscle-sparing or minimally invasive plane for exposure of the knee joint between the posterior border of the vastus muscle and the intermuscular septum. The space is bounded anteriorly by the vastus medialis and laterally by the femur. The posterior boundary is made up of the intermuscular septum and the adductor magnus. As a route to the knee joint, the space extends proximally as far as the adductor hiatus. The contents of the space are the descending genicular artery and the saphenous nerve. The mobilization of the vastus muscle is limited proximally by the passage of the femoral artery and vein through the adductor hiatus to the posterior aspect of the thigh [20].

Technique

The knee is flexed and an anterior midline skin incision is made. A medial incision is not recommended because the majority of the blood flow to the skin passes from medial to lateral and so with a medial incision the length of the undermined lateral flap may be quite large and increase the risk of a skin slough. A standard midline incision is preferred in order to preserve as much blood flow to the lateral flap as possible. This is particularly important in valgus knees where a more extensive lateral exposure is needed to facilitate the required releases, needed to balance the knee. The length of the skin incision can be varied according to the preferences of the surgeon. However, if the patella is to be dislocated, the incision should go from the medial edge of the tibial tubercle to a point at least two patellar lengths above the superior pole of the patella. It is critically important that the skin incision be carried down through the deep facia in order to preserve the anastomotic vessels which lie on the deep side of the facia and supply the superficial skin vessels.

After the facia is incised, it is usually quite easy to elevate the deep facial layer from the extensor mechanism by simply sliding a finger into the interval between the facia and the vastus muscle and bluntly separating the two. The facia may be intimately attached to the underlying distal vastus medialis obliquous (VMO) and require a small amount of sharp release. The size of the flaps varies depending on the pre-operative deformity of the knee. In the more common varus knee the medial side of the extensor mechanism is exposed along with an area of lateral retinaculum about half as wide as the patella to allow eversion for easier bone preparation. In the valgus knee, the lateral flap is undermined out to the inferior border of the illiotibial band. This allows the surgeon to gain adequate exposure for selective soft-tissue releases to correct tight lateral soft tissues.

The arthrotomy is begun by bluntly elevating the inferior border of the muscle off of the intramuscular septum. The index finger of the more cefelad hand is placed under the lower edge of the vastus muscle a few centimeters proximal to the joint line (Fig. 9.12). The surgeon then can use his free hand to push the dissecting finger proximally, sliding the vastus off of the intermuscular septum. The muscle should be elevated for 6–10 cm proximally to obtain adequate freedom to dislocate the patella if so desired. This is accomplished by pushing the dissecting hand as far proximal as possible. After elevating the muscle, the retinacular exposure is begun.

The capsulotomy is begun at the tibial tubercle about 2 mm into the patellar tendon cutting a gently curved incision running proximally and staying 1 cm or more medial to the patella to avoid the circumflex anastomotic vessels. The distal incision is beveled slightly medially so that the infra-patellar fat pad is left with the tendon. This capsular incision is carried up through the medial patella-femoral ligament taking care not to penetrate deeply which could result in a laceration of the medial collateral ligament. Proper depth of the incision can be easily judged by placing tension on the elevated vastus muscle (Fig. 9.13). It

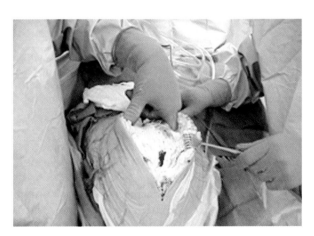

 Fig. 9.12. The surgeon slides the index finger between the lower edge of the vastus and then bluntly strips the muscle off of the intermuscular septum

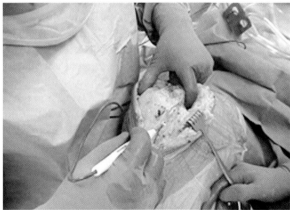

 Fig. 9.13. The capsulotomy is carried proximally past the medial patella-femoral retinaculum as seen here. The incision is a centimeter medial of the patella avoiding the anastomotic ring feeding the bone

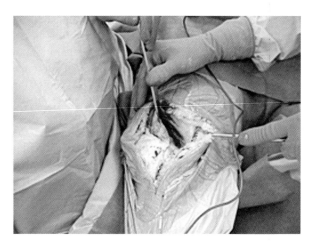

Fig. 9.14. The Hohmann retractor is used like a periosteal elevator to aide in the release of the supra patellar pouch from the surface of the femur

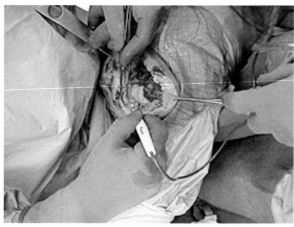

Fig. 9.15. Both the supra patellar pouch and the infra patellar fat pad are released from their respective bony attachments to the femur and the tibia as seen here

is not necessary to enter the synovium at this time. When the capsular incision has extended proximally enough, the patella will slide laterally as part of a continuous extensor sleeve.

The knee is now extended and the arthrotomy is completed. A Hohmann retractor is placed onto the anteromedial surface of the femur about 2 or 3 cm above the proximal articular margin. The Hohmann is advanced laterally under the suprapatellar pouch like a periosteal elevator allowing the pouch to be released from the femur (Fig. 9.14). The release of the intact pouch is completed sharply with electrocautery from the articular margin. It is also necessary to release the attachment of the infrapatellar fat pad from the anterior surface of the tibia to facilitate the elevation of the pouch so that the extensor sleeve becomes more freely mobile (Fig. 9.15).

After the extensor sleeve has been adequately released, the patellar tendon is reinforced with a tibial tubercle pin as described by Engh [5]. A 0.062 mm pin is placed into the medial edge of the patellar tendon at the level of its insertion (Fig. 9.16). The pin is directed laterally so that it will not interfere with an intramedullary guide or the stem of a tibial component. After the pin has been advanced approximately 2 cm into the tibia, it is cut at 3–4 cm proud, then bent 90° twice so that the cut end can be buried in the soft tissue to reduce the risk of injury to the surgical team. The knee can now be flexed with a very slight risk of extensor injury. The patella is easily everted and the remaining lateral attach-

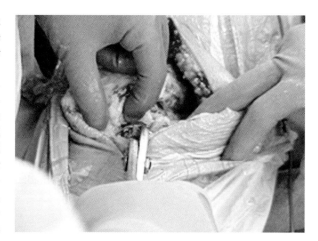

Fig. 9.16. The tibial tubercle pin is inserted into the medial border of the patellar tendon at the level of its attachment and angled laterally to avoid blocking access to the tibial canal. After the pin is cut, it is easily bent twice with a pair of pliers to bury the sharp end in the soft tissue

ment of the fat pad can be elevated from the anterolateral surface of the tibia to allow for easy placement of cutting jigs (Fig. 9.17).

Closure is begun by reattachment of the suprapatellar pouch to the anterior surface of the femur. This is accomplished with a single absorbable suture placed between the medial border of the pouch and the periosteum of the medial femur. The capsule is then closed with interrupted absorbable sutures under no tension.

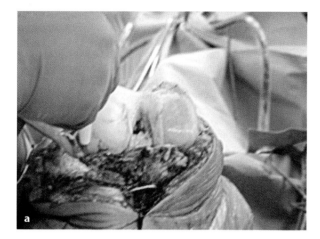

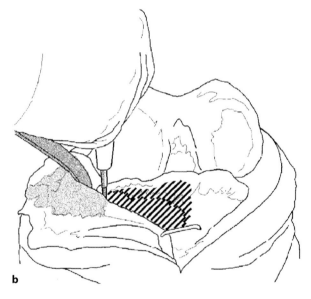

Fig. 9.17. **a** The entire anterior aspect of the tibia is easily visualized for placement of tibial cutting jigs. **b** The shaded area represents the fat pad release zone

Technical Tips

The most common problems encountered when attempting this approach are the result of inadequate soft-tissue releases. Many authors talk about the upper limit of vastus elevation being 10 cm above the knee at the adductor hiatus. Although the hiatus is the safe upper limit of dissection, its location varies and in many patients the muscle can be safely released much further

proximally. The release has been safely accomplished by the author in over 3000 cases by simply pushing the dissecting finger as far proximally as possible without entering the hiatus or damaging the femoral artery.

The suprapatellar pouch must also be fully released from the anterior surface of the femur. The lateral attachment of the pouch extends beyond the anterior lateral femoral flange and must be released subperiosteally. The second tether commonly overlooked is the lateral attachment of the infrapatellar fat pad to the tibia. This attachment extends around the front corner of the lateral tibia and must also be completely released subperiosteally to freely mobilize the extensor mechanism. In some cases with a very large quadriceps muscle or patella baja, eversion may be difficult and may result in a longitudinal fracture of the patella. In these cases where eversion seems difficult with the knee extended, the lateral patellar retinaculum can be subperiosteally elevated off the surface of the lateral third of the patella to facilitate eversion. If this problem is encountered in a case with a tight lateral retinaculum, a lateral release may make eversion easier. In cases of an extremely difficult exposure, the approach can be extended utilizing a tibial tubercle osteotomy.

Results

From 1989 to 2004 the subvastus approach has been used in every primary total knee replacement performed by the author (>3100), and in over 90% of knee revisions. In contrast to the recommendations of Hoffman [11], our indications for the muscle-sparing or subvastus approach are identical to those for the median parapatellar approach.

Over 50% of the primary patients undergoing knee replacements using the subvastus approach are able to straight leg raise by the morning after surgery. Eighty percent of inpatients have required parenteral narcotics for less than 48 h after surgery. The average hospital stay has been 3.2 days since 1991. In an electromyographic evaluation we have noted a return to normal levels of muscle activation by one month after surgery [16].

The rate of complications associated with this surgical approach has been few. Early on the author experienced difficulty, obtaining an adequate exposure in two cases which required a tibial tubercle osteotomy. In both cases the course of treatment and the outcomes were otherwise unaffected. There have been no patellar tracking problems, and only one case of patellar loosening. One patient underwent patellectomy approximately 3 years after the index procedure due to stress fracture. There have been no other patellar fractures in the absence of significant trauma. Mild skin sloughs have occurred in 12 patients, three of whom required subsequent irrigation and debridement followed by delayed primary closure. The rest healed secondarily.

The occurrence of heterotopic ossification has been lower than the 5% to 26% reported in the literature for the median parapatellar approach in total knee arthroplasty [8, 10, 17]. During 1998 we performed a series of 150 cases in which we did not reattach the suprapatellar pouch to the anterior femur and 9% of those patients developed small areas of heterotopic bone around the distal femurs. None of these was felt to be clinically significant, but this finding did prompt us to resume repairing the attachment of the pouch which returned our rate of asymptomatic heterotopic ossification to less than 5%.

There have been four cases of patellar tendon rupture or avulsion in this primary series within 3 months of the index procedure. In each case the patients had some contributing problem such as renal failure, lupus, or morbid obesity. Prior to our use of the tibial tubercle pin in 2001, there were intra-operative partial patellar tendon avulsions in almost 20% of cases. These avulsions comprised less than one third of the total tendon in all cases, and appeared to have no clinical manifestations or consequence. With the use of the tibial tubercle pin this occurrence has been reduced to less than 1% in this series.

References

1. Abbott LC, Carpenter WF (1945) Surgical approaches to the knee joint. J Bone Joint Surg 27(2): 277–310
2. Bindelgias DF, Vince KG (1996) Patellar tilt and subluxation following subvastus and parapatellar approach in total knee arthroplasty: implication for surgical technique. J Arthroplasty 11 (8): 507–511
3. Chang CH, Chen KH, Yang RS, Liu TK (2002) Muscle torques in total knee arthroplasty with subvastus and parapatellar approaches. Clin Orthop 398: 189–195
4. Cila E, Guszel V, Ozalay M, Tan J, Simsek S (2002) Subvastus versus medial parapatellar approach in total knee arthroplasty. Arch Orthop Trauma Surg 122: 65–68
5. Engh GA (2001) Complications after total knee arthroplasty: Prevention and management. AAOS, San Francisco
6. Erkes F (1929) Weitere Erfahrungen mit physiologischer Schnittführung zur Eröffnung des Kniegelenks. Bruns Beitr Klin Chir 147: 221–232
7. Faure BT, Benjamin JB, Lindsey B, Volz RG, Shutte D (1993) Comparison of the subvastus and paramedian surgical approaches in bilateral knee arthroplasty. J Athroplasty 8(5): 511–516
8. Furia JP, Pelligrini VD (1995) Heterotopic ossification following primary total knee arthroplasty. J Arthroplasty 10(4): 413–419
9. Gustke K, Smigielski M (1989) The southern approach to the knee. Journal of the Florida Orthopedic Society, Summer 1989
10. Hasegawa M, Ohashi T, Uchida A (2002) Heterotopic ossification around distal femur after total knee arthroplasty. Arch Orthop Trauma Surg 122(5): 274–278
11. Hoffman AA, Plaster RL, Murdock LE (1991) Subvastus (Southern) approach for primary total knee arthroplasty. Clin Orthop 269: 70–77
12. Kayler DE, Lyttle MB (1988) Surgical interruption of patella blood supply by total knee arthroplasty. Clin Orthop 229: 221
13. Matsueda M, Gustilo RB (2000) Subvastus and medial parapatellar approaches in total knee arthroplasty. Clin Orthop 371: 161–168
14. Ogata K, Ishinishi T, Hara M (1997) Evaluation of patellar retinacular tension during total knee arthroplasty: special emphasis on lateral retinacular release. J Arthroplasty 12(6): 651–656
15. Peters PC, Kenezevich S, Engh GA, Preidis FE, Dwyer KA (1992) Comparison of subvastus quadriceps-sparing and standard quadriceps-splitting approaches in total and unicompartmental knee arthroplasty. Orthop Trans 16: 146
16. Petrella JK, Cress ME, Bickel CS, Ferrara MS, Mahoney OM, Dudley GA (2004) Knee joint pain, quadriceps femori, and physical function 3 months after total knee arthroplasty. In press
17. Rader CD, Barthel T, Haase M, Setzeider M, Eulert J (1997) Heterotopic ossification after total knee arthroplasty. Acta Orthop Scand 68(1): 46–50
18. Roysam GS, Oakley MJ (2002) The subvastus approach for total knee arthroplasty resulted in better short term outcomes. JBJS 84A(2): 325
19. Roysam GS, Oakley MJ (2001) Subvastus approach for total knee arthroplasty. J Arthroplasty 16(4): 454–457
20. Scheibel MT, Schmidt W, Thomas M, von Sulis Soglin G (2002) A detailed anatomical description of the subvastus region and its clinical relevance for the subvastus approach in total knee arthroplasty. Surg Radiol Anat 24: 6–12
21. Whiteside LA, Ohl MD (1990) Tibial tubercle osteotomy for exposure of the difficult total knee arthroplasty. Clin Orthop 260: 6–9

Lateral Approach to Total Knee Arthroplasty: Minimal Soft Tissue Invasion

M.A. Mont, P.M. Bonutti, S.K. Chauhan, S. Axelson, A. Canonaco, P. Krijger,
M. Nemec, J.W. Raistrick, G. Walsh, E. Rugo, P. Treacy, T. Hoeman

Introduction

Utilizing standard approaches to total knee replacements have led to excellent short-term and long-term results with survival rates over 95% at 10 years and greater in multiple studies [2, 5, 6, 8, 12, 14, 16]. However, in the short term, these procedures lead to tremendous amount of morbidity with rehabilitative efforts that may take 3 months or more. There is a tremendous amount of pain associated with this procedure and patients will often need 1–2 h of physical therapy per day for the first 6 weeks after these procedures to lead to optimal results. In addition, some patients will need further operative procedures, i.e. manipulations, to obtain optimal results. Furthermore, the functional outcomes of patients with these procedures may not be as optimal as what has been reported in the literature. In a number of papers looking at patient-related outcomes, it appears that between 20 and 40% of patients are not completely satisfied with their total knee replacement [3, 4, 18]. The total knee replacement limits various functional activities. Multiple studies have described a discrepancy between how the surgeons perceive total knee replacement outcomes and how patients believe they have done. In a study by Dickstein et al. [4], one-third of respondents felt dissatisfaction with their operation, evaluated at 6 and 12 months post-operatively. This concept was iterated in an article by Bullens et al. [4], who concluded "it appears that surgeons are more satisfied than patients after total knee arthroplasty". In another study of the functional limits of total knee arthroplasty of patients that high Knee Society objective scores (greater than 90 points) at one year, only 35% of these patients had no limitations with activity [11]. It was worse for patients under 60 years of age where only 13% believed

they had no activity limitations [11]. Thus, the total knee replacement may be an even less viable option for young patients, despite excellent objective Knee Society scores.

The authors believe that the reasons for these less than optimal results are multifold, but may have to do with the operative surgical approach in performing total knee replacements. The procedures are often performed with large incisions (16–30 cm) and are not muscle-sparing. The quadriceps is cut into and this may lead to permanent muscle damage. This is a concern as some studies show persistent negative EMG changes even a year after the procedure. Other features that may lead to this long rehabilitative process and permanent knee damage include the dislocation of the knee joint which invariably affects posterior capsular structures. It is with all of these factors in mind that this present lateral approach for performing a total knee replacement was conceived as a minimally invasive method of performing a knee replacement with an attempt to minimize soft-tissue damage when performing knee replacements.

The features of the lateral approach that have been developed to date and successfully used in patients include the following:

1. Small-incision approach: The incisions have been done with incisions less than 10 cm. However, it is certainly possible to do this approach through a larger incision and this may make it easier to perform as the authors are not sure what the specific effect of incision size, if any, there is on outcome. This may be only a cosmetic effect that patients prefer.

2. The procedure is muscle-sparing. This approach goes through the iliotibial band only and does not necessitate any invasion of the quadriceps muscle

whatsoever. As opposed to other approaches where there are at best small amounts of muscle that are split, this is not needed in the lateral approach.

3. The patella is not everted in this procedure. Patellar preparation just involves cutting the patella *in situ* on top of the femoral trial component or minimal subluxation of the patella to make the cuts and preparation. It is believed that the full eversion of the patella may cause much of the damage found in standard total knee replacements.

4. The knee joint is not dislocated or subluxed during the procedure. The lateral approach allows for the cuts to be made on the femur and the tibia as well as the patella *in situ*. The tibia does not have to be dislocated in front of the femur as for most total knee replacements. This is facilitated by the method and the order of the cuts as well as the small keel on the tibial component.

5. Another feature of this procedure is that patients from the front do not see their incision as it is made from the lateral side. Although this is a cosmetic feature, it is certainly appreciated by patients. In addition, it is found that there is less of a nerve plexus on the lateral side of the skin than anteriorly and, therefore, patients have much less pain through their skin afferents. Related to this, is the fact that it is very painful in a standard knee to bend your knee from the front of an incision, which is necessary for rehabilitation. In this approach, the patient bends their knee in the front of the knee is not affected, but rather there is no problem when you bend your knee and the incision is placed on the side of your knee. This experience has been found from previous studies of patients who underwent peroneal nerve palsies where they were able to go home the same day without pain from the lateral side of their knee.

6. Use of navigation that avoids intramedullary instrumentation. Intramedullary rods can lead to embolic showering of the lungs. It may be extremely advantageous to avoid these rods.

In summary, all of these features the authors believe are important for the lateral approach and distinguish it from standard approaches to total knee replacements. These are certainly evolutionary and are further being refined, but the authors believe that these methods will change the way patients perceive the results of knee replacement. These methods should translate into not

only short-term advantages with less morbidity and rehabilitative efforts needed, but also may lead to better long-term functional outcome because of the muscle-sparing nature of this approach. This is a procedure that allows patients to be finished with rehabilitation fairly soon with minimal pain.

Surgical Technique

General Comments

The surgical technique utilizes a number of unique features including:

1. Down-sized and unique instrumentation: Cutting blocks have been down-sized 40% from traditional blocks. Certain blocks facilitate the ability to cut the knee from the side rather than the front of the knee.

2. Use of navigation: Cutting blocks have been designed for use with navigation to avoid intramedullary instrumentation.

3. The position of the leg allows for exposure of different parts of the knee. For example, flexion of the knee facilitates exposure of posterior structures and extension of the knee allows visualization of anterior structures. Retractors are used symbiotically to facilitate exposure of the medial or lateral part of the knee.

4. Bone platforms can be used to take out bone in a piece-meal manner when necessary.

Specific Details

The patient is first placed supine on a standard operating table. A tourniquet is applied with standard skin preparation and draping undertaken. It is important to keep the medial and lateral malleoli free, as well as the medial side of the knee free, so that appropriate navigational mapping can be undertaken. The tibia rest can be placed against the distal lateral thigh to allow for opening of the medial part of the joint.

The initial surgical exposure involves marking the patient's patella, patellar tendon, lateral tibial plateau, Gerdy's tubercle, fibular head, and distal femur. This allows for a 8–10 cm incision made from slightly below Gerdy's tubercle to the lateral epicondyle lateral to the patella (◘ Fig. 9.18). The skin and underlying subcutaneous tissue is then incised revealing the iliotibial band. The surgeon can then easily expose the proximal tibia as well as the distal femur from the lateral side. Through the lateral arthrotomy wound, the fat pad is excised together with the anterior horn of the lateral meniscus. This releases the anterolateral knee capsule from the anterior surface of the tibia. Dissection is then continued by putting soft-tissue retractors underneath the patellar tendon and across to the medial side of the tibia, releasing any soft tissue that is necessary. The surgeon can then visualize the anteromedial surface of the tibia and the anterior horn of the medial meniscus which can be removed under direct vision. Attention can then be directed to the proximal soft tissue and again the selective use of retractors with the knee in extension allows visualization of the suprapatellar pouch. The fat and synovial tissue from the anterior surface of the distal femur can be removed, including any plical bands, to free the lateral as well as the medial gutter. At this point, it should be very easy to displace the patella medially.

At this point, the navigation steps are set up (◘ Fig. 9.19). A tracker is set up 10–12 cm proximal to the distal femur and angled approximately 45° placed from lateral to medial. Likewise, a similar retractor is placed at approximately 10 cm below the tibial joint line. Once the femoral and tibial anchors are made, navigation software is used to map the hip center as well as the various landmarks of the femur (both epicondyles, center of knee, AP axis [Whiteside's line]), as well as the tibial landmarks (condylar surfaces, tibial spine center, tibia) and the ankle is mapped concerning the center of the ankle and the medial and lateral malleoli.

The distal femoral resection is made by positioning the resection guide in relation to three axes of freedom: varus/valgus, flexion/extension, and distal resection depth. Once this has been done, the distal femoral cut is made (◘ Fig. 9.20). The tibial resection is made again with a similar guide baring the three axes of freedom and the proximal tibial cut is made (◘ Fig. 9.21). It is certainly possible to do only three-quarters of the cut initially to avoid risking cutting the medial collateral ligament.

Attention is then directed to the femur where a T-bar device is used to re-map the femoral rotation landmarks. At this point with the distal femur and proximal tibial cut, it is easy to use the epicondylar rotation guide

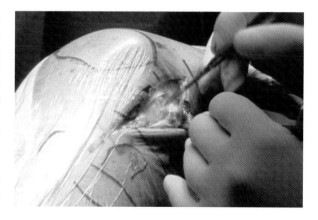

◘ **Fig. 9.18.** An incision is made from slightly below Gerdy's tubercle to the lateral epicondyle lateral to the patella

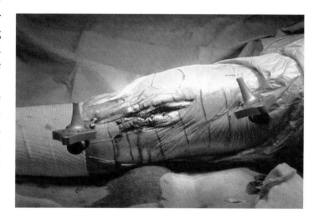

◘ **Fig. 9.19.** The two navigation trackers have been set up on the distal femur and the proximal tibia above and below the incision

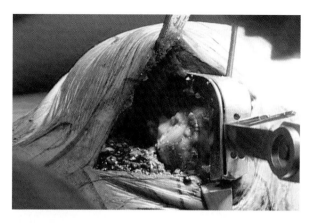

◘ **Fig. 9.20.** Distal femoral cut being made through a special femoral guide after appropriate axes of freedom (varus/valgus, flexion/extension, and distal resection depth) have been confirmed by navigation

which is based on the 90° relationship between Whiteside's AP axis and the surgical trans-epicondylar axis. The long arm of this alignment guide is placed along Whiteside's AP axis with the tip of the lateral arm aligned with the lateral epicondyle. These points are marked which allows for accurate assessment of rotation for the next step.

The final preparation of femur occurs first by using templates from radiographs and a femoral sizing guide. The anterior femur is then made with a special guide which is linked a navigation unit ensuring the appropriate rotation (◘ Fig. 9.22). Once this cut is made, the femoral four in one cut can be used to finish the appropriate cuts on the femur.

The surfaces can be checked to ensure appropriate alignment with the navigation devices and the femur as well as tibia is then trialed. Tibial rotation can be checked with the navigation unit and the appropriate sized tibia is checked, then a tibial punch guide can be made. Distal femoral holes can also be made and then the patella is cut without everting the patella (◘ Fig. 9.23). Trial components are then inserted with soft-tissue assessment made.

Simplex™ cement is used for component implantation. Typically in this approach, the tibia is implanted first. A separate step is made to ensure appropriate removal of any excess cement, especially medially. After this is performed, the femur and patella can then be cemented in place. The final tibial insertion is then made, with a final analysis of the kinematics of the knee from extension to deep flexion using the navigation tools.

The joint is then thoroughly irrigated. A single drain is used, typically put out through the medial side. The lateral arthrotomy site is closed with interrupted 1–0 vicryl sutures followed by 2–0 vicryl sutures for the subcutaneous tissue with the skin closed with 3–0 vicryl sutures or staples.

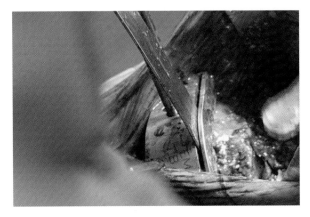

◘ **Fig. 9.21.** The tibial resection is being performed through a guide similar to the distal femoral guide

Results

The results on the initial cohort of patients being studied with an IRB prospective study have shown that patients have had minimal anterior knee pain and have

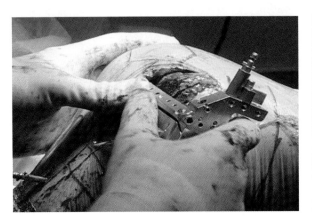

◘ **Fig. 9.22.** Special femoral guide to complete femoral cuts is being applied to distal femur

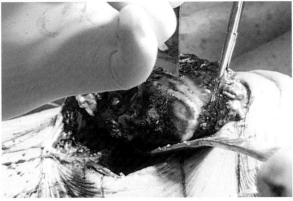

◘ **Fig. 9.23.** The patella is being cut while avoiding eversion of the quadriceps mechanism

been able to straight leg raise immediately after surgery. This is quite different from patients with standard knee replacement approaches that are being compared.

Discussion

Many of the techniques for this approach have evolved from a minimally invasive approach that was first developed by Peter Bonutti, who has performed over 400 knee replacements with a medial approach which involves a small amount of muscle-splitting with incisions typically less than 10 cm long [1, 9, 11, 17]. Dr. Bonutti's principles included the symbiotic use of retractors with appropriate flexion and extension of the leg without eversion of the patella and the piece-meal approach to removing bone when using the small incisions. Because of the excellent results that he obtained in over 400 knee replacements and the reproducibility that was obtained in a multi-center study using this approach, we felt that it was worthwhile to further expand some of these techniques and apply them to the lateral approach to the knee. Patients that have had this new lateral technique have so far had superior short-term results when compared to patients with standard total knee arthroplasty techniques. Patients have all been able to straight leg raise almost immediately post-operative or earlier than with standard total knee arthroplasty techniques. Patients have no pain in the anterior part of their knees. At the present time, the authors are looking at various modalities such as gait analyses to see the true effects of this approach and are eager to know if the short-term gains in using this approach will be also beneficial in the long term. Patients have been quite happy with the small size of their incision as well as the cosmetic nature of placing the incision laterally.

Some of this experience can be compared to the experience of unicompartmental knee arthroplasty [7, 13, 15]. This has recently been developed as a minimally invasive technique, popularized over the past few years. The advantages of unicompartmental knee replacements are that these are small incisions with minimal soft-tissue destruction and can be done with minimal muscle damage. The disadvantages are that they are very often hard to achieve alignment and the results may not be durable in the long term. The authors believe that the present lateral approach to full total knee replacement offers all of the advantages of a unicompartmental knee arthroplasty (small incision, minimal soft-tissue damage) and may not have the disadvantages of decreased longevity or lack of the ability to always reproduce alignment. Because of the limited nature of our present approach to knee arthroplasty, we would often prefer this possibly long-term durable approach than utilizing unicompartmental knee arthroplasty, which may be only a temporary procedure.

In summary, this lateral approach has tremendous advantages over standard total knee arthroplasty approaches. It is a small laterally based incision which may reduce immediately pain for post-operative patients. The approach does not involve any degree of muscle-splitting which has many advantages. In addition, the knee is not dislocated nor is the patella everted, which also should be advantageous. The use of navigation avoids the potential side effects of an IM rod. For all of these reasons, we think that this can be a tremendous approach that can be utilized for most patients undergoing a total knee arthroplasty. Further refinements will allow its general use for any surgeon.

References

1. Bonutti PM, Neal, DJ, Kester MA. Minimal incision total knee arthroplasty using the suspended leg technique. Orthopedics 2003; 26: 899–903
2. Buechel FF Sr. Long-term follow-up after mobile-bearing total knee replacement. Clin Orthop 2002; 404: 40–50
3. Bullens PH, van Loon CJ, de Waal Malefijt MC, Laan RF, Veth RP. Patient satisfaction after total knee arthroplasty: a comparison between subjective and objective outcome assessments. J Arthroplasty 2001; 16: 740–747
4. Dickstein R, Heffes Y, Shabtai EI, Markowitz E. Total knee arthroplasty in the elderly: patients' self-appraisal 6 and 12 months postoperatively. Gerontology 1998; 44: 204–210
5. Font-Rodriguez DE, Scuderi GR, Insall JN. Survivorship of cemented total knee arthroplasty. Clin Orthop 1997; 345: 79–86
6. Hanssen AD, Rand JA. A comparison of primary and revision total knee arthroplasty using the kinematic stabilizer prosthesis. J Bone Joint Surg Am 1988; 70: 491–499
7. Iorio R, Healy WL. Unicompartmental arthritis of the knee. J Bone Joint Surg Am 2003; 85: 1351–1364
8. Keating EM, Meding JB, Faris PM, Ritter MA. Long-term follow-up of nonmodular total knee replacements. Clin Orthop 2002; 404: 34–39
9. Kolisek F, Bonutti P, Hozack W, Purtill J, Sharkey P, Zelicof S. A prospective, randomized comparison of total knee arthroplasties performed by the MIS technique compared to standard technique. (unpublished data)

10. Mont MA, Ragland P. Functional results of patients with total knee replacements with excellent Knee Society Scores (unpublished data)

11. Mont MA, Stuchin SA, Paley D, Sharkey PF, Parvisi J, Tria AJ Jr, Bonutti PM, Etienne G. Different surgical options for monocompartmental osteoarthritis of the knee: high tibial osteotomy versus unicompartmental knee arthroplasty versus total knee arthroplasty: indications, techniques, results, and controversies. Instr Course Lect 2004; 53: 265–283

12. Rand JA, Ilstrup DM. Survivorship analysis of total knee arthroplasty: Cumulative rates of survival of 9200 total knee arthroplasties. J Bone Joint Surg Am 1991; 73: 397–409

13. Repicci JA. Mini-invasive knee unicompartmental arthroplasty: bone-sparing technique. Surg Technol Int 2003; 11: 280–284

14. Scott WN, Rubinstein M, Scuderi G. Results after knee replacement with a posterior cruciate-substituting prosthesis. J Bone Joint Surg Am 1988; 70: 1163–1173

15. Sculco TP. Orthopaedic crossfire – can we justify unicondylar arthroplasty as a temporizing procedure? In opposition. J Arthroplasty 2002; 17 [Suppl 1]: 56–58

16. Stern SH, Insall JN. Posterior stabilized prosthesis: Results after follow-up of nine to twelve years. J Bone Joint Surg Am 1992; 74: 980–986

17. Stryker-Howmedica-Osteonics Technical Monograph on MIS TKA

18. Trousdale RT, McGrory BJ, Berry DJ, Becker MW, Harmsen WS. Patients' concerns prior to undergoing total hip and total knee arthroplasty. Mayo Clin Proc 1999; 74: 978–982

9.3

Clinical Experiences with the Unicondylar Knee Arthroplasty

A.J. Tria, Jr.

Introduction

Unicondylar knee arthroplasty (UKA) was introduced in the early 1970s by Marmor [1]. There were many subsequent designs for the prostheses and many clinical studies were published in the late 1980s and the early 1990s [2–5]. Unfortunately, the results were not satisfactory, especially when they were compared to the results of total knee arthroplasty (TKA) [6–8]. In the early 1990s, Repicci developed the UKA as a minimally invasive surgery (MIS) [9]. Through his efforts, interest in the UKA increased, and the MIS technique became the common mode of surgery. The surgical approach was changed so that the UKA was no longer performed as a modified TKA. UKA does not include ligament releases, over-correction of the knee, or excessive flexion and extension gap tightness. With these modifications, UKA is now a well-accepted procedure for the properly chosen patient.

Preoperative Evaluation

The patient should be evaluated through a good history along with a thorough physical examination and proper X-ray studies. The patient's pain should be localized to the medial or lateral tibiofemoral compartment. The symptoms should be reproducible and there should be no patellofemoral pain. It is often helpful to compare the pain with walking on level surfaces and on stairs or inclines. If the patient notices a difference in the intensity of the pain or the location with stair climbing, the patellofemoral joint is probably involved and the UKA is contra-indicated.

The physical examination should confirm the same location of the pain with tenderness on the joint line and no tenderness elsewhere. The ligaments of the knee should be intact; however, anterior cruciate ligament insufficiency is not an absolute contra-indication to UKA as long as a fixed bearing implant is chosen. The knee should have no deformity greater than 10° of varus, 15° of valgus, or a 10° flexion contracture. Ideally, the varus or valgus deformity should correct to neutral for greater ease of performing the surgery and obtaining proper laxity in flexion and extension with the UKA implant. The range of motion should be at least 110°.

The X-ray evaluation should include a standing anteroposterior view (◘ Fig. 9.24) along with a lateral and patellofemoral view, such as a Merchant X-ray. It is ideal to have a full-length view of the limb from the hip to the ankle, but it is not mandatory. The standing X-ray is important for evaluation of the degree of medial or lateral narrowing along with any possible translocation of the tibial beneath the femur. Translocation indicates that there is some arthritic involvement of the opposite compartment and correlates with a thrust of the femur on the tibia through the stance phase of gait on the physical examination (◘ Fig. 9.25). Translocation is a relative contra-indication to UKA. The standing X-ray should be used to measure the anatomic alignment of the limb. If the varus exceeds 10° or the valgus exceeds 15°, the UKA is contra-indicated. Argenson emphasizes that the deformity should be correctable to neutral and performs stress X-rays pre-operatively [10]. Almost all X-rays of the knee will show some involvement of the opposite compartment and of the patellofemoral joint. Insall stated that only 6% of knees would satisfy the requirements for UKA and that may indeed be true [11]. The author will accept some moderate involvement (Ahlback 1 or 2) [12] of the two other compartments of the knee, especially in the older population (age >80 years). However,

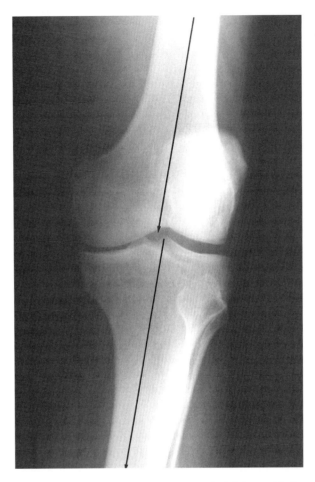

Fig. 9.24. Standing anteroposterior X-ray of a left knee with the anatomic axis of the femur and the tibia outlined

in the younger age group, it is best to adhere to strict criteria for the best results. The remaining compartments should have minimal arthritic changes.

Operative Technique

The author performs all of the UKA surgeries with an MIS technique. The medial approach uses an incision from the top of the patella to the tibial joint line (◘ Fig. 9.26). If there is any need to extend this incision, it is best to do so proximally. The capsule is opened in a parallel technique to the skin incision, avoiding the vastus medialis and the quadriceps tendon. The deep medial collateral ligament is released from the tibial joint line for the purposes of exposure only and not for correction of the existing varus. The medial joint is debrided and the intramedullary hole is made on the femoral side just above the roof of the intercondylar notch. The intramedullary guide is inserted and the distal cutting guide is attached (◘ Fig. 9.27). The standard cut removes 6 mm of bone which matches the thickness of the femoral implant. The angle of this cut is determined by the difference between the anatomic and biomechanical axis of the limb. For most clinical purposes, the varus knee requires a 4° angle and the valgus knee uses a 6° angle. The tibial cutting guide is extramedullary and aligns with the tibial tubercle and the prominence of the tibial shaft (◘ Fig. 9.28). The horizontal cut is made 2–3 mm below the lowest surface, perpendicular to the tibial shaft, and sloped from anterior to posterior to

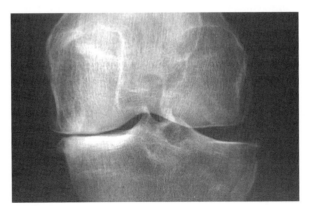

Fig. 9.25. Anteroposterior X-ray of the left knee with translocation of the lateral tibial spine touching the lateral femoral condyle

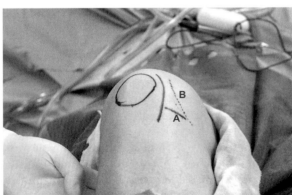

Fig. 9.26. The medial MIS incision for UKA replacement extends from the top of the patella to just below the tibial joint line (*A*). *B* is the outline of the femoral condyle

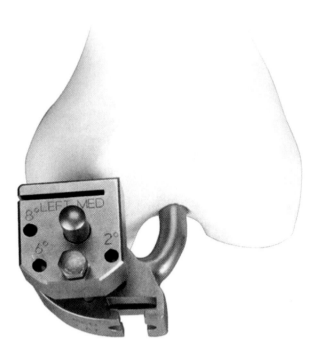

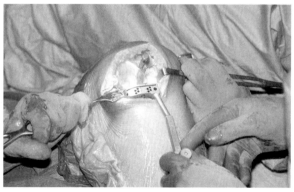

Fig. 9.28. The extramedullary tibial guide references the tibial tubercle and the ankle

Fig. 9.27. The intramedullary guide is in the femoral canal and the cutting guide for the distal femur is set at 4°. This will resect a total of 6 mm of bone, equal to the thickness of the femoral implant

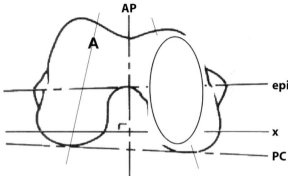

Fig. 9.29. The femoral runner should be placed to cover the distal cut surface of the femoral condyle but should be perpendicular to the tibial surface in 90° of flexion. On occasion, this may require that the femoral runner overlaps the intercondylar notch

match the pre-existing slope of the tibia that has been measured on the pre-operative lateral X-ray of the knee. Once the proximal tibial cut has been completed, the distal femur is easier to approach and the surface is sized for the correct cutting block. If the bone surface is between two sizes, it is always best to use the smaller size to avoid impingement on the patellofemoral surface. The femoral component should be set perpendicular to the tibial cut surface in full extension and in 90° of flexion. If the femoral condyles have an increased divergence angle, the component should not be placed anatomically on the cut surface because this will lead to edge loading of the femoral runner on the polyethylene. The runner should still be placed perpendicular to the tibial surface even if this leads to slight overhang into the femoral notch (Fig. 9.29). The final femoral cuts and peg holes are completed and, then, the tibial surface can be sized. External rotation of the knee at 90° of flexion brings the tibia forward and makes the exposure much easier. The tibial tray should cover the entire surface to rest on the remaining cortical rim for good support but should not

overhang, especially medially, where it can cause irritation of the medial collateral ligament and pain. Once all of the cuts are completed, a trial reduction should be performed. The knee should come to full extension and full flexion with 2 mm of laxity at full extension and 90° of flexion (Fig. 9.30). The pre-operative varus or valgus should be partially corrected but not fully. That is, if the pre-operative knee has 6° of varus it will commonly have about 2° of varus after the surgery. A 15° valgus knee should have about 10–12° of valgus after the operation.

During the course of the surgery, the extension and flexion gaps are compared similarly to TKA. The laxity in the two positions should be 2 mm. After all of the cuts have been completed in the UKA, it is easiest to correct on the tibial side. If the extension gap is too tight, the tibial cut can be deepened anteriorly and left the same pos-

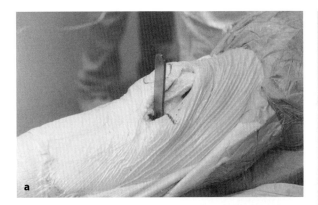

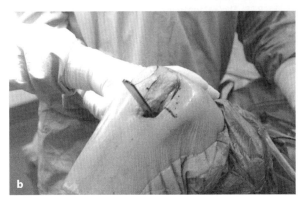

Fig. 9.30a,b. The UKA should have 2 mm of laxity, measured with this type of tongue depressor, in full extension (**a**) and in 90° of flexion (**b**)

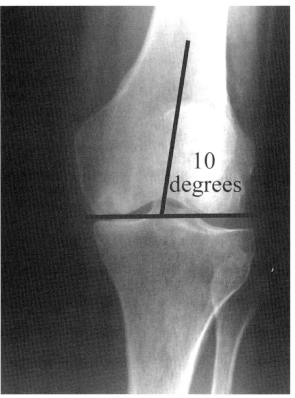

Fig. 9.32. The anatomic valgus of this distal femur is 10°. If the knee had a flexion contracture, an additional 2 mm of bone could be resected from the femur correcting the contracture and decreasing some of the excess distal femoral valgus

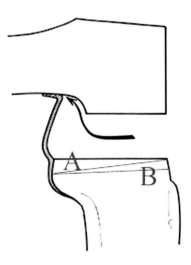

Fig. 9.31. Line *A* is the standard slope cut and line *B* is the cut slightly deeper at the anterior aspect with the same depth posteriorly. Line *B* will increase the extension space, correcting a flexion contracture, without affecting the flexion gap

teriorly by changing the slope of the original cut. This will give more room in extension and the same space in flexion. If the gap in flexion is too tight, the slope of the tibial cut can be increased to give more space in flexion and the same gap in extension (**Fig. 9.31**).

Flexion contractures of up to 10° can be corrected in the varus knee. The author measures the anatomic valgus of the distal femur on the pre-operative standing X-ray (**Fig. 9.32**). If the valgus is 6° or more, an additional 2 mm of bone can be resected from the distal femur. This corrects the flexion contract even though the cut is only made on one condyle and it reduces some of the excess femoral valgus. If the femoral valgus is 5° or less, the flexion contracture is corrected by making the tibial cut slightly deeper anteriorly with less slope posteriorly. In the valgus knee, modification of the cuts is not applicable, and the standard operative approach should be applied with a vertical, lateral MIS incision.

The capsule is closed with a drain in the knee joint. Proper tracking of the patella is confirmed after the closure.

Physical therapy is instituted a few hours after the surgery and the patients are discharged home the next day. Fondaparinux (Arixtra) [13, 14] is used for anticoagulation starting at 8 a.m. the day after surgery. The pentasaccharide is continued for 10 days and bilateral Doppler ultrasounds are performed before discontinuing the agent. Outpatient physical therapy is continued for about 6 weeks after the surgery.

Results

The author has performed more than 300 UKAs over the past 4 years. The first 63 knees are now 3 years after surgery. The average age of the entire group is 67 with 25% below the age of 60 and 25% above the age of 75. The medical complications for the entire group include one fatal pulmonary embolism (prompting us to move from aspirin to fondaparinux for anticoagulation) and one proximal femoral DVT (also on aspirin at the time). The orthopedic complications include: two tibial fractures that occurred after the surgery and did not displace or require re-operation, one femoral loosening secondary to sizing, one patellar subluxation leading to revision TKA, and two knees with persistent patellofemoral pain leading to revision TKA. There have been no manipulations or knees with decreased range of motion.

Approximately 2 years ago, the author switched anticoagulation from aspirin to fondaparinux. The TKAs are usually anticoagulated with a low-dose coumadin technique. It was difficult to anticoagulate the UKAs with coumadin because of the early discharge protocol with the MIS surgery. Initially, aspirin was the chosen agent. However, the early fatal pulmonary embolism caused us to re-evaluate our routine for DVT protection. 55 consecutive patients have been anticoagulated with fondaparinux over the past 20 months and all of the bilateral Doppler ultrasound studies performed at 10 days after the surgery have been negative for any clot at all. The TKAs anticoagulated with low-dose coumadin have a positive DVT incidence of 18% below the knee and 7% in the thigh.

The incidence of re-operation, thus far, is 1.3% (4 knees in 300). It is interesting that all four of the knees that required revision had symptoms within the first 12 months of the initial surgery. No knee has developed new symptoms of pain after the first year. It appears that a successful UKA that is 18 months to 2 years after surgery will last for many years to come.

References

1. Marmor L: The modular knee. Clin Orthop 94: 242–248, 1973
2. Insall JN, Aglietti P: A five to seven-year follow-up of unicondylar arthroplasty. J Bone Joint Surg (Am) 62: 1329–1337, 1980
3. Bernasek TL, Rand JA, Bryan RS: Unicompartmental porous coated anatomic total knee arthroplasty. Clin Orthop 236: 52–59, 1988
4. Magnussen PA, Barlett RJ: Cementless PCA unicompartmental joint arthroplasty for osteoarthritis of the knee: A prospective study of 51 cases. J Arthroplasty 5: 151–158, 1990
5. Scott RD, Cobb AG, McQueary FG, Thornhill TS: Unicompartmental knee arthroplasty. Eight- to 12-year follow-up evaluation with survivorship analysis. Clin Orthop 271: 96–100, 1991
6. Ranawat CS, Boachie-Adjei O: Survivorship analysis and results of total condylar knee arthroplasty. Eight to eleven year follow-up. Clin Orthop 226: 6–13, 1988
7. Rand JA, Ilstrup DM: Survivorship analysis of total knee arthroplasty. Cumulative rates of survival of 9,200 total knee arthroplasties. J Bone Joint Surg 73: 397–409, 1991
8. Stern SH, Insall JN: Posterior stabilized prosthesis: Results after 9–12 years follow-up. J Bone Joint Surg 74: 980–986, 1992
9. Repicci JA, Eberle RW: Minimally invasive surgical technique for unicondylar knee arthroplasty. J South Ortho Assoc 8: 20–27, 1999
10. Argenson JN, Chevrol-Benkeddache Y, Aubaniac JM: Modern unicondylar knee arthroplasty with cement: A three to ten year follow-up study. J Bone Joint Surg 84: 2235–2239, 2002
11. Stern SH, Becker MW, Insall JN: Unicondylar knee arthroplasty: An evaluation of selection criteria. Clin Orthop 286: 143–148, 1993
12. Ahlback S: Osteoarthrosis of the knee. A radiographic investigation. Acta Radiol Diagn 277 [Suppl]: 7–72, 1968
13. Eriksson BL, Bauer KA, Lassen MR, Turpie AG: Fondaparinux compared with enoxaparin for the prevention of venous thromboembolism after hip-fracture surgery. N Engl J Med 345(18): 1298–1304, 2001
14. Bauer KA, Eriksson BL, Lassen MR, Turpie AG. Fondaparinux compared with enoxaparin for the prevention of venous thromboembolism after elective major knee surgery. N Engl J Med 345(18): 1305–10, 2001

Unicondylar Minimally Invasive Approach to Knee Arthritis

J.A. Repicci, J.F. Hartman

Introduction

The technological advancement in total knee arthroplasty (TKA) of the 1980s and subsequent favorable results [14, 41, 45, 50, 52, 55] led to the recognition of TKA as the ultimate knee-salvage procedure for the treatment of osteoarthritis. When considering treatment options, however, the pathology and progression of the disease must be considered. Past studies examining osteoarthritis of the knee have revealed that the disease is slowly progressive and typically limited to the medial tibiofemoral compartment [1, 7, 19, 61]. Furthermore, the erosion of cartilage in the medial compartment is almost always limited to the anterior half of the medial tibial plateau and the corresponding contact area on the distal portion of the medial femoral condyle [61]. White and colleagues coined the phrase anteromedial osteoarthritis to describe this distinct clinicopathological condition [61]. A sclerotic layer of bone, or medial tibial buttress, is formed in response to this characteristic pattern of cartilage destruction. The widening of the medial tibial plateau and increased bone density compensate for articular cartilage loss. Although this may appear to be an inefficient solution, this layer of sclerotic bone assists the medial compartment in withstanding joint loading, supporting weight, and permitting continued ambulation for 10–19 years after initiation of osteoarthritis [19]. The resulting plastic deformation and ligament imbalance, however, produce pain and loss of function.

The clinical presentation of this early unicompartmental form of osteoarthritis must be differentiated from that of patients with more advanced osteoarthritis. For patients with the tricompartmental variant of the disease, the pain often is so debilitating that activities of daily living are severely restricted, independence is lost, and ambulatory aids, such as crutches, a walker, or wheelchair, are required. In such cases, TKA is the most appropriate surgical option to relieve pain and to restore some degree of independence. Fortunately, however, unicompartmental osteoarthritis is far more prevalent than the more advanced tricompartmental form of the disease, as demonstrated by previous studies [1, 19]. Patients with unicompartmental osteoarthritis usually are not disabled by the disease, but typically are inconvenienced by pain. In general, these patients are more active than their tricompartmental counterparts and, therefore, will not be satisfied with simple pain relief. Because most patients also desire restoration of function and a return to activities of daily living, unicondylar knee arthroplasty (UKA) is a viable option for many of these patients. Furthermore, when patients exhibiting osteoarthritis limited to one tibiofemoral compartment are presented with a choice between UKA and TKA, they tend to choose the less invasive procedure [48].

Based on this understanding of the disease process, treatments such as UKA that address the single diseased compartment, preserving bone and soft tissue, seem appropriate. Unlike the other conservative treatment options, such as arthroscopic debridement and high tibial osteotomy, UKA specifically addresses the pathology of unicompartmental osteoarthritis by combining realignment, replacement of the single damaged tibiofemoral compartment, and ligamentous balancing [44].

The use of UKA in the United States continues to increase as more orthopedic surgeons become aware of the enhanced low morbidity and rapid rehabilitation associated when a minimally invasive surgical technique is combined with the procedure [44]. The popularity of UKA also is rising in response to patient demand [44]. The conservative nature of this procedure, combined with the low morbidity, rapid rehabilitation, and desirable level of post-operative function, appeals to many patients suffering from unicompartmental osteoarthritis of the knee. The steadfastness of patient choice regarding UKA use, whether educated through word-of-mouth or through various media sources, should not be underestimated.

Surgical Technique

The surgical technique for performing minimally invasive UKA using a resurfacing design has been described previously [43] and is reviewed, focusing on medial implantation, which is the most common indication for UKA. Patient preparation and closure are performed, using standard protocols and, thus, will not be discussed.

Prior to commencing the UKA procedure, diagnostic arthroscopy is performed to corroborate the pre-operative diagnosis of unicompartmental osteoarthritis by verifying that the contralateral compartment is unaffected. The status of the contralateral meniscus also is evaluated, which cannot be accomplished during the open procedure, as the meniscus cannot be visualized through the flexion gap. The UKA procedure itself may proceed, provided that the osteoarthritis is limited to one tibiofemoral compartment and the contralateral meniscus is functional. If, however, the disease is more progressive, the surgeon must be prepared to perform a TKA, of which the potential should be pre-operatively discussed and consented to by the patient.

The following steps summarize the minimally invasive UKA procedure using a resurfacing design as performed by the senior author.

Exposure with Posterior Femoral Condyle Resection (◘ Fig. 9.33)

A 3- to 4-inch incision is created from the superomedial edge of the patella to the proximal tibial region. A subcutaneous dissection producing a 1- to 2-inch skin flap surrounding the entire incision improves skin mobility and visualization. A medial parapatellar capsular incision from the superior pole of the patella to the tibia is produced. A one-inch transverse release of the vastus medialis tendon is performed to further aid in visualization.

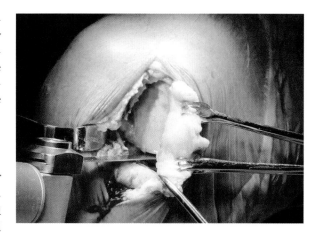

◘ **Fig. 9.33.** Exposure with posterior femoral condyle resection

Avoiding patellar dislocation is critical to the minimally invasive technique, as the suprapatellar pouch must remain intact. The suprapatellar pouch is a unique structure that unfolds four times in length when the knee is flexed 90° [24]. When the patella is dislocated, as is performed in traditional open TKA and UKA procedures, the suprapatellar pouch is damaged. Extensive physical therapy then is required to reverse the iatrogenic damage to this structure.

Next, the posterior femoral condyle is resected 5–8 mm. This resection is necessary to create space in the flexion gap to accommodate the UKA prosthesis, as medial compartmental osteoarthritis is an extension gap disease (◘ Fig. 9.34). The articular defect is located at the distal femur and the anterior tibia. When the knee is flexed 90°, the femur rolls back onto the tibia to an area of preserved articular cartilage. Because there is no defect present in the flexion gap, the joint line in the area of retained articular cartilage is an excellent reference point for reconstruction.

Distraction with Tibial Inlay Preparation and Resection (◘ Fig. 9.35)

To improve tibial visualization, curved distractor pins are placed at the femoral and tibial levels and are attached to a joint laminar distractor. Approximately 10 mm space must be created in the flexion gap to accommodate the UKA prosthesis. Because 5–8 mm has been resected previously from the posterior

Flexion Gap

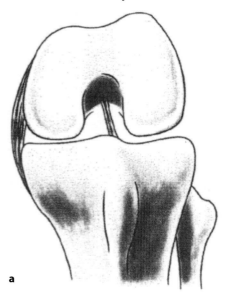

a

Extension Gap

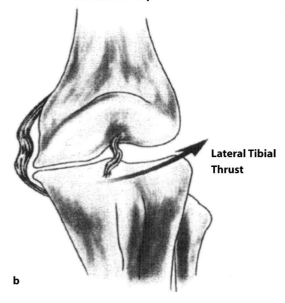

Lateral Tibial Thrust

b

◘ **Fig. 9.34a,b.** Medial unicompartmental osteoarthritis is an extension gap disease. **a** There is no articular surface loss in the flexion gap. **b** In contrast, a loss of approximately 5 mm is present in the extension gap. This narrowing of the medial compartment joint space is evident on radiographic evaluation and is responsible for ACL and MCL laxity, the lateral tibial thrust, or varus deformity, present in the extension gap, and the absence of deformity in the flexion gap, which are all clinical observations characteristic of medial unicompartmental osteoarthritis (From [44])

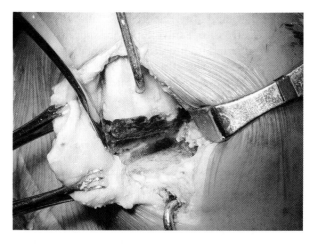

◘ **Fig. 9.35.** Distraction with tibial inlay preparation and resection

femoral condyle, the additional 5 mm necessary for prosthetic implantation is created by burring 5 mm into the tibia adjacent to the posterior tibial rim. This resection, combined with the previous 5- to 8-mm resection of the posterior femoral condyle, provides adequate space in the flexion gap. The burr then is buried at a half-depth (only 3 mm) at the anterior tibial region, which corresponds to the area of articular cartilage loss and sclerotic bone formation. This creates the proper depth for tibial component insertion. A crosshatch is created at the anterior tibial level, which is the natural location of femoral weight transfer. Bulk bone is removed in quadrants. Preservation of a 2- to 3-mm circumferential rim of tibial bone and maintenance of the sclerotic layer of bone is crucial to stabilize the component. The tibial inlay then may be fitted and adjusted as necessary.

This resurfacing inlay technique preserves the layer of sclerotic bone to provide a stable platform for the component and to minimize medial tibial bone loss, which is a major cause of UKA revision [3, 38]. The importance of protecting this medial tibial buttress may be likened to the preservation of the posterior acetabular rim in total hip arthroplasty in that, when lost, future reconstruction is severely compromised. Unlike other UKA designs, the resurfacing, inlay tibial component preserves the medial tibial buttress. The amount of bone resected for UKA implantation of resurfacing UKA designs compared to that resected for saw-cut UKA designs is depicted in ◘ Fig. 9.36. Because the medial

9.5

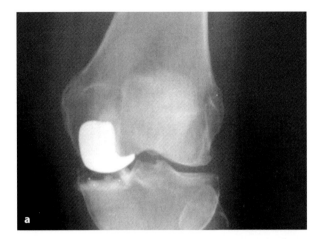

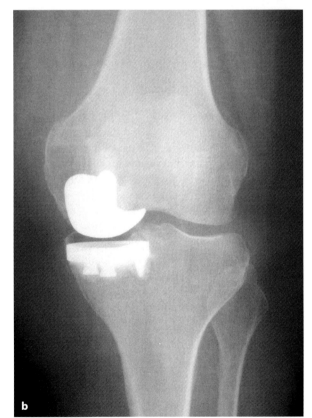

tibial buttress is preserved, the senior author considers resurfacing UKA as the last reconstruction procedure for a patient, but classifies any technique in which the medial tibial buttress is sacrificed, whether it may be other UKA techniques or TKA, as the first salvage procedure.

Femoral Preparation and Resection (■ Fig. 9.37)

At the femoral level, the 5.5 mm round burr is used to drill to a depth of 3 mm into the femoral extension gap surface, which serves as a depth gauge. An additional full-burr depth (5 mm) is created at the junction of the previous saw cut and the distal femoral surface, which allows the curved portion of the femoral prosthesis to set midway between the flexion and extension gaps (45° flexion position). Bone bulk is removed with the burr. This resection permits adequate spacing of the femoral component, while preventing settling.

Femoral-Tibial Alignment (■ Fig. 9.38)

Methylene blue marks are used to indicate the desired center of rotation, or contact point, of the femoral component in relation to the tibial component and to indicate the desired center point of the femoral component. A femoral drill guide, manufactured with a large central slot to visualize component alignment, is inserted

■ **Fig. 9.36a,b.** Inlay all-polyethylene versus saw-cut tibial component. AP weight-bearing post-operative radiographs of knee joints exhibiting Ahlback III osteoarthritis with complete loss of medial joint space. **a** Limited bone resection and preservation of the medial tibial buttress associated with the use of the inlay all-polyethylene tibial component. **b** More aggressive bone resection and corresponding medial tibial buttress sacrifice required with the use of saw-cut metal-backed designs

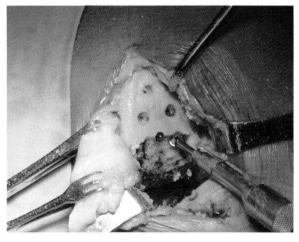

■ **Fig. 9.37.** Femoral preparation and resection

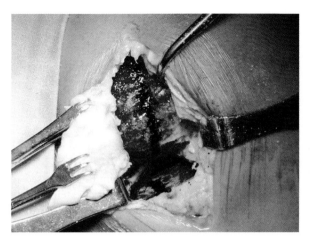

Fig. 9.38. Femoral-tibial alignment

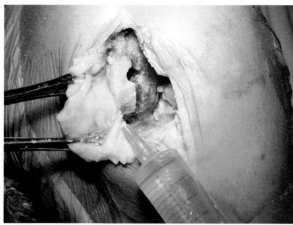

Fig. 9.39. Local anesthetic injection

to assist aligning the femoral contact with adequate tibial support. A sagittal saw or side-cutting burr may be used to create a keel-slot for the fin of the femoral component. Femoral preparation is concluded by inserting the trial femoral component using the femoral inserter.

Trial Reduction and Local Anesthetic Injection (■ Fig. 9.39)

Trial reduction is performed by implanting the trial components to evaluate range of motion through 115° of flexion and to assess soft-tissue balance. Ligament balancing is achieved primarily by the insertion of a properly sized and fitted implant. If the ligaments are tight in only the extension gap, tension may be adjusted by further bone removal at the distal femoral level. If, however, tension exists in both the flexion and extension gaps, tibial bone resection as previously described should be repeated in 1 mm increments. The round femoral surface permits easy adjustment.

Once range of motion and soft-tissue balancing are satisfactory, the trial components are removed, the joint is irrigated thoroughly, and a dry field is established. The femoral and tibial preparations will be visible. Prior to component insertion, all incised tissues are infiltrated with anesthesia (0.25% bupivacaine and 0.5% epinephrine solution) for post-operative pain relief and hemostasis.

Component Insertion and Final Preparation (■ Fig. 9.40)

All components are inserted using methylmethacrylate cement. After insertion of each component, excess cement is removed with a dental pick. Range of motion should be performed a final time to evaluate the flexion–extension gaps. The cement is cured with the knee in full extension. Once the cement mantle is hardened, it may be necessary to remove any remaining osteophytes, contour the patella, or perform notch plasty. The procedure is completed by irrigating the joint with sterile saline. A tube drain then is inserted into the contralateral compartment via a stab wound. Sterile dressing, a circumferential ice cuff, a pneumatic compression device, and an immobilizer are placed on the knee prior to exiting the operating room.

Potential Pitfalls

The 3-inch minimally invasive surgical approach described above provides appropriate visualization to effectively perform UKA. If, however, visualization or technique is compromised at any point in the technique, it may be converted to an open procedure, with full dislocation of the patella, at which time the procedure would not be considered minimally invasive.

Although many UKA failures may be attributed to implant design, technical errors are often a result of human judgment. Over-correction may lead to aseptic

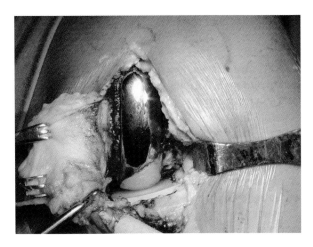

Fig. 9.40. Implantation of UKA resurfacing prosthesis

loosening and/or subsidence, as well as secondary degeneration of the contralateral compartment. These failure modes stress the importance of proper training, experience, and strong surgical technique. Because of the steep learning curve associated with developing accurate surgical technique [5, 6, 27, 31, 32, 35, 37, 44, 59], instructional training is highly advised to avoid the early failure that may result if UKA is attempted without proper training.

Christensen emphasized the need for such training by contending that TKA systems with good instrumentation may be implanted using only written instructions, while UKA technique is best taught in the operating room [13]. In addition, Robertsson et al. stressed that skill, patient-selection decisions, and operative routine are assumed to be influenced by the number of procedures performed by the surgeon [47]. Indeed, centers performing UKA on a regular basis demonstrate better results than those centers where the procedure is occasionally performed [32, 46]. To successfully perform UKA, orthopedic surgeons, therefore, must seek appropriate instructional training prior to attempting UKA and be cognizant of the learning curve that must be overcome to avoid the technical errors that are well-established failure modes of UKA.

Results

A retrospective study comprised of 136 UKA cases conducted by the senior author using broad selection criteria demonstrated an overall 7% revision rate requiring

TKA among Ahlback stage-2, -3, and -4 patients at 8 years [48]. Among the 20 Ahlback stage-4 cases, 5 (25%) required revision at 8 years [48]. The Repicci II unicondylar knee system (Biomet, Inc., Warsaw, IN) was utilized in all cases. Within 4 h after surgery, all patients ambulated with a walker and most (98%) were discharged from the hospital within 23 h [48]. Most patients, however, ambulate with a walker within 2 h post-operatively and are discharged home within 4–6 h. Hospitalization for 48 h was required for refractory nausea in one case and telemetry observation for new onset atrial fibrillation in another case [48]. In the 8 cases requiring revision to TKA, primary designs were utilized with good (25%) or excellent (75%) Knee Society clinical ratings at follow-up [48]. The results from this study highlight the safety and efficacy of the minimally invasive surgical technique, demonstrate the decreased recovery and rehabilitation time, and support the relative ease of conversion to TKA, if required, of this particular UKA device.

Discussion

Although recognized as a safe and efficacious procedure for the treatment of osteoarthritis, TKA has a finite longevity. An effective procedure, such as UKA, is needed to address treatment of the earlier, non-advanced cases of osteoarthritis, postponing or delaying the need for TKA. Given the slow, progressive nature of osteoarthritis [1, 7, 19, 61], UKA, which addresses the single-diseased compartment and preserves bone and soft tissue, is an appropriate treatment option for the unicompartmental form of the disease. Not only is there a clinical need for such a treatment, but also patient demand for such a procedure is quite strong [44, 48].

The senior author uses UKA under broad selection criteria to supplement TKA, extending the spectrum of knee prosthetic survivability and decreasing the likelihood that a complex revision procedure will be required in a patient's lifetime. As previously summarized [44, 48], all patients between 50 and 90 years, of age diagnosed with osteoarthritis of the knee limited to a single tibiofemoral compartment who have failed non-operative treatment, are considered for UKA if presenting with weight-bearing pain that significantly impairs quality of life. Patients with Ahlback stage 2, 3, or 4 [1] are candidates if range of motion is at least 10–90°.

Although an attenuated or ruptured anterior cruciate ligament (ACL) is an absolute contra-indication to lateral UKA, instability, including a compromised ACL, is a relative contra-indication to medial UKA [12, 13, 22, 53, 54, 56]. When presented with a choice between UKA and TKA, UKA candidates tend to choose the less invasive procedure [48].

Combining a minimally invasive surgical technique with UKA is appealing to both surgeons and patients, as morbidity and rehabilitation time are reduced [44]. A successful minimally invasive technique, regardless of its application, must meet the following goals:

- minimal physiologic disruption;
- minimal interference in patient lifestyle;
- minimal hindrance to future treatment options.

In 1992, the senior author implemented a minimally invasive UKA program [43] that is significantly different from simply the use of a small skin incision or implementation of only a minimally invasive surgical approach. The following concepts, which are all minimally invasive by nature, were combined into a single program to meet the above goals:

- minimally invasive surgical approach avoiding patellar dislocation;
- adjunct use of arthroscopy;
- resurfacing UKA design with an inlay tibial component;
- pain management with local anesthetic and without the use of narcotics.

The utilization of arthroscopy in conjunction with UKA reduces the morbidity of the procedure and enhances survivorship by identifying patients with advanced osteoarthritic involvement and/or a compromised meniscus in the contralateral compartment whom otherwise may not have been excluded based on pre-operative radiograph evaluation and traditional surgical inspection alone. The pre-planned UKA procedure should be abandoned for these patients in favor of TKA, the procedure of choice for more advanced cases of osteoarthritis. A fully functioning, intact contralateral meniscus, which cannot be verified through traditional surgical exposure, is a significant factor affecting UKA survivability, as the surface area of load bearing and the stability of the knee joint are enhanced by intact menisci [16, 18, 20, 23, 28, 51, 57]. When the menisci are intact, the average surface contact area of the tibia is 765–1150 mm²;

however, the tibial contact with the femur is reduced to approximately 520 mm² when the menisci are removed [17, 25, 29]. Based on these findings, Kuster et al. concluded that a contact area of approximately 400 mm² is required to avoid polyethylene stress and to prevent cold flow in knee prostheses [29]. Although a certain amount of cold flow is expected in UKA designs, due to lower tibiofemoral contact surface area compared to TKA designs, an absent contralateral meniscus will result in an inadequate amount of tibiofemoral contact. This lack of tibiofemoral contact, coupled with the concurrent continued osteoarthritic process, may hasten the rate of degeneration of the untreated contralateral side and may also lead to early failure of the UKA device [33]. Therefore, although eliminating over-correction has reduced the incidence of UKA failures in recent years [2, 4, 8, 10–12, 15, 18, 34, 49, 53, 58, 60], contralateral compartment degeneration and early UKA failure remain a concern if the status of the contralateral meniscus is not assessed.

The minimally invasive surgical approach utilized by the senior author must be differentiated from a "mini incision," which is merely a small hole. The use of a "mini incision" may cause significant distortion of soft tissue. This minimally invasive surgical approach preserves tissue and maintains the function of the suprapatellar synovial pouch, the quadriceps tendon, and the patella. Traditional TKA and UKA surgical techniques, on the other hand, involve dislocation of the patella, which, in turn, destroys the suprapatellar pouch and requires extensive physical therapy. The advantages of this minimally invasive approach include reduction in post-operative morbidity, reduction in post-operative pain, decreased rehabilitation time without the need for formal physical therapy, and the ability to perform the procedure on a same-day or short-day basis [9, 15, 26, 36, 40, 43, 48]. Several studies have demonstrated a faster rate of recovery, defined as the time required to achieve straight leg raises, knee flexion, and independent stair climbing, and discharge in minimally invasive UKA, when the patella is not dislocated and when the suprapatellar pouch remains intact, compared to traditional open UKA or TKA [36, 39, 40]. In addition, studies have documented that UKA may be performed as reliably with a minimally invasive approach as through a wide incision, without compromising proper component placement or long-term results [9, 26, 36, 40]. The preservation of the quadriceps tendon and suprapatellar pouch, rather than the short skin incision itself, is most likely responsible for the diminished post-operative pain and decreased rehabilitation time associated with the minimally invasive surgical technique [40].

Because medial tibial bone loss is a major problem in converting a UKA to TKA [3, 38], a significant advantage of using an inlay all-polyethylene tibial component compared to modular components requiring a saw-cut tibial technique is that such resurfacing designs require less bone resection and preserve the medial tibial buttress, increasing the likelihood that conversion to TKA may be more easily accomplished with less bone resection should future revision become necessary, as illustrated in ◘ Fig. 9.41. Modular saw-cut tibial components are much thicker than their inlay counterparts and require sacrifice of the medial tibial buttress. In addition, resection designs often require full exposure of the joint for jig instrumentation and involve resection of larger amounts of bone. Such saw-cut components frequently utilize peg or fin fixation, which further compromises tibial bone upon implant removal and may require the use of bone grafts, special custom devices, or metal-wedge tibial trays to stabilize the tibia if conversion is necessary, further complicating the revision surgery [3, 21, 30, 38, 42].

Outpatient status requires a structured pain-management program. Spinal or general anesthesia is used in all cases. Patient education, avoidance of cerebral-depressing injectable narcotics, infiltration of all incised tissues with long-acting local anesthetics, and the pre-emptive use of scheduled oral 400 mg ibuprofen every 4 h and oral 500 mg acetaminophen/5 mg hydrocodone bitartrate every 4 h for the first 3 days post-operatively, all aid in controlling pain. In addition, 30 mg ketoroloc tromethamine (15 mg for patients over 65 years of age) is administered either intramuscularly or intravenously during surgery and is repeated after 5 h in patients with normal renal function. This pain-management program results in fully alert patients in the recovery room with no local knee pain. When pain is absent, patients are able to perform straight leg raises and to actively participate in their post-operative rehabilitation process. In addition to the minimally invasive surgical approach, the use of the local anesthetic and avoidance of narcotics are credited for shortening the recovery and rehabilitation time, permitting the procedure to be performed on an outpatient basis.

In summary, by utilizing arthroscopy, patients with more advanced stages of osteoarthritis are excluded

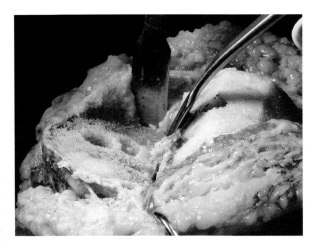

◘ **Fig. 9.41.** Intra-operative photograph depicting the conversion of a bone sparing, resurfacing medial UKA to TKA. After 10 years, revision to a primary TKA was required due to advanced disease of the lateral compartment. With the use of an inlay tibial component, the medial tibial buttress is preserved and the amount of tibial bone loss at revision is minimal, allowing a relatively easy conversion to TKA

from UKA and, instead, may receive the more appropriate TKA. The use of arthroscopy to assist in proper patient selection reduces morbidity and increases survivorship. By avoiding patellar dislocation and nonessential tissue dissection, interference in physiology is avoided and lower morbidity and rapid rehabilitation are achieved. The minimally invasive surgical approach, combined with the specific pain-management program, allows UKA to be performed on an outpatient basis, with full independence achieved by 4 h post-operatively. This rapid rehabilitation and return to activities of daily living addresses patient satisfaction regarding minimizing interference of lifestyle. The use of a resurfacing UKA design diminishes bone resection compared to other UKA designs. Consequently, future treatment options are not interfered with and UKA use is permitted in a broader range of patients, including younger, heavier or active patients. These individual concepts, combined by the senior author into a multi-pronged minimally invasive program, work in unison to meet the goals of a minimally invasive technique: minimal interference in physiology, lifestyle, and future treatment options.

Finally, whereas TKA marks the end of a disease process and the beginning of a new predictable construct, UKA is implanted into the middle of a less predictable disease process and is considered an extension of conservative management. Long-term survivorship of UKA is affected by many factors, including the stage of the disease at insertion, limited tibial bone support, and material limitations, such as polyethylene deformity and wear. A minimally invasive surgical technique adds a significant variable; therefore, surgeons who choose to utilize this technique would greatly benefit from instructional training. In this context, UKA is feasible as a minimally invasive, bone-sparing outpatient procedure with low morbidity.

References

1. Ahlback S (1968) Osteoarthrosis of the knee. A radiographic investigation. Acta Radiol Diagn 277 [Suppl]: 7–72
2. Ansari S, Newman JH, Ackroyd CE (1997) St. Georg sledge for medial compartment knee replacement. 461 arthroplasties followed for 4 (1–17) years. Acta Orthop Scand 68(5): 430–434
3. Barrett WP, Scott RD (1987) Revision of failed unicondylar unicompartmental knee arthroplasty. J Bone Joint Surg Am 69(9): 1328–1335
4. Berger RA, Nedeff DD, Barden RM, Sheinkop MM, Jacobs JJ, Rosenberg AG, et al (1999) Unicompartmental knee arthroplasty. Clinical experience at 6- to 10-year follow-up. Clin Orthop 367: 50–60
5. Bohm I, Landsiedl F (2000) Revision surgery after failed unicompartmental knee arthroplasty. A study of 35 cases. J Arthroplasty 15(8): 982–989
6. Bourne RB (2001) Reevaluating the unicondylar knee arthroplasty. Orthopedics 24(9): 885–886
7. Brocklehurst R, Bayliss MT, Maroudas A, Coysh HL, Freeman MA, Revell PA et al. (1984) The composition of normal and osteoarthritic articular cartilage from human knee joints. With special reference to unicompartmental replacement and osteotomy of the knee. J Bone Joint Surg Am 66(1): 95–106
8. Broughton NS, Newman JH, Baily RA (1986) Unicompartmental replacement and high tibial osteotomy for osteoarthritis of the knee. A comparative study after 5–10 years' follow-up. J Bone Joint Surg Br 68(3): 447–452
9. Brown A (2001) The Oxford unicompartmental knee replacement for osteoarthritis. Issues Emerg Health Technol 23: 1–4
10. Cartier P, Cheaib S (1987) Unicondylar knee arthroplasty. 2–10 years of follow-up evaluation. J Arthroplasty 2(2): 157–162
11. Cartier P, Mammeri M, Villers P (1982) Clinical and radiographic evaluation of modular knee replacement. A review of 95 cases. Int Orthop 6(1): 35–44
12. Cartier P, Sanouiller JL, Grelsamer RP (1996) Unicompartmental knee arthroplasty surgery. 10-year minimum follow-up period. J Arthroplasty 11(7): 782–788
13. Christensen NO (1991) Unicompartmental prosthesis for gonarthrosis. A nine-year series of 575 knees from a Swedish hospital. Clin Orthop 273: 165–169
14. Dennis DA, Clayton ML, O'Donnell S, Mack RP, Stringer EA (1992) Posterior cruciate condylar total knee arthroplasty. Average 11-year follow-up evaluation. Clin Orthop 281: 168–176
15. Deshmukh RV, Scott RD (2001) Unicompartmental knee arthroplasty: long-term results. Clin Orthop 392: 272–278
16. Fithian DC, Kelly MA, Mow VC (1990) Material properties and structure-function relationships in the menisci. Clin Orthop 252: 19–31
17. Fukubayashi T, Kurosawa H (1980) The contact area and pressure distribution pattern of the knee. A study of normal and osteoarthritic knee joints. Acta Orthop Scand 51(6): 871–879
18. Grelsamer RP (1995) Current concepts review. Unicompartmental osteoarthrosis of the knee. J Bone Joint Surg Am 77(2): 278–292
19. Hernborg JS, Nilsson BE (1977) The natural course of untreated osteoarthritis of the knee. Clin Orthop 123: 130–137
20. Ihn JC, Kim SJ, Park IH (1993) In vitro study of contact area and pressure distribution in the human knee after partial and total meniscectomy. Int Orthop 17(4): 214–218
21. Insall J, Dethmers DA (1982) Revision of total knee arthroplasty. Clin Orthop 170: 123–130
22. Jackson RW (1998) Surgical treatment. Osteotomy and unicompartmental arthroplasty. Am J Knee Surg 11(1): 55–57
23. Johnson RJ, Kettelkamp DB, Clark W, Leaverton P (1974) Factors affecting late results after meniscectomy. J Bone Joint Surg Am 56(4): 719–729
24. Kapandji IA (ed) (1987) The physiology of joints. 5th edn, vol. 2. Churchill Livingston, New York, pp 64–246
25. Kettelkamp DB, Jacobs AW (1972) Tibiofemoral contact area – determination and implications. J Bone Joint Surg Am 54(2): 349–356
26. Keys GW (1999) Reduced invasive approach for Oxford II medial unicompartmental knee replacement- a preliminary study. The Knee 6(3): 193–196
27. Kozinn SC, Scott R (1989) Unicondylar knee arthroplasty. J Bone Joint Surg Am 71(1): 145–150
28. Kurosawa H, Fukubayashi T, Nakajima H (1980) Load-bearing mode of the knee joint: physical behavior of the knee joint with or without menisci. Clin Orthop 149: 283–290
29. Kuster MA, Wood GA, Stachowiak GW, Gachter A (1997) Joint load considerations in total knee replacement. J Bone Joint Surg Br 79(1): 109–113
30. Lai CH, Rand JA (1993) Revision of failed unicompartmental total knee arthroplasty. Clin Orthop 287: 193–201
31. Lewold S, Knutson K, Lidgren L (1993) Reduced failure rate in knee prosthetic surgery with improved implantation technique. Clin Orthop 287: 94–97
32. Lindstrand A, Stenstrom A, Lewold S (1992) Multicenter study of unicompartmental knee revision. PCA, Marmor, and St. Georg compared in 3,777 cases of arthrosis. Acta Orthop Scand 63(3): 256–259
33. Marmor L (1977) Results of single compartment arthroplasty with acrylic cement fixation. A minimum follow-up of two years. Clin Orthop 122: 181–188
34. Marmor L (1988) Unicompartmental knee arthroplasty. Ten- to 13-year follow-up study. Clin Orthop 226: 14–20
35. Marmor L (1988) Unicompartmental knee arthroplasty of the knee with a minimum ten-year follow-up period. Clin Orthop 228: 171–177
36. Murray DW (2000) Unicompartmental knee replacement: now or never? Orthopedics 23(9): 979–980
37. Murray DW, Goodfellow JW, O'Connor JJ (1998) The Oxford medial unicompartmental arthroplasty: a ten-year survival study. J Bone Joint Surg Br 80(6): 983–989

38. Padgett DE, Stern SH, Insall JN (1991) Revision total knee arthroplasty for failed unicompartmental replacement. J Bone Joint Surg Am 73(2): 186–190

39. Price A, Webb J, Topf H, Dodd C, Goodfellow J, Murray D (2000) Oxford unicompartmental knee replacement with a minimally invasive technique. J Bone Joint Surg Br 82 [Suppl 1]: 24

40. Price AJ, Webb J, Topf H, Dodd CA, Goodfellow JW, Murray DW (2001) Rapid recovery after Oxford unicompartmental arthroplasty through a short incision. J Arthroplasty 16(8): 970–976

41. Ranawat CS, Boachie-Adjei O (1988) Survivorship analysis and results of total condylar knee arthroplasty. Eight- to 11-year follow-up period. Clin Orthop 226: 6–13

42. Rand JA, Bryan RS (1988) Results of revision total knee arthroplasties using condylar prostheses. A review of fifty knees. J Bone Joint Surg Am 70(5): 738–745

43. Repicci JA, Eberle RW (1999) Minimally invasive surgical technique for unicondylar knee arthroplasty. J Southern Orthop Assoc 8(1): 20–27

44. Repicci JA, Hartman JF (2003) Unicondylar knee replacement: the American experience. In: Fu FH, Browner BD (eds) Management of osteoarthritis of the knee: an international consensus. American Academy of Orthopaedic Surgeons, Rosemont, IL, pp 67–79

45. Ritter MA, Campbell E, Faris PM, Keating EM (1989) Long-term survival analysis of the posterior cruciate condylar total knee arthroplasty. A 10-year evaluation. J Arthroplasty 4(4): 293–296

46. Robertsson O, Borgquist L, Knutson K, Lewold S, Lidgren L (1999) Use of unicompartmental instead of tricompartmental prostheses for unicompartmental arthrosis in the knee is a cost-effective alternative. 5,437 primary tricompartmental prostheses were compared with 10,624 primary medial or lateral unicompartmental prostheses. Acta Orthop Scand 70(2): 170–175

47. Robertsson O, Knutson K, Lewold S, Lidgren L (2001) The routine of surgical management reduces failure after unicompartmental knee arthroplasty. J Bone Joint Surg Br 83(1): 45–49

48. Romanowski MR, Repicci JA (2002) Minimally invasive unicondylar arthroplasty. Eight-year follow-up. Am J Knee Surg 15(1): 17–22

49. Schai PA, Suh JT, Thornhill TS, Scott RD (1998) Unicompartmental knee arthroplasty in middle-aged patients: a 2- to 6-year follow-up evaluation. J Arthroplasty 13(4): 365–372

50. Scuderi GR, Insall JN, Windsor RE, Moran MC (1989) Survivorship of cemented knee replacements. J Bone Joint Surg Br 71(5): 798–803

51. Shrive NG, O'Connor JJ, Goodfellow JW (1978) Load-bearing in the knee joint. Clin Orthop 131: 279–287

52. Stern SH, Insall JN (1992) Posterior stabilized prosthesis. Results after follow-up of nine to twelve years. J Bone Joint Surg Am 74(7): 980–986

53. Stockelman RE, Pohl KP (1991) The long-term efficacy of unicompartmental arthroplasty of the knee. Clin Orthop 271: 88–95

54. Thornhill TS, Scott RD (1989) Unicompartmental total knee arthroplasty. Orthop Clin North Am 20(2): 245–256

55. Vince KG, Insall JN, Kelly MA (1989) The total condylar prosthesis. 10- to 12-year results of a cemented knee replacement. J Bone Joint Surg Br 71(5): 793–797

56. Voss F, Sheinkop MB, Galante JO, Barden RM, Rosenberg AG (1995) Miller-Galante unicompartmental knee arthroplasty at 2- to 5-year follow-up evaluations. J Arthroplasty 10(6): 764–771

57. Walker PS, Erkman MJ (1975) The role of the menisci in force transmission across the knee. Clin Orthop 109: 184–192

58. Weale AE, Newman JH (1994) Unicompartmental arthroplasty and high tibial osteotomy for osteoarthrosis of the knee. A comparative study with a 12- to 17-year follow-up period. Clin Orthop 302: 134–137

59. Weale AE, Halabi OA, Jones PW, White SH (2001) Perceptions of outcomes after unicompartmental and total knee replacements. Clin Orthop 382: 143–153

60. Weale AE, Murray DW, Baines J, Newman JH (2000) Radiological changes five years after unicompartmental knee replacement. J Bone Joint Surg Br 82(7): 996–1000

61. White SH, Ludkowski PF, Goodfellow JW (1991) Anteromedial osteoarthritis of the knee. J Bone Joint Surg Br 73(4): 582–586

Unicondylar Minimally Invasive

C.M. McAllister

Introduction

Unicompartmental knee arthroplasty has been and remains controversial. Poor results reported in early reviews established the opinion that total knee replacement was a more reliable and durable operation. More recent reports have demonstrated 10-year survivorship after unicondylar knee replacement that is comparable to total knee arthroplasty [1, 14, 22, 24, 25]. It is generally felt that these reports reflect improved patient selection, surgical technique, component design, and instrumentation. "Unicompartmental knee arthroplasty now is characterized as a procedure with a reliable 8- to 10-year outcome in improperly selected patients with osteoarthritis who receive a skillfully implanted, proper design" [5].

The advantages of unicompartmental knee replacement are well documented. Compared to total knee arthroplasty, unicondylar knee arthroplasty is less invasive, with less blood loss, less post-operative pain, and a lower infection rate [6]. The range of motion and kinematics are more normal [19, 24, 25]. It is an attractive alternative for patients who seek rapid return of function and normal lifestyle regardless of age [3]. Unicondylar knee replacement is a bone conserving, soft-tissue-friendly operation that sets the stage for an easier, and more successful revision arthroplasty, making it an important option for the younger, low demand patient who seeks to put off their first total knee replacement [6, 11, 13, 15].

To help guarantee long-term results that are comparable to total knee replacement, it is important to understand the unique elements of unicompartmental knee replacement. Component design and instrumentation for unicondylar knee replacements allow improved alignment, decreased polyethylene wear, and improved long-term results. Minimally invasive surgical techniques allow easier recovery and less morbidity. But unicondylar knee replacement is not simply a downsized total knee. Surgeons who rely on their experience in total knee arthroplasty as the foundation for unicondylar knee arthroplasty will certainly be disappointed, as will their patients. This chapter focuses on essential principles of knee arthroplasty, component design, instrumentation, and surgical techniques that constitute a skillfully implanted, proper unicondylar knee replacement.

Angular Alignment

Angular alignment directly influences long-term failure rates and is at least as important in unicondylar knee replacement as it is in total knee replacement. Most surgeons experienced in unicondylar knee replacement advocate under-correcting the mechanical axis by about 2–3° [2, 4, 5, 21, 25]. Giou et al. reviewed a multi-hospital registry of implant and explant information with emphasis on reasons for revision of unicondylar knee replacements [7]. The major reasons for revision were **opposite side degeneration** (51%), **aseptic loosening** (25%), and **polyethylene wear** (21%). Over-correction of a varus knee (HKA angle >180°) leads to opposite compartment degeneration [25]. Severe under-correction (HKA <170°) leads to loosening and polyethylene wear. Hernigou's work demonstrates that angular alignment directly influences these failure modes [8]. Ideal alignment after unicondylar knee replacement should fall between 179° and 171°. Accurately correcting alignment with unicondylar knee replacement greatly reduces opposite compartment degeneration. It also improves patellofemoral mechanics and helps reduce patellofemoral degeneration and pain [4, 14, 25].

Component Design

Component design influences surgical technique and determines long-term results. Early unicondylar designs frequently involved too much constraint, high contact stresses, thin polyethylene, and rudimentary instrumentation [5, 10, 12, 16]. Freehand techniques encouraged poor implant placement, rim loading, impingement, polyethylene wear, loosening, and subsidence [10, 12, 24, 25]. Tibial components with large lugs and deep fixation methods created difficult revisions requiring structural graft, stems, and custom implants [1]. It is no surprise that surgeons eventually opted for the more reliable results of total knee replacement over the less invasive unicondylar knee replacement. However, recent unicondylar design improvements address these issues.

Tibial Component Design: Onlay vs. Inlay

An inlay tibial component is cemented into a defect that is surgically created within the rim of the tibia. Freehand burring techniques are used, and the tibia is simply resurfaced with little emphasis on alignment. The component is placed within the cortical rim of the tibia on denser, subchondral bone. This technique has the theoretic advantage of preserving bone the medial tibial rim [11, 18]. However, the overall position of the tibial component, cement technique, limb alignment, and tibiofemoral kinematics are heavily influence by the native anatomy of the diseased tibia (◘ Fig. 9.42).

An onlay tibial system starts with an L-cut tibial osteotomy that emphasizes a conservative resection, rim purchase, optimal bone coverage, and proper component position and size (◘ Fig. 9.43). Other advantages include thicker polyethylene, instrumentation systems that establish and reproduce proper alignment, and improved cement technique [1, 5, 21]. Extramedullary guide systems can be used to eliminate freehand techniques, and instrumentation is used to achieve ligament balancing, alignment, and kinematics [4].

One of the main reasons for the poor results in early unicondylar knee replacements has been tibial loosen-

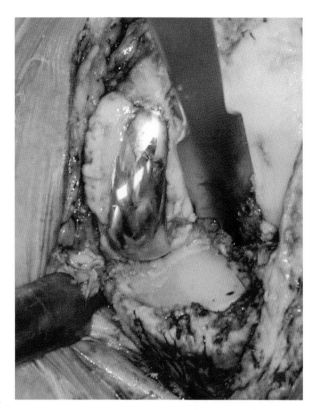

◘ **Fig. 9.42.** Taken from a revision of an inlay tibial component. The tibial component is contained within the rim of cortical bone. Large femoral osteophytes are growing over the femoral component and are articulating with the tibial rim, and eccentric loading is associated with polyethylene cracking and tibial component loosening at one year post operation

ing and polyethylene wear attributed to the use of thin polyethylene. Bartel et al. demonstrated a 6-fold increase in the stress seen in polyethylene when implants are less than 6 mm thick [2]. Marmor's experience with a 6 mm polyethylene insert showed accelerated wear, loosening, and subsidence [12]. The Food and Drug Administration now requires a minimum thickness of 6 mm, and most modern tibial inserts include at least 8 mm of plastic [5].

Most unicondylar systems include all polyethylene tibial components. Deep fixation lugs have been eliminated in favor of smaller fixation keels and designs that allow interdigitation between cement and polyethylene insert. This improves torsional strength and resistance to lift off forces. These all-polyethethylene tibial designs allow the same precision and fixation as metal-backed designs without requiring added bone resection

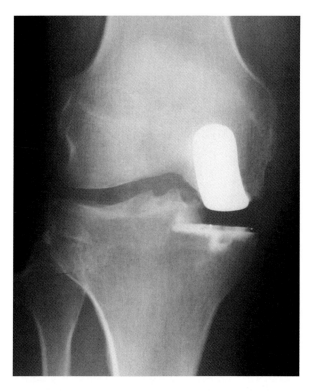

Fig. 9.43. The onlay tibial component covers the medial tibial bone with optimal rim purchase. Cement intrudes 2 mm into ideal cancellous bone. Because of the symmetric outer cross-section, the femoral component can be oriented to fit the native femoral anatomy without edge-loading

9.5.1

or the risk of component dislocation. Adding metal backing will either reduce the polyethylene thickness or increase bone resection. Thinner polyethylene promotes wear, breakage, and subsidence [2, 9]. Deeper bone resections create a larger tibial defect and place the implant on inferior bone. Metal backing also increases shear and tensile stresses at the cement/bone and the cement/implant interfaces [4, 9]. Metal backing also adds cost, and no clinical studies have demonstrated improved results due to metal backing.

Femoral Component Design

Modern unicondylar femoral components are designed to be bone-conserving while fully capping the femoral condyle. Ideally, the entire femoral condyle is covered by the implant, and the anterior lip of the component is recessed to avoid patellar impingement. The geometry, shape and size of the implant should match the native femoral condyle. The femoral condyle may be "resurfaced" (burred) or resected (flat-cut), or a combination. In a flat cut system, an oscillating saw is used with cutting jugs. Any error with these systems tends to cause gaps, and it can be difficult to precisely resect bone. A resurfacing system uses high-speed burs that can be used with milling guides. This combination creates a precise and reproducible fit with very little bone resection.

In the EIUS system, a flat-cut resection of the posterior femur is combined with distal femoral burring. The femoral posterior resection is linked to the tibial resection through the use of tensioning blocks combined with femoral cutting jigs. Flexion space tension and tibio-femoral kinematics are addressed systematically. Femoral component shape and sizing insures adequate capping and avoids impingement. The EIUS component designed also includes an I-beam construction with a symmetric outer cross-section. The symmetric outer cross-section enhances tibio-femoral conformity within a 10° variation of positioning. The I-beam construction adds strength to this thin, low-profile component. The beam and the macro-textured surface also add to cement fixation.

Conformity Without Constraint

The tibio-femoral interface of the unicondylar knee replacement sees complex stresses throughout the knee's range of motion. Conformity throughout a range of motion helps avoid edge loading and polyethylene wear. Minimizing constraint helps avoid loosening, and maximizing implant-to-bone contact helps avoid subsidence [16].

The Oxford design utilizes a meniscal-bearing tibial implant that allows increased conformity without increasing constraint [12]. The Oxford experience has shown improved long-term results largely attributed to improve wear characteristics seen in a highly congruous tibio-femoral articulation. However, the implantation of a meniscal-bearing design is technically demanding and unforgiving [24, 25]. Meniscal-bearing designs introduce an additional wear surface and added bone loss. More recent designs achieve conformity without constraint in a fixed bearing design [9].

Patient Selection

Minimally invasive surgical techniques begin with patient selection. As medial compartment osteoarthritis becomes progressively severe, the knee develops increasing deformities:
- patello-femoral arthrosis and osteophytes,
- tibial osteophytes,
- medial capsular contracture,
- tibial erosion,
- fixed varus deformity,
- tibio-femoral subluxation,
- posterolateral capsular laxity,
- flexion contracture.

Some of these deformities can be managed within the scope of minimally invasive unicondylar knee replacement. Low-grade patellofemoral arthrosis does not preclude successful unicondylar knee replacement [18, 23, 25]. Still, patellofemoral osteophytes can interfere with exposure and can impinge on the femoral implant. A partial patellar facetectomy and careful sizing and positioning of the femoral component can address both of these issues.

To some extent, varus deformity, medial contracture, and flexion contracture can be addressed by removing tibial osteophytes and releasing the coronary ligament [5]. However, varus deformities of greater than 10° from neutral can make unicondylar knee replacement complicated. Flexion contractures of greater than 10–15° are difficult to manage without removing excessive amounts of tibial bone. This places the tibial implant on weaker bone with poor load carrying capabilities and can create difficult revision situations. Tibio-femoral subluxation and posterolateral laxity cannot be addressed with unicondylar knee arthroplasty.

Minimally Invasive Surgical Techniques for Unicondylar Knee Replacement

Minimally invasive surgical techniques for unicondylar knee replacement are well established [4, 17, 19]. These techniques utilize a small incision and avoid eversion of the extensor mechanism. This allows less post-operative pain, early return of function (stair climbing and straight-leg raising), more normal range of motion, and the potential for outpatient surgery. Modern unicondylar instrumentation is well suited to minimally invasive surgery. These methods utilize more precise dissection, and most of the dissection is tailored to each patient. These techniques differ substantially from standard knee arthroplasty, and surgeons need to adapt accordingly. Minimally invasive surgical techniques for unicondylar knee replacement involve patient positioning, skin incision, arthrotomy, extensor mechanism, deep dissection, and cement technique.

Patient Positioning

Ideally, the patient is positioned with the knee at 90°. However, optimal exposure through a small incision requires moving and stressing the knee in a variety of positions. It also requires ranging the knee from full extension to full flexion throughout the operation. The leg should be set up with a buttress and draped so that the surgeon can apply valgus and varus stresses as needed.

The skin-incision location is important, especially if small incision length is essential. Most medial unicondylar knee replacements can be done through an 8-to 10-cm incision located just medial to the mid-pole of the patella and extending to tibial tubercle. It is helpful to undermine the subcutaneous tissues and mobilize the skin. The deep dissection can be extended beyond this skin incision so that the arthrotomy can extend from the quadriceps tendon to the tibial tubercle.

There is no need to evert the extensor mechanism, which greatly eases post-operative recovery. After the skin incision and subcutaneous mobilization is completed, the arthrotomy is extended from the superior pole of the patella to the tibial tubercle. With the knee in extension, the fat pad is partially resected and the medial corner of the patella is examined. Very little retropatellar fat pad is resected. Medial patellar osteophytes are removed, and the partial patellar facetectomy can be performed if necessary. Patellar mobility is assessed. The extensor mechanism needs to be mobilized so that the patella can be shifted laterally. If extensor mechanism cannot be adequately lateralized, the arthrotomy can be extended proximally into the quadriceps tendon. A small Z retractor can be levered against the lateral side of the medial femoral condyle and the medial side of the patella in order to shift the extensor mechanism laterally (◻ Fig. 9.44). The deep dissection is then continued

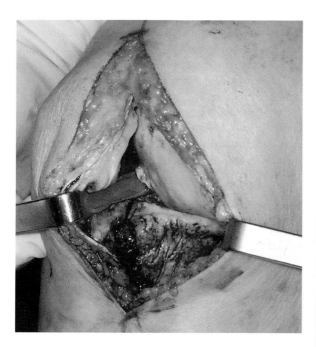

Fig. 9.44. The incision extends from the mid-pole of the patella to the tibial tubercle. After fat-pad and extensor release, a retractor is levered against the lateral aspect of the medial femoral condyle. The medial capsule release allows a retractor to be levered around the posterior medial corner of the tibia, protecting the medial collateral ligament during tibial osteotomy

postero-medially along the tibia. Releasing the coronary ligament and placing an angled Hohmann's retractor exposes tibial osteophytes. This step corrects medial contracture and aids in the removal of the tibial bone after tibial osteotomy. With his type of exposure, a modified Hohmann's can be placed along the medial tibial bone, protecting the medial collateral ligament and retracting the soft tissues out of the way during the transverse tibial osteotomy.

Tibial Osteotomy

The tibial osteotomy is one of the pivotal steps in unicondylar knee arthroplasty. It determines tibial slope, angular alignment, tibiofemoral mechanics, flexion and extension gaps, range of motion, and stability. It is important to take all of these elements into consideration as the osteotomy is performed. The osteotomy is begun by localizing the most deficient part of the diseased tibial condyle and placing an external tibial guide

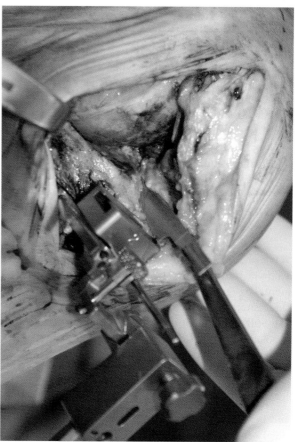

Fig. 9.45. The external tibial guide system localizes the sulcus of deficient tibial bone and is oriented correctly in all planes. A reciprocating saw blade is left in place after the sagittal cut

system. The surgeon needs to consider axial alignment, rotational alignment, the position of the tibial tubercle, and tibial slope. For a medial unicondylar tibial implant, the proper rotation can be referenced from tibial flare of the spine and the lateral side of the medial femoral condyle. A reciprocating saw is used to perform a the sagittal osteotomy. That saw blade can be left in place to prevent undercutting of the tibial spine during the transverse osteotomy (**Fig. 9.45**).

Once tibial alignment, slope, and rotation have been set, the tibial osteotomy is done using the most conservative resection possible. The difference between the thickness of the tibial bone resected and the thickness of an onlay tibial insert determines angular alignment. Varus knees that can be corrected with a valgus stress and have a full range of motion will need very little bone

9.5.1

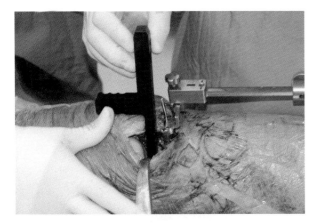

Fig. 9.46. The tibial osteotomy has been completed, and an 8-mm tensor block is used to evaluate ligament balancing. Alignment rods can be combined with the tensor blocks to assess the impact of thicker tibial implants on alignment

resected. Knees with a fixed varus deformity and a fixed flexion contracture will require more bone resection in order to accommodate an 8-mm polyethylene insert. It is difficult to accurately estimate the ideal amount of tibial bone to be resected based on standard bony landmarks. After an initial, 2-mm resection, a tensor block is combined with alignment rods to evaluate ligament balancing and alignment in flexion and extension. With the knee in full extension, increasing thickness of the tensor block creates a more valgus alignment, and the alignment rod projects further and further away from the femoral head (■ Fig. 9.46).

Fitting the Femoral Component

Preparing the femoral condyle and placing a unicondylar femoral component differs greatly from total knee arthroplasty. Sizing and positioning of the femoral component begins with identifying the tidemark and the medial-to-lateral width and contour of the femoral condyle. Since the fit is very precise, removing all osteophytes helps to avoid over-sizing and medial overhang. The femoral cutting guide can be combined with a flexion space tensioner. This instrumentation "links" the femoral posterior resection to the tibial cut and ensures appropriate ligament balancing. The positioning of the instrumentation needs to be evaluated for flexion space tensioning, femoral sizing, and femoral fit (■ Fig. 9.47).

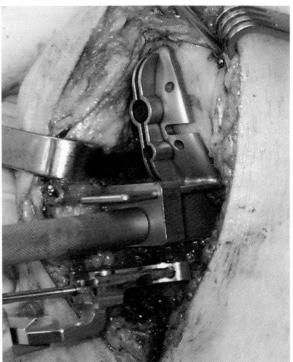

Fig. 9.47. A flexion space tensioner is linked to the femoral posterior resection guide. Final position of this guide is based on the tibial osteotomy, the flexion space, and the femoral condylar anatomy

Unicondylar knee replacements preserve native femoral anatomy, and the femoral component is essentially fitted to that anatomy. Angular alignment is determined by the tibial osteotomy and thickness of the tibial component. Conversely, the coronal rotation and placement of the femoral component has little impact on angular alignment. Fortunately, the femoral component is designed to allow 10° of variation in the varus/valgus plane without edge-loading. Therefore, femoral component positioning can be determined according to the shape of the femur. Femoral component design and instrumentation allows for small adjustments in the sagittal, coronal, and axial planes in order to achieve maximum capping without medial overhang or lateral impingement. Once the position of the posterior resection has been linked to the tibial cut, it is appropriate to make minor adjustments in the axial rotation in order to optimize the fit. After the posterior resection is completed, a tensioner can be used to confirm the accuracy of the cut and flexion space balancing.

Placement of the distal femoral bur guide is another pivotal step in a resurfacing, unicondylar knee replacement. It determines coronal rotation of the implant and the depth and completeness of the distal femoral resection. There is significant variation in shape from one normal femoral condyle to the next, and these variations need to be considered as the bur guide is placed. Errors in this step can lead to medial overhang, lateral impingement, and incomplete distal resections.

A unicondylar femoral component resurfaces the femur distal and posterior and does not capture the femur anterior the way total knee femoral components do. Unicondylar femoral components cannot allow any gaps. Gaps, especially posterior, will create tension forces on the component/cement interface and ultimately lead to failure. Femoral cutting jigs, milling guides, and tensor blocks can be sequenced and utilized so that gaps are not created. The distal femoral bone in the knee with medial compartment osteoarthritis is typically deficient. If the bur guide is positioned appropriately on the posterior resection, this femoral deficiency creates an apparent gap distal. If the gap is eliminated by simply impacting the guide, a posterior gap is created. Therefore, the distal gap should be managed by systematically improving the fit of the bur guide. This is done by eliminating the apex of the bone between the posterior resection and the distal femoral condyle and the removing anterior osteophytes using the high-speed bur (□ Fig. 9.48). Finally, it is very helpful to overstuff the flexion space with tensioning blocks as the bur guide is positioned and impacted (□ Fig. 9.49). Eliminating posterior gapping and managing the fit distally creates a precise and accurate fit between the femoral component and host bone. Since unicondylar femoral components are not captured, this is a critically important nuance of unicondylar technique.

Cement Technique in Unicondylar Knee Replacement

Cementing techniques for unicondylar knee replacement are different from those of total knee replacement. The main differences stem from bone quality, the more limited exposure of unicondylar knee replacement, and the potential to develop retained cement posterior. Bone resections on the tibial and femoral side are quite conservative, leaving dense, sclerotic bone for cement surfaces. A bur can be used to penetrate sclerotic bone, and applying cement before it begins to set up helps as well.

It is critical to avoid excess cement. Using an implant to pressurize mounded-up cement leads to extrusion

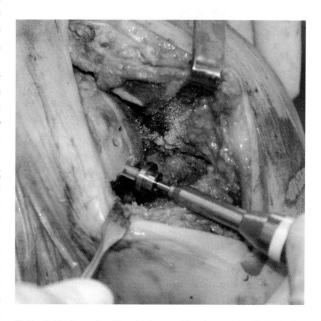

□ **Fig. 9.48.** An end cutting, high-speed bur is used to eliminate the apex between the posterior femoral resection and the deficient distal femur as well as anterior femoral osteophytes. This improves the fit between the milling guide and the native femoral anatomy

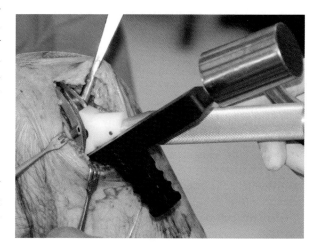

□ **Fig. 9.49.** After optimizing the fit between the host bone and the milling guide, a tension block is placed in flexion space to force the milling guide against the posterior femoral resection. The milling guide is gently impacted into position

and poor penetration of cement into bone. Intrusion without extrusion is achieved by using a cement tool to pressurize small amounts of cement. Excess cement can easily be removed, and additional increments of cement can be pressurized until the bone surface is fully impregnated. Once this process of intrusion without extrusion is completed, cement is evenly pressurized over the entire cancellous bed and little or no cement is seen above the bone surface.

Cement is then thoroughly but carefully preloaded onto the implant. In the case of the tibial implant, cement is carefully packed into the dovetail insets. Again, little or no excess cement is used. The cement is already pressurized, and any mounded cement only serves to create extrusion. The tibial component can be seated in an a posterior-to-anterior direction, forcing extruded cement anterior. A soap sponge can be packed into the popliteal space prior to cementing. This restricts cement that may extrude. Excess cement can be removed as the sponge is removed. This same basic technique is useful for the femoral side. It is easy to safely preload femoral bone over the distal femoral condyle. The posterior femoral resection should be preloaded carefully and conservatively with a cement tool. Any preloading posterior must leave the cement flush with bone so that cement is not piled posterior as the implant is placed. Instead, preload cement on the implant. This will help keep extruded cement out of the popliteal space.

Conclusions

Unicondylar knee replacement can be much more than a minimally invasive resurfacing of worn out tibial and femoral joint surfaces. This procedure can and should adhere to the basic principles that have established total knee replacements as one of the most successful, reliable and durable operations available. Authors have shown that results of unicondylar knee replacement can be comparable to those of total knee replacement. However, other reports have shown that poor implant design, surgical technique, and patient selection can lead to disappointing results [20]. The use of an onlay tibial component enables precise management of component position, flexion and extension spaces, alignment, and tibio-femoral kinematics. Modern component design combined with precise and conservative bone resections provides stable, reliable, and durable fixation. Instrumentation and surgical techniques that enable accurate restoration of ideal alignment will help prevent opposite-compartment degeneration, polyethylene wear, loosening, and subsidence. In an era when total knee replacement is becoming less invasive and more reliable, unicondylar knee replacement must achieve comparably reliable, long-term results.

References

1. Barrett WP, Scott RD (1987) Revision of failed unicondylar knee arthroplasty. J Bone Joint Surg 69: 1328–1335
2. Bartel DL, Bicknell VL, Wright TM (1986) The effect of conformity, thickness, and material on stress in ultra high molecular weight components for joint replacements J Bone Joint Surg 68: 1041
3. Böhm I, Landsiedl F (2000) Revision surgery after failed unicompartmental knee arthroplasty. J Arthroplasty 15: 982–989
4. Cartier P, Sanouiller J, Grelsamer RP (1996) Unicompartmental knee arthroplasty: ten year minimum follow-up. J Arthroplasty 11: 782–788
5. Deshmukh RV, Scott RD (2001) Unicompartmental knee arthroplasty: long-term results. CORR 392: 272–278
6. Engh GA (2002) Can we justify unicondylar arthroplasty as a temporizing procedure? J Arthroplasty 17 [Suppl 1]: 54–55
7. Giou T, Killeen K, Hoeffel D, Bert J, Comfort T, Scheltema K, Mehle S (2003) Analysis of unicompartmental arthroplasty in a community-based implant registry. 70th Annual Meeting Proceedings, AAOS, p 561
8. Hernigou P, Deschamps G, le Fort, D (2003) Unicompartmental knee arthroplasty: Influence of post-operative alignment on wear, loosening, and recurrence of deformity. The 70th Annual Proceedings, AAOS: p 561
9. Hyldahl HC, Regner L, Carlsson L, Carrholm J, Heidenhielm L (2001) Does metal backing improve fixation of tibial component in unicondylar knee arthroplasty? A randomized radiostereometric analysis. J Arthroplasty 16: 174–179
10. Laskin RS (2001) Unicompartmental knee replacement: some unanswered questions. CORR 392: 267–271
11. Levine WN, Ozuna RM, Scott RB, Thornhill TS (1996) conversion of failed modern unicompartmental arthroplasty to total knee arthroplasty. J Arthroplasty 11: 797–801
12. Marmor L (1988) Unicompartmental knee arthroplasty: Ten to 13 year follow up study CORR 226: 14
13. McAuley JP, Engh GA, Ammeen DJ (2001) Revision of failed unicompartmental knee arthroplasty. CORR 392: 279–282
14. Murray DW, Goodfellow JW, O'Connor JJ (1998) The Oxford Medial Unicompartmental Arthroplasty: a ten-year survival study. J Bone Joint Surg 8-B: 983–989
15. Padgett, DE, Stern SH, Insall, JN (1991) Revision total knee arthroplasty for failed unicompartmental replacement. J Bone Joint Surg 73: 186

16. Palmer SH, Morrison PJ, Ross AC (1998) Early catastrophic tibial component wear after unicompartmental knee arthroplasty. CORR 350: 143, 148
17. Repicci JA, Eberle RE (1999) Minimally invasive surgical technique for unicondylar knee arthroplasty. J Southern Orthop Assoc 8: 20–27
18. Romanowski MR, Repicci JI (2002) Minimally invasive unicondylar arthroplasty: eight-year follow-up. J Knee Surg 15: 17–22
19. Rougraff BT, Heck DA, Gibson EE (1991) A comparison of tricompartmental and unicompartmental arthroplasty for treatment of gonarthrosis. Clin Orthop 273: 157–164
20. Sculco TP (2002) Can we justify unicondylar arthroplasty as a temporizing procedure? J Arthroplasty 17 [Suppl 1]: 56–58
21. Stockelman RE, Pohl KP (1991) Long-term efficacy of unicompartmental arthroplasty of the knee. CORR 271: 88–95
22. Squire MW, Callaghan J, Goetz D, Sullivan PM, Johnston RC (1999) Unicompartmental knee replacement: a minimum 15-year follow-up study. CORR 367: 61–72
23. Tabor OB, Tabor OB (1998) Unicompartmental arthroplasty: A long term follow-up study. J Arthroplasty 13: 373–379
24. Weale AE, Halabi, OA, Jones PW, White SH (2001) Perceptions of outcome after unicompartmental and total knee replacements. CORR 382: 143–153
25. Weale AE, Murray DW, Baines J, Newman JH (2000) Radiological changes five years after unicompartmental knee replacement. J Bone Joint Surg 8-B: 996–1000

9.5.1

Part IV   Minimally Invasive total Joint Arthro-
plasty and Computer Assisted Surgery

10

How Can CAOS Support MIS TKR and THR? – Background and Significance

A. Wolf, A.B. Mor, B. Jaramaz, A.M. DiGioia III

Many areas of surgery have been revolutionized by the development of minimally invasive surgical (MIS) procedures enabled by the introduction of fiberoptic technology (i.e. arthroscopy, endoscopy, laparoscopy, etc.) The clinical benefits to patients are profound when an "open" procedure can be made minimally or less invasive. By definition, performing any procedure less invasively results in less soft-tissue and bone disruption, which reduces pain, speeds healing and the recovery of patients, and potentially reduces complications. However, there are also new challenges that surgeons face when trying to develop techniques that are minimally invasive. For instance, if a less invasive technique limits the surgeon's ability to achieve the surgical goal, then the procedure cannot be considered a success. In addition, if the surgeon's view of the work area is limited, then the procedure could potentially be less accurate or damage surrounding structures, which would also result in a less than optimal outcome for the patient.

Compared to other surgical disciplines, adult reconstructive orthopedic surgery has fallen behind the trend to make procedures minimally invasive because of several unique challenges. For example, in the area of total joint-replacement (TJR) surgery, surgeons focus on both bone and joint surfaces. However, many of the complications that develop during or following surgery are directly related to the way surgeons handle the soft tissues, rather than the bone. The current techniques require extensive soft-tissue dissections to accurately prepare the bone and insert the implant. In addition, the tools that surgeons use to plan and execute TJR have not significantly changed in over 30 years of joint-replacement surgery.

There are many inherent benefits of developing MIS techniques for TJR, including: reduced soft-tissue and bone dissections, less bleeding, fewer infections and dislocations, less damage to surrounding muscles, ligaments, nerves or blood vessels, less pain and a faster recovery for the patient. There will also be less disruption of the blood supply to bone and surrounding soft tissues, resulting in better overall healing, which will be especially important as we develop new biologic based tissue-engineered joint-replacement surfaces.

The surgical goals in joint reconstruction procedures and TJR are to relieve pain by reconstructing or replacing the diseased joint surfaces with a new surface. Currently, we use man-made artificial replacement surfaces. In the future, though, surgeons will likely be able to replace a damaged surface with a tissue-engineered composite graft, consisting of bone and cartilage grown in vitro from the patient's own tissues. Key to the success of any reconstructive joint surgery, whether using man-made or biologic materials, is to obtain an accurate fit and fixation of the implants to the prepared surfaces and to achieve good overall limb alignment. In addition, the interaction between the bones and soft tissues like ligaments, muscles and capsular restraints is another large contributor to the functioning of the joint after reconstruction. Adding to the challenge, both natural and reconstructed joints are subjected to extremely large forces requiring relatively rigid implants of significant bulk, making introduction of the artificial or biologic component in a less invasive way difficult. Satisfying these requirements – proper fixation, joint alignment, and soft-tissue balancing – is critical to the successful performance of the reconstructed joint and positive patient outcomes.

Because of these challenges, current surgical exposures are large and require extensive soft-tissue dissections to access, visualize and prepare the bone surfaces for implantation and to insert the new artificial joint surface. Surgeons and clinical researchers also lack sensitive measurement devices that can be used both during surgery and post-operatively to accurately gauge factors like alignment, soft-tissue balancing, load transfer, implant wear, loosening or implant migration.

In general, there are three main components of most adult reconstructive surgical procedures: bone preparation, soft-tissue balancing, and the insertion and fixation of the new (artificial or biologic) surface. Adult reconstructive surgeons undertake several interdependent and sequential tasks in order to achieve the surgical goals:

— Soft-tissue dissection and surgical exposure in order to visualize the bone and joint surfaces to be reconstructed.
— Evaluate interaction of bone and soft-tissue constraints (ligaments, capsular, muscular).
— Preparation and shaping of the bone surface.
— Insertion and fixation of the implant or resurfacing material.
— Evaluation of composite bone/implant/soft-tissue system (range of motion, balancing, stability, etc.).
— Closure and repair of the surgically altered soft tissues.
— Post-operative follow up and evaluations.

By addressing each of these steps, we can identify several clinical and technical challenges to overcome in order to perform truly minimally invasive joint-reconstructive surgery and provide the post-operative tools to gauge and quantify surgical outcomes. For instance, on the purely clinical side, minimally invasive procedures should utilize surgical exposures that reduce the trauma on the patient's soft tissue and bone, not only the incision length, which could reduce rehabilitation time for the patient. CAOS, though, can help improve surgical performance in all these areas.

Advanced visualization methods that allow surgeons to view models of the underlying anatomy through the skin have been developed (❑ Fig. 10.1), and are being improved upon. CAOS systems, such as

surgical navigation tools, can assist in the evaluation of the interaction between bone and soft tissue through a combination of tracking of the patient's pre- and intraoperative motion and prediction based on biomechanical models of the patient's anatomy. Tracking and displaying the patient's actual motion, and simulating possible outcomes based on surgical plans can improve the surgeon's understanding of the surgical outcome (❑ Fig. 10.2). This can improve prediction accuracy

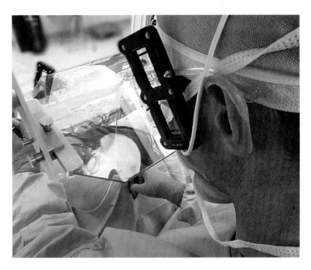

❑ **Fig. 10.1.** Advanced visualization with Image Overlay, where virtual models are overlaid onto patient anatomy

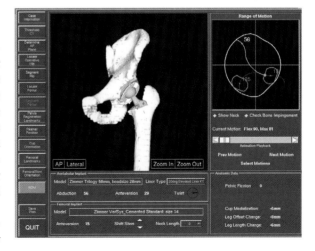

❑ **Fig. 10.2.** Prediction of post-operative outcome for total hip arthroplasty

compared to models solely based on pre-operative images, due to additional information and constraints introduced by tracking patient motion. Evaluation of the patient's motion can be used pre-operatively, intra-operatively, and post-operatively to accurately characterize the patient's biomechanics. Navigation systems to assist the surgeon in accurately locating and placing cutting tools, cutting guides, and implants are already available commercially. More advanced robotic or semi-active devices which will help the surgeon cut more precisely (☐ Fig. 10.3), and to actually cut the implant cavity directly with a small robotic platform (☐ Fig. 10.4), are currently being developed. These small active and semi-active robotic systems will help motivate the development of smaller implant components that conform more closely to the natural anatomical shape, rather than the large bulky implants currently in use designed to be inserted onto flat surfaces. Post-operative follow-up is also being improved with CAOS tools, allowing accurate determination of implant component positions from a standard post-operative radiograph (☐ Fig. 10.5).

In order to perform less or minimally invasive surgery, adult reconstructive surgeons will need to perform more accurate and precise pre-operative planning coupled with simulations of their actions before the actual patient's surgery. Surgical techniques will need to be radically modified. Technically, less invasive surgical tools and more powerful intra-operative visualization devices that can provide updated images of the bone surfaces and soft tissues being manipulated in a less invasive way are needed. These tools also require high fidelity and accurate pre-operative planners and surgical

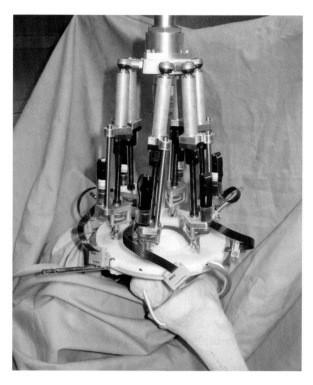

☐ Fig. 10.4. Miniature Bone-Attached Robotic System (MBARS) that directly attaches to the bone before milling the implant cavity

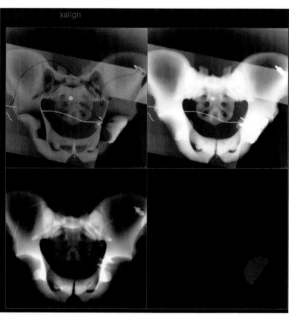

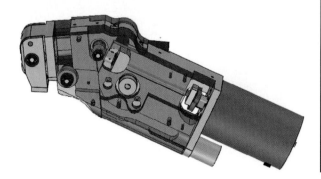

☐ Fig. 10.3. Precision Freehand Sculptor (PFS) that only cuts in areas with tissue to be removed

☐ Fig. 10.5. Accurate evaluation of post-operative radiograph using Xalign

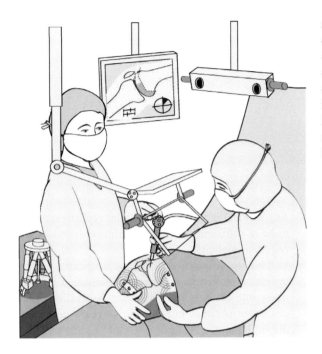

■ **Fig. 10.6.** Next-generation CAOS/MIS surgical tool suite

simulators. Then, in order to address the wide spectrum of clinical challenges faced by surgeons, various enabling technologies will need to be integrated into a complete MIS system (■ Fig. 10.6). This next generation of tools will include surgical planners and simulators, image-guided navigation systems, image overlay visualization, micro-electromechanical systems (MEMS) sensors and actuators, micromanipulators and other robotic surgical devices.

CT-based Navigation for Knees and Hips in Minimally Invasive Surgery

F. Langlotz, L.-P. Nolte

Introduction

The use of a surgical navigation system improves intra-operative visibility into the surgical situs and has therefore been believed to provide the means towards less or even minimally invasive interventions. However, these expectations have usually not been met during the experimental or routine application of navigation systems for total knee or total hip arthroplasty. In contrast, the increased accuracy and safety of this technology had often to be paid for with larger incisions, increased blood loss, prolonged operation times, or additional trauma.

This article tries to highlight the reasons for this apparent discrepancy and summarizes current developments that aim at overcoming the dilemma. The basic principles and concepts of surgical navigation in the domain of orthopedics have been presented in detail before [1, 2] and will therefore not be covered by this paper.

Invasiveness of Surgical Interventions

The treatment of pathologies that are situated deep inside a patient's body such as arthritis or other joint diseases requires the direct access to these anatomical structures. Established surgical approaches grant this access through superjacent layers of soft tissue. In general, three reasons [3] can be identified why orthopedic surgery has to be invasive in the first place:

- Instruments that are employed to treat pathologies need to have contact to the diseased structures. Such contact can obviously be realized in an invasive manner only.
- During total joint replacement, implant components need to be anchored into the bone, and these components need to be delivered to the anchoring sites.

Any surgical incision for total joint replacement has to be of sufficient size to enable introduction of the required implants.

- Last but not least, visual feedback is essential for the operating surgeon, and the optic sensation is definitely one of the most important impressions that guarantee optimal intra-operative performance of the surgeon.

Obviously, optimizing surgical skills and the development of dedicated surgical approaches [4] are means to minimize invasiveness as induced by the first reason given above. Implant manufacturers are constantly advancing their instruments and implants to enable less invasive techniques of arthroplasty [5]. Improving the insight into the surgical action that takes place in the situs is potentially a third way to reduce the invasiveness of surgical interventions while maintaining precision. Although mechanical aiming devices have been proposed as tools to achieve this goal, their accuracy has been highly questioned [6].

Computer Assistance to Reduce Invasiveness

With the introduction of CT-based computer-assisted navigation systems in the mid-nineties of the last century [2] a technology became available that was believed to pave the road for less invasive or even minimally invasive surgical procedures [7–9]. However, the enthusiasm and optimism of these pioneers did not turn out to become reality except for a very limited number of selected applications [10–12].

This apparent discrepancy lies in the additional steps that are required for CT-based navigation [1]. The unavoidable relative motion of the operated bony structures needs to be compensated [13] by means of one or

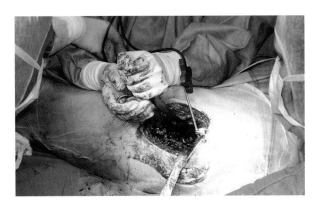

□ Fig. 11.1. During navigated total hip replacement, a dynamic reference base is attached to the pelvis through the standard surgical access

more so-called dynamic reference bases (DRB) [9]. These devices require a rigid and stable connection to the bone to be operated on. In the case of total hip replacement one DRB is affixed to the pelvic crest [10] and/or the femur [14] through the existing (□ Fig. 11.1) or even additional incisions. During total knee replacement, DRBs are inserted into the distal femur and the proximal tibia [15]. Early implementations of surgical navigation for TKR required even the placement of a DRB to the pelvis [16, 17] in order to enable precise acquisition of the mechanical axis of the limb.

Using any pre-operative image data such as a CT scan as the virtual object of a navigation system requires a registration between the patient's anatomy and this image [1]. Many mathematical methods have been presented [18] to achieve registration between the underlying coordinate spaces, but all early implementations relied upon the direct digitization of features such as anatomical landmarks on the bony surfaces of the operated structures. It is obvious that such a data collection using a tracked pointer [9] prohibits the introduction of minimally invasive procedures.

In order to overcome the described obstacles, alternative, less or non-invasive methods for registration and/or referencing were required and a large variety of different approaches have been proposed.

Alternative Ways of Registration

Intra-operative and interactive registration of the patient's anatomy with a pre-operative image-data set is

obviously not required when using intra-operatively acquired image data for navigation purposes [14, 19]. However, this aspect of computer-assisted total knee and hip arthroplasty is beyond the focus of this article and shall therefore not be addressed.

The probably most obvious approach to minimally invasive registration is to use a different method of point-data acquisition which will eventually permit the established mathematical algorithms to be applied that have been developed for pointer-based registration. Calibrated ultrasound has been proposed as a means to accurately determine deeply located bone contours. First applications using A-mode ultrasound probes in the context of navigation were presented for neurosurgical interventions [20] and are still being applied in the area of the skull [21]. However, inherent difficulties proved this method to be non-applicable during orthopedic surgery, in particular when applied for the registration of deep structures such as the pelvis or femur [22]. Especially the linear reflection of the sound pulse causes problems, since it requires the ultrasound probe to be oriented perpendicularly to the surface to be assessed. B-mode ultrasound technology overcomes this disadvantage. The acquired images are two-dimensionally and show bone boundaries that can be determined. As a result, the location of points along such a surface line may be fed into a registration algorithm. However, B-mode ultrasound images are usually very noisy, and the automated determination of bone contours is non-trivial. Tonetti et al. [23] therefore presented an approach involving the interactive intra-operative segmentation of the acquired ultrasonic images. They could demonstrate a sufficient accuracy of their approach when used at the pelvis. The problem of reliable, automatic bone-contour detection from B-mode ultrasonography has meanwhile been solved experimentally [24, 25] as shown in □ Fig. 11.2, but has not been used clinically in a broad way so far.

Another method to acquire the locations of points without accessing them directly is provided by calibrated C-arm fluoroscopy [26]. If two or more two-dimensional projection images are acquired of an anatomical location from different directions, three-dimensional locations can be calculated with the help of a triangulation approach. The spot to be reconstructed is identified on each of the images resulting in a set of lines in 3D space along the respective projection direction. The associated 3D point can then be found at the intersection of these lines. This method involves the interactive

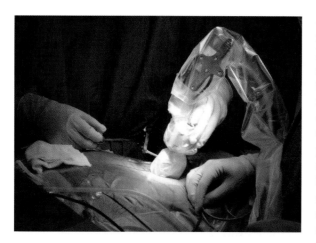

◩ **Fig.11.2.** In a prototype setup, a calibrated and tracked ultrasound probe is used to acquire bone contours in a minimally invasive manner. Behind the probe, a dynamic reference base is visible that is fixated through a stab incision

digitization of landmarks in the acquired images, which can be accomplished in an operating-room-compatible manner [14]. However, this procedure is rather time-consuming and tiresome. It is thus difficult to be promoted for the acquisition of larger quantities of points as needed for exact intra-operative registration.

The logically next step in the development of fluoroscopy-based registration techniques was the automated feature extraction from the recorded images to enable a less cumbersome intra-operative application of this technology. This "fluoromatching" method has been implemented for navigated spinal surgery. First, the surgeon needs to specify the vertebra to be registered. The associated CT data is then presented in a lateral and anteroposterior view, and corresponding fluoroscopic images need to be acquired with the DRB in place. To initialize the registration algorithm, the surgeon manually aligns both images with the CT views, and the system tries to refine this coarse registration. Despite the considerable amount of interactivity that this approach requires, the concept is still lacking perfect reliability [27].

Alternative Ways of Referencing

Referencing is essential for any kind of surgical navigation [13]. It is of particular importance when pre-operative images are used as virtual objects since there is no

correspondence between the patient's position during image acquisition and during the actual operation. Robotically-assisted surgery achieves referencing by means of a mechanical link between the robot and the bone to be operated on [28] or by mounting a miniature robot directly onto the bone [29]. These approaches often result in an increased invasiveness when compared to the respective conventional techniques. However, the placement of dynamic reference bases during total knee and total hip replacement also involves steps of increased invasiveness in the very most cases. DiGioia et al. anchored the DRB through a small additional incision "near the wing of the ilium" [10], while DRB fixation during total knee replacement is usually possible through the standard surgical approaches.

Hardly any research has been performed with the aim to reduce the invasiveness of DRB placement. Lund et al. presented a prototype system for navigated spine surgery [30] in which they reduced the incision for fixing the reference base to a minimum. However, a portion of their reference base (◩ Fig. 11.3) had to be implanted

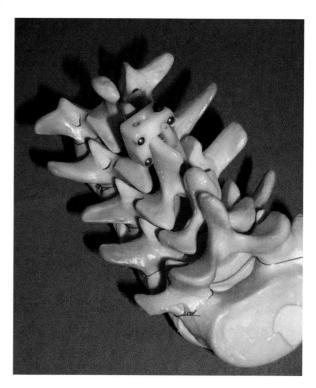

◩ **Fig. 11.3.** This base block of a spinal dynamic reference base (DRB) is put into place prior to pre-operative CT scanning. It then enables DRB attachment without any further exposure

prior to CT scanning, i.e. pre-operatively, which was found to be unacceptable for routine use. Apparently, there is no technique available for referencing of the operated anatomy that does not rely upon the physical attachment of a reference base. Hence, approaches towards less or minimally invasive referencing have to focus on the development of associated fixation techniques for DRBs or come up with entirely different solutions. If, for instance, ultrasound registration could be realized in real-time and in a fully automatic way, the resultant matching transformation could be constantly re-calculated during navigation, essentially eliminating the need for any separate referencing.

Conclusions

CT-based surgical navigation provides means to improve visual perception during total joint replacement. In this sense, the technique has the potential to contribute to a reduction of the invasiveness. Current approaches, however, usually require invasive access to the operated bone for the acquisition of registration data and the fixation of dynamic reference bases. A major focus of research was and is the desire to implement alternative registration methods. Referencing – up to now – has received less attention potentially due to the absence of complementary ways to compensate for motion of the patient relative to the tracking system. At present least invasive navigation support can be achieved using computer-assisted systems that use intra-operative [31] rather than pre-operative image data. However, one important positive aspect of CT-based navigation must not be underestimated: only a three-dimensional scan of the pre-operative pathologic situation of a joint allows planning the operation sterically and enables the sophisticated simulation of the post-operative performance of the prosthesis [10].

References

1. Langlotz F, Nolte LP. Technical approaches for computer-assisted orthopaedic surgery. Eur J Trauma 30: 1–11, 2004
2. Sugano N. Computer-assisted orthopaedic surgery. J Orthop Sci 8: 442–448, 2003
3. Langlotz F, Keeve E. Minimally invasive approaches in orthopaedic surgery. Minim Invasiv Ther 12: 19–24, 2003
4. Berger RA. Total hip arthroplasty using the minimally invasive two-incision approach. Clin Orthop 417: 232–241, 2003
5. Sherry E, Egan M, Warnke PH, Henderson A, Eslick GD. Minimal invasive surgery for hip replacement: a new technique using the NILNAV hip system. Aust NZ J Surg 73: 157–161, 2003
6. Digioia AM 3rd, Jaramaz B, Plakseychuk AY, Moody JE Jr, Nikou C, Labarca RS, Levison TJ, Picard F. Comparison of a mechanical acetabular alignment guide with computer placement of the socket. J Arthroplasty 17: 359–364, 2002
7. Kalfas IH, Kormos DW, Murphy MA, McKenzie RL, Barnett GH, Bell GR, Steiner CP, Trimble MB, Weisenberger JP. Application of frameless stereotaxy to pedicle screw fixation of the spine. J Neurosurg 83: 641–647, 1995
8. Merloz P, Tonetti J, Pittet L, Coulomb M, Lavallée S, Traccaz J, Cinquin P, Sautot P. Computer-assisted spine surgery. Comput Aided Surg 3: 297–305, 1998
9. Nolte LP, Visarius H, Langlotz F, Schwarzenbach O, Berlemann U, Rohrer U. Computer-assisted spine surgery – a generalized concept and early clinical experiences. Int Soc Comput Aided Surg 3: 1–6, 1996
10. DiGioia AM III, Jaramaz B, Nikou C, LaBarca RS, Moody JE, Colgan BD. Surgical navigation for total hip replacement with the use of HipNav. Oper Techn Orthop 10: 3–8, 2000
11. Grützner PA, Vock B, Zheng G, Kowal J, Nolte LP, Wentzensen. Minimalinvasive, computerassistierte Plattenosteosynthese bei Frakturen langer Röhrenknochen. In: Kirschner P, Sturmer KM (eds) Hefte zu "Der Unfallchirurg", Vol. 283. Berlin, Heidelberg: Springer, p 160, 2001
12. Grützner PA, Rose E, Vock B, Holz F, Nolte LP, Wentzensen A. Computer-assistierte perkutane Verschraubung des hinteren Beckenrings – Erste Erfahrungen mit einem Bildwandler basierten optoelektronischen Navigationssystem. Unfallchirurg 105: 254–260, 2002
13. Glossop N, Hu R. Effects of tracking adjacent vertebral bodies during image guided pedicle screw surgery. In: Troccaz J, Grimson E, Mösges R (eds) CVRMed-MRCAS 97. Berlin, Heidelberg: Springer, pp 531–540, 1997
14. Zheng G, Marx A, Langlotz U, Widmer KH, Buttaro M, Nolte LP. A hybrid CT-free navigation system for total hip arthroplasty. Comput Aided Surg 7: 129–145, 2002
15. Perlick L, Bäthis H, Tingart M, Grifka J. Implementation of a CT-based navigation system in two-stage reimplantation for infected total knee arthroplasty. Acta Orthop Belg 69: 355–360, 2003
16. Jenny JY, Boeri C. Computer-assisted implantation of total knee prostheses: a case-controlled comparative study with classical instrumentation. Comput Aided Surg 6: 217–220, 2001
17. Sparmann M, Wolke B, Czupalla H, Banzer D, Zink A. Positioning of total knee arthroplasty with and without navigation support. A prospective, randomised study. J Bone Joint Surg Br 85B: 830–835, 2003
18. Maintz JBA, Viergever MA. A survey of medical image registration. Med Image Anal 2: 1–36, 1998.
19. Stulberg SD, Loan P, Sarin V. Computer-assisted navigation in total knee replacement: results of an initial experience in thirty-five patients. J Bone Joint Surg Am 84A Suppl 2: 90–98, 2002
20. Schreiner S, Galloway RLJ, Lewis JT, Bass WA, Muratore DM. An ultrasonic approach to localization of fiducial markers for interactive, image-guided neurosurgery – part II: implementation and automation. IEEE Trans Biomed Eng 45: 631–641, 1998
21. Amstutz C, Caversaccio M, Kowal J, Bächler R, Nolte LP, Häusler R, Styner M. A-mode ultrasound-based registration in computer-aid-

ed surgery of the skull. Arch Otolaryngol Head Neck Surg 129: 1310–1316, 2003

22. Hüfner T, Oszwald M, Kfuri M Jr., Rosenthal H, Citak M, Krettek C. A-mode ultrasound registration in computer assisted pelvic surgery. In: Langlotz F, Davies BL, Bauer A (eds) Computer-assisted orthopaedic surgery – 3rd Annual Meeting of CAOS-International (Proceedings). Darmstadt: Steinkopff, pp 148–149, 2003

23. Tonetti J, Carrat L, Blendea S, Merloz P, Troccaz J, Lavallée S, Chirossel JP. Clinical results of percutaneous pelvic surgery – computer-assisted surgery using ultrasound compared to standard fluoroscopy Comput Aided Surg 6: 204–211, 2001

24. Amin DV, Kanade T, DiGioia AM 3rd, Jaramaz B. Ultrasound registration of the bone surface for surgical navigation. Comput Aided Surg 8: 1–16, 2003

25. Kowal J, Amstutz CA, Nolte LP. On B-mode ultrasound-based registration for computer assisted orthopaedic surery. Comput Aided Surg 6: 47, 2001

26. Hofstetter R, Slomczykowski M, Krettek C, Koppen G, Sati M, Nolte LP. Computer-assisted fluoroscopy-based reduction of femoral fractures and antetorsion correction. Comput Aided Surg 5: 311–325, 2000

27. Verheyden AP, Glasmacher S, Hölzl A, Katscher S, Josten C. First experiences with CT-fluoromatching navigation of transoral C1 instrumentation in displaced atlas fractures using the ENT headset. In: Langlotz F, Davies BL, Bauer A (eds) Computer-assisted orthopaedic surgery. Darmstadt: Steinkopff, pp 386–387, 2003

28. Jakopec M, Harris SJ, Rodriguez y Baena F, Gomes P, Cobb J, Davies BL. The first clinical application of a "hands-on" robotic knee surgery system. Comput Aided Surg 6: 329–339, 2001

29. Ritschl P, Machacek Jr. F, Fuiko R. Computer-assisted ligament balancing in TKR using the Galileo system. In: Langlotz F, Davies BL, Bauer A (eds) Computer-assisted orthopaedic surgery – 3rd Annual Meeting of CAOS-International (Proceedings). Darmstadt: Steinkopff, pp 304–305, 2003

30. Lund T, Schwarzenbach O, Jost B, Rohrer U. On minimally invasive lumbosacral spinal stabilization. In: Nolte LP, Ganz R (eds) Computer-assisted orthopedic surgery (CAOS). Seattle: Hogrefe & Huber, pp 114–120, 1999

31. Jenny JY, Boeri C. Unicompartmental knee prosthesis implantation with a non-image-based navigation system with either conventional or mini-invasive approach. Tech Orthop 18: 167–173, 2003

11

Direct Anterior Approach Using Image-Free Navigation

M. Nogler, F. Rachbauer, J. Schaffer

Introduction

As described in an earlier chapter, the direct anterior approach is a single-incision approach. The skin incision is made two fingerbreadths distal to the anterior superior iliac spine at the ventral border of the tensor fasciae latae muscle. The surgical portal lies between the lateral border comprised of the tensor muscle and the sartorius and rectus femoris muscle medially. The entire length of the incision will vary slightly depending on body habitus, but 8 cm is the typical incision length in our patient population. Special retractors developed for this procedure allow for excellent access to the acetabulum. With angulated reamer handles and cup introducers, acetabular preparation and cup implantation can be accomplished without the need for a larger incision. Femoral preparation and implantation are facilitated using special retractors that elevate the femur to a position that permits satisfactory access for stem preparation and using instruments with an anterior offset.

When utilizing the small incision for a minimally invasive surgery approach, visualization of the operative field is decreased as compared to the traditional approach. More importantly, the instruments have angulated or curved handles that give the surgeon less intuitive information on the axis of the instrument. To date, the potential for positioning error using non-axial instruments has not been evaluated. The use of an electronic navigation system would negate or significantly decrease any potential positioning error. Such a system calculates the position of an instrument irrespective of the handle configuration and can direct the surgeon's efforts during preparation and implantation. The value of navigation for cup placement and orientation has been proven in multiple studies [1–4]. In a study by the authors' group, conventional cup implantation was compared to navigated cup implantation with the Hip Navigation System (Stryker-Leibinger, Freiburg, Germany). In this study, no pre-operative or peri-operative imaging study was necessary and the 90th percentile for inclination and anteversion of the conventionally operated group (15.7° inclination – 18.5° anteversion) demonstrated a significantly larger range of results than the navigated group (4.3° inclination – 7.1° anteversion). It was also shown that leg-length change could be minimized (<0.3 mm median leg-length change). These findings indicate that the use of navigation systems in total hip arthroplasty can positively impact the accuracy of implant position.

Implant-design and material combinations are consistent topics in hip arthroplasty, but recent advances have focused the current discussion on minimally invasive approach and the navigation systems. These recent developments will re-focus the implant design and material discussion such that implant designs specific to MIS will be forthcoming. The early results from our institution indicate that the combination of the direct anterior approach and the Stryker hip-navigation system has been successful in permitting accurate implantation of the total hip components and earlier mobilization of the patient.

The Imageless Concept

A surgical navigation system translates a patient's anatomy into a visual display of the implant position and orientation relative to that anatomy throughout the surgical procedure. There are currently two major navigation paradigms with regard to the acquisition of the relevant patient anatomy. The patient's anatomic structures can be defined either through pre-operatively (MRI, CT) or intra-operatively (fluoroscopy) acquired images or intra-operative digitization of anatomical landmarks that is not dependent on image acquisition. Such intra-operative digitization is performed with tactile probes percutaneously or through the open approach placing the probes directly at the anatomic point of interest. These navigation systems are known as imageless systems. Attempts to digitize bony landmarks with ultrasound probes have been made but are not yet clinically relevant [5–7].

An imageless navigation system that enables the surgeon to intra-operatively define anatomic landmarks and control instrument and implant position has several advantages:

1. No additional pre- or intra-operative radiation (an additional "invasiveness" that is not necessary),
2. All reference frames are acquired intra-operatively and can be checked and changed intra-operatively,
3. Pre-operatively preparation time is not increased waiting for the imaging study.

Tracking

Tracking of anatomic structures is the navigation system's responsibility and is done such that all bones are tracked independently. Currently, tracking is performed by all navigation systems with rigidly fixed bodies, that are either passive or active devices, such as those used with the Stryker Hip Navigation System. The trackers are fixed to the bone, using either screws or wires. The active devices are battery-powered electronic devices that are visible to the navigation system's cameras. Although fixation of these trackers can affect the minimally invasive nature of the approach we anticipate that solutions will eventually be found which permit non-invasive tracking. At the present, attaching the trackers should be undertaken using as minimally invasive an approach as possible.

Orientation and Landmarks

The orientation of the acetabular and femoral implants is based on intra-operatively determined landmarks and consecutively calculated reference frames that are updated in real-time. With the hip-navigation system (Stryker-Leibinger, Freiburg, Germany), these landmarks are acquired either precutaneously or – as in the case of the acetabular points – through the incision. ◻ Figure 12.1 gives an overview of the reference frames that are constructed intra-operatively by the system's software:

1. Acetabular component orientation is navigated, based on a pelvic reference frame defined by the two anterior superior iliac spines and a midpoint between the two pubic tubercles. Alternatively, a single point, the pubic symphysis, can be chosen. These points are digitized by the surgeon percutaneously with the pistol-grip pointer. The system calculates the cup position relative to the pelvic reference plane (PRP) according to DiGioia's definition of a "surgical alignment" [2]. Coordinates of these points are recorded relative to the pelvic tracker pin. The distance between the two pubic tubercles and the midpoint is calculated.
2. The orientation of the femoral component is determined relative to a femoral reference plane which is defined by the entry point of the anatomic femoral axes, the popliteal fossa, and the Achilles tendon midpoint, thus resembling the figure-of-four position of the leg.
3. Acetabular landmarks consist of the fovea – with the deepest point giving an estimation of the desired cup-placement depth –, the articular surface and the acetabular rim. Additionally, the articular surface points that are collected provide a graphical representation of the acetabulum during reaming and subsequent implantation.
4. The proximal shaft axes are measured intramedullarly for varus-valgus alignment of the stem.
5. The center of rotation of the hip is determined kinematically by moving the leg through a circumducted range of motion. New centers of rotation are defined later in the procedure after cup implantation and final reduction.

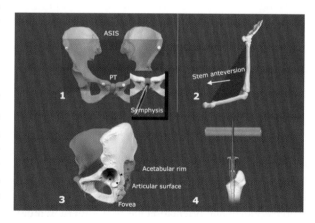

◻ **Fig. 12.1.** Indirect or direct digitization of anatomic landmarks is performed on the pelvic and femoral anatomic landmarks

System and Surgical Setup

The Stryker Hip Navigation System is equipped with up to three boom-mounted infrared cameras, which are able to track active, battery-powered instruments with LEDs communicating with the camera's localizing system. The system's software runs on a standard laptop (■ Fig. 12.2).

An active pistol-grip pointer is used as a software controller and to percutaneously digitize the anatomic

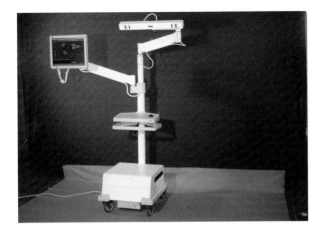

■ **Fig. 12.2.** The system with flat screen and a camera boom, containing three infrared cameras. The laptop is covered and installed in the box on bottom of the cart

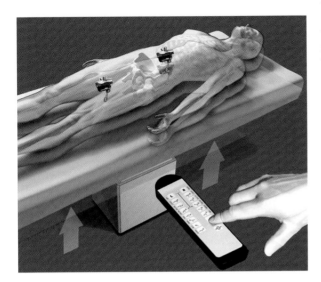

■ **Fig. 12.3.** The patient is placed in the supine position and draped such that both legs are moveable intra-operatively

landmarks. The specific geometric data of the instruments, such as length and configuration, and of the specific implants is known to the software through the user controls. The reaming process and implant impaction are navigated in real-time, showing the instrument's position and orientation on the screen as well as the numerical values of cup inclination and version.

For the direct anterior approach, the patient is placed in the supine position on the operative table and bilateral draping is performed such that both legs can be moved intra-operatively. One tracker is mounted on the screw which was percutaneously placed in the area of the ASIS. The distal screw is placed in the anterior aspect of the distal femur, approximately 15 cm proximally to the joint line of the knee. A device is available to use three K-wires instead of the distal screw, giving the same stability but offering better protection of the soft tissues (■ Fig. 12.3).

Navigation of the Femoral Neck Resection

In an open approach, resection of the femoral neck can be accomplished without the use of navigation. In the direct anterior approach, resection of the femoral neck is far more difficult due to the limited exposure of the proximal femur and the narrow workspace. Consequently, a resection-guidance module was implemented in the system that is based on the anatomic axes of the femur (■ Fig. 12.4). Current development work in our lab bases the resection model on digitized landmarks, such as the most distal point of the piriformis fossa as well as the border of the femoral neck.

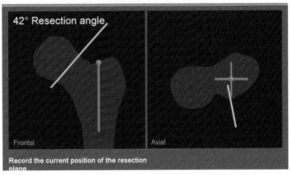

■ **Fig. 12.4.** Neck resection navigation is based on the anatomic axes

Cup Navigation

Based on the digitized pelvic PRP, the process of acetabular preparation and cup implantation is navigated in real-time. In addition to orientation of the reamers and the final component, the depth of the acetabulum is a major issue. In systems that are not image-based there is no knowledge about the thickness of the acetabular floor. The image-free navigation system permits the user to digitize the fovea and takes the deepest point along the acetabular entrance axis as the bottom of the acetabulum. During the reaming process, this point is defined as zero point. After preparation of the bone, the system establishes a new definition of the deepest point, e.g. the point which the deepest point of the acetabular implant reaches during impaction. Distance to the defined zero point is displayed in real-time (□ Fig. 12.5).

As depicted in □ Fig. 12.5 for the reaming and implantation of the acetabular component is monitored by the navigation system. Cup inclination and anteversion are displayed relative to the pelvic reference plane. After implantation, the final position of the acetabular component is recorded to define a new center of rotation. Throughout the process, the effects of the real-time cup position on leg length and offset are calculated and displayed on the screen. Results that are out of range are considered mal-placements and are displayed in red.

Stem Navigation

In order to define a femoral reference frame, a tracker screw or 3-wire fixation is placed in the distal femur. As discussed earlier in this chapter, both methods require additional incisions outside the surgical area. To date, however, no non-invasive alternatives are available. The anatomic reference frame is calculated based on the rotational center of the hip and the digitized landmarks. From these landmarks, the mechanical axis, anatomical shaft axes and a femoral reference plane (see □ Fig. 12.4) are calculated assuming that a normal vector of this plane directs to 0° of anteversion on the femoral neck (see □ Fig. 12.1). As neither the mechanical axes nor the anatomic shaft axes provide a valid orientation for the varus/valgus alignment of the femoral component, an additional step measures the proximal shaft axes intra-medullarly. These proximal shaft axes confound the references axes to which broaches and implant are aligned. As in the case of cup positioning, the system supports the navigation of reaming, broaching and placement of trial and final implants. Real-time display of the varus/valgus angle, rotation and depth are visualized on screen, based on position information of the trackable instruments relative to the femur (□ Fig. 12.6).

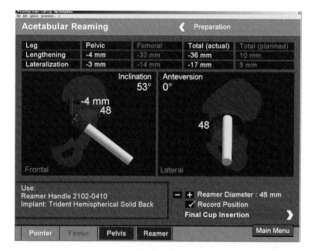

□ **Fig. 12.5.** The navigation screen for acetabular reaming, giving the position of the reamer relative to the PRP as well as the depth within the acetabulum. The effects of the cup placement on leg length and offset are displayed

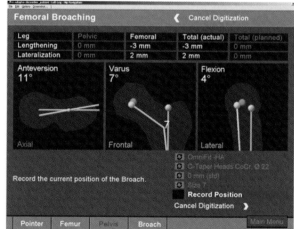

□ **Fig. 12.6.** The femoral navigation screen provides information on broach and stem position and rotation as well as the effects of the implant position as it changes on leg length and offset

Control over Leg Length and Offset

Equalizing a patient's leg length is an important outcome parameter in THA. Using a navigation system, the real-time changes in leg length during the process of cup- and femur preparation are calculated and a visual evaluation offered to the surgeon. The real-time implant position is calculated in part, based on the configuration information for the implants chosen for the procedure and contained in the system's database. In a traditional surgical approach, the surgeon is used to orienting the components in relation to anatomic landmarks such as the tip of t he greater trochanter or the depth of the fossa. During a procedure with a limited view of the surgical field, the navigation system provides the surgeon with the data to precisely control these crucial parameters leading to optimal implant position and orientation.

After the trial implants have been implanted, the navigation system provides for a trial reduction and evaluation of leg length and resulting offset as compared to the values calculated during the surgery. Through changes in implant position and implant size or type – depending on the modularity of the implant design – the surgeon has the opportunity to address each of these parameters and evaluate the resulting range of motion and the stability and potential for impingement during a kinematic motion test (☐ Fig. 12.7).

Conclusions

In our desire to provide our patients with the accelerated healing that is potential with a minimally invasive hip arthroplasty, we have focused our efforts on the direct anterior approach. As with all of the different anatomic routes to the hip joint, the initial results are encouraging, but long-term outcome studies will provide the validation that is ultimately needed. For the surgeon, the direct anterior approach has proven to be feasible when used with instruments that have been developed to facilitate the exposure while offering maximally soft-tissue protection. These instruments enable the surgeon to operate within a limited surgical field, limited only by the implant size (☐ Fig. 12.8). The anatomic foundation of the direct anterior approach provides for minimizing damage to the muscular structures. The location and tracks of the vascular and neural structures in that field of the anterior approach have been extensively evaluated in our laboratory to determine the element of risk that may exist during the operative procedure (see earlier in this book). To date, the cosmetic results are impressive (see ☐ Fig. 12.8) and an ongoing prospective randomized study will demonstrate the level of benefit to our patients. For surgeons performing this approach in either the supine or later decubitus position – as in any MIS approach – it is more

▼

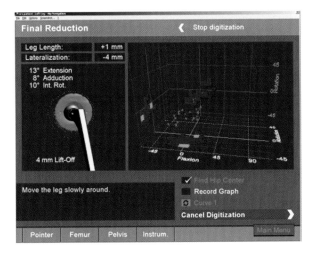

☐ Fig. 12.7. This screen shows the real-time measurements of the reduced hip, giving leg length and offset data as well as range of motion: red points indicate lift-off and dislocation

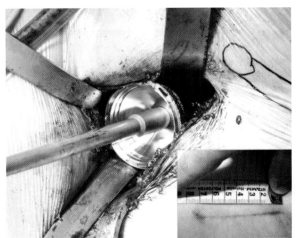

☐ Fig. 12.8. Special retractors protect the soft tissue during cup impaction. The minimally invasive procedure produces scars that are small, typically 8 cm

demanding than a traditional procedure. The learning curves associated with the minimally invasive hip approaches have not been satisfactorily described and often run contradictory to the decades of experience of many arthroplasty surgeons. The intra-operative navigation systems that can assist the surgeon in optimizing implant position and orientation are a requirement for those approaches in which the operative field is limited. However, combining the minimally invasive approach with the use of a navigation system can present a significant challenge to many arthroplasty surgeons until the learning curve is overcome. Moreover, the navigation systems are associated with a slight increase in operative time for the intra-operative digitization process until the user gains significant experience. The imageless navigation system does offset this increased time to some extent as pre-operative imaging is not required. Our investigations have proven the system to be valuable in controlling and optimizing cup position, orientation and leg length, which should ultimately result in improved clinical outcomes.

A navigated minimally invasive hip arthroplasty through the direct anterior approach can provide the patient with a viable alternative to the traditional approach. Further improvements in the navigation software will ensure optimal neck resection based on the anatomic landmarks of the proximal femur. Providing navigated instrumentation, such as the MIS saw used for neck resection, would provide the surgeon with real-time instrument position and orientation. Perfecting the use of anatomic reference points without the invasive placement of a wire or screw should also continue the development to the least invasive surgical approach for total hip arthroplasty.

References

1. Digioia AM III, Plakseychuk AY, Levison TJ, Jaramaz B: Mini-incision technique for total hip arthroplasty with navigation. J Arthroplasty 18(2): 123–128, 2003
2. DiGioia AM et al.: The Otto Aufranc Award. Image guided navigation system to measure intraoperatively acetabular implant alignment. Clin Orthop 355: 8–22, 1998
3. Sherry E, Egan M, Warnke PH, Henderson A, Eslick GD: Minimal invasive surgery for hip replacement: a new technique using the NILNAV hip system. ANZ J Surg 73(3): 157–161, 2003
4. Cameron HU: Mini-incisions: visualization is key. Orthopedics 25(5): 473, 2002
5. Amin DV, Kanade T, DiGioia AM III, Jaramaz B: Ultrasound registration of the bone surface for surgical navigation. Comput Aided Surg 8(1): 1–16, 2003
6. Amstutz C, Caversaccio M, Kowal J, Bachler R, Nolte LP, Hausler R, Styner M: A-mode ultrasound-based registration in computer-aided surgery of the skull. Arch Otolaryngol Head Neck Surg 129(12): 1310–1316, 2003
7. Winter S, Brendel B, Rick A, Stockheim M, Schmieder K, Ermert H: Registration of bone surfaces, extracted from CT-datasets, with 3D ultrasound. Biomed Tech (Berl) 47 [Suppl 1]: 57–60, 2002
8. Keggi K, Nao M, Zatorski LE: Anterior approach in hip prosthesis. Khirurgiia (Mosk) 2: 42–48, 1995

Double-Incision and Mini-Posterior Total Hip Arthroplasty Using Imageless Navigation

B. Donnelly

Introduction

The recent surge in interest in minimally invasive approaches for total hip arthroplasty has captured the attention of both surgeon and patient and resulted in a proliferation of new surgical techniques. Simultaneously we are experiencing the introduction of computerized navigation systems for total hip arthroplasty that enables the surgeon to more accurately and reproducibly perform bone preparation and component insertion. Both of these new technologies are still in their infancy and will continue to evolve markedly over forthcoming years, with surgeon experience and most importantly the results of appropriately constructed and performed clinical trials directing their path. The use of computerized navigation in total hip replacement allows the advantages of minimally invasive surgery to be combined with the safety of anatomical and other information available to the surgeon previously only afforded by more invasive exposures.

Total hip arthroplasty has long been accepted as one of the most successful and cost-effective operations of the 20th century following its widespread introduction in the 1960s. Over recent decades, technological advances in this field have been directed towards aspects of component design, articular surface tribology and interface materials with little emphasis on the technique of implantation, soft-tissue handling and exact component positioning. Our assessment parameters have largely based outcomes and success upon Kaplan-Meyer survival graphs with revision or radiological failure as the end point [1].

Despite the overall success of total hip arthroplasty, one must not become complacent as there is always room for improvement. The eventual failure of the pros-

thetic-bone interface with aseptic loosening and articular interface wear remain ongoing long-term challenges. The short-term complications include infection, dislocation, leg-length discrepancy and impingement to name just a few [2–8].

Recently we have seen a strong push in two new areas not previously widely acknowledged in arthroplasty surgery: muscle-sparing (minimally invasive) surgery and computerized navigation techniques. The latter are able to aid the surgeon with the accurate placement of both acetabular and femoral components and provide precise leg-length measurements.

Minimally invasive surgery allows total joint arthroplasty to be performed through smaller incisions with potential early rehabilitation benefits to the patient. This trend goes against the grain of our conservative orthopedic education where we were taught that "wounds heal from side to side, not end to end" and the "big surgeon, big cut" philosophy. The reasoning behind these teachings was that a larger incision firstly allowed the surgeon to visually obtain more bony landmarks thus aiding with "eyeballing of the component position" and secondly to allow better inspection of the interfaces for component insertion, whether it be cemented or press-fit. Despite using accepted standard incisions, component position has been found to be extremely variable and poor positioning related to a decreased overall survival [9–11].

There has been a growing trend towards the implementation of minimally invasive surgical techniques throughout the western world, with wide publicity and patients frequently presenting to their surgeons, printed internet pages clutched in hand, requesting these new procedures. The factors involved with this type of introduction, namely in financed training centers and significant printed and electronic media coverage have initially created a "market-driven demand" initially bypassing the scientific approach of publication in peer-reviewed journals. The published literature on the benefits and potential risks of these procedures has, to date, been conspicuous by its low volume [12–17] although many adequately designed prospective studies are currently underway. This I believe leaves many responsible surgeons in a difficult position with regards to when and if it is safe to employ these exciting new techniques.

The combination of minimally invasive surgery with navigation has been described as the "silver bullet" application with the minimally invasive total hip arthroplasty, providing the patient the benefits of early rehabilitation and the navigation ensuring the accuracy of component placement given the limitations of exposure [18, 19]. In this chapter the practical aspects, advantages and limitations of using navigation with the double-incision and mini-posterior total hip arthroplasty are discussed.

Computerized Navigation Units for THR

Although not yet routinely used, computerized navigation systems have become accepted in total knee arthroplasty with an increased accuracy of component placement and limb alignment being reported in the literature [20–22]. Following this initial success, a number of hip-navigation systems have been released to the market [19, 23–25]. The navigation systems all employ certain similar components;

1. **Patient trackers:** Individual trackers are fixed to the pelvis and femur. This allows the navigation unit to "see" the pelvis and femur and record dynamic movements and changes of position. The trackers may be infra-red optical or electromagnetic. The trackers may either be wired (connected by cable to the host computer), or wireless where they are battery-powered and actively transmit information via IR.

2. **Camera:** A stereoscopic camera is mounted in the operating theater within a functional range of the trackers and feeds information to the navigation computer. Newer generation machines are currently being developed with multiple cameras to provide a greater effective operating field.

3. **Navigation computer:** A laptop P4 notebook or similar computer controls the systems and provides output to the operating surgeon on a screen. The computer is usually docked into a housing station on the navigation machine, providing the interface to all components of the navigation unit.

The navigation systems differ in their need for pre-operative or intra-operative imaging. Image-based systems may either require a pre-operative CT scan with a 3-D reconstruction or intra-operative fluoroscopy for image acquisition. At our institution the time and expense of a routine pre-operative CT scan on each patient undergoing routine total hip arthroplasty was unjustifiable on a cost and resources basis and the use of intra-operative fluoroscopy was unappealing to the surgeon. Intra-operative fluoroscopy involves the use of a C arm in the operative field which may be cumbersome and requires the surgeon to wear a lead gown which is definitely undesirable!

At our institution we have chosen an imageless Stryker-Leibinger Navigation System running Hip Navigation V1.1 software module. This system requires no extra-imaging than that which the surgeon would routinely perform (routine pre-operative radiographs for diagnostic purposes). Using this system, the surgeon is required to register the frontal plane of the pelvis and sagittal plane of the femur by identifying a number of bony landmarks. This pelvic reference frame is calculated after the surgeon registers both anterior superior iliac spines and the pubic symphysis. The femoral reference frame is calculated following registration of the piriformis fossa, popliteal fossa and midpoint of the achilles tendon. A small number of ancillary anatomical points are then required to be registered throughout the procedure. The navigation system is then able to create two dynamic relational reference frames that give the surgeon anatomical information in the following:

- Acetabular reaming:
  - inclination and version of reamer,
  - depth to fovea.
- Acetabular component (Fig. 13.1):
  - inclination and version of component,
  - depth to fully seated.
- Femoral broaching:
  - predictive changes in leg length and offset not requiring trial reduction,
  - varus/valgus alignment of broaching.

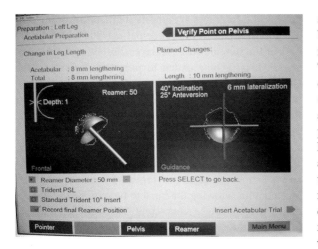

Fig. 13.1. Screenshot of the Stryker Hip Navigation Unit, during acetabular preparation showing inclination, version and depth to base of the fovea

- Femoral stem insertion:
  - predictive change in leg length and offset at the current position of the stem,
  - varus/valgus alignment of stem,
  - all permutations and combinations of head size and neck length.
- Range of motion and stability:
  - both at trial reduction and finalreduction range of motion and stability are real-time 3-D modeled and recorded graphically with the graph turning red at areas of lift-off.

Surgical Technique: Minimally-Invasive Approaches for Navigated THR

The Double-Incision Approach with Navigation

As this surgical approach is covered elsewhere in this volume, only a brief summary is presented here as a reference for navigation. The Trident acetabular component (fully navigated) and the Accolade femoral stem have been chosen in our unit for double incision minimally invasive hip arthroplasties. The Accolade stem was chosen for its low profile and the suitability of instrumentation for this approach. Currently the loading of the geometric data from the Accolade stem into the navigation program is being completed. The full features of navigation of the broaching and femoral

stem insertion are presently not available, but will have been released prior to publication of this book. In the following description of navigated double-incision MIS THR for broaching and femoral stem insertion the characteristics that the system will possess are outlined (as are currently available for the secure-fit femoral stem). Presently the navigation software provides complete information on acetabular cup insertion, overall leg length and femoral offset as well as joint stability and range of movement information. We currently continue to use the image intensifier for insertion of the femoral stem. In the next version of the software (Stryker Hip Navigation V1.2) the Accolade stem will be fully navigated and the use of intra-operative fluoroscopy will become obsolete.

The patient is placed on the operating table in a supine position with a one-liter sandbag on the ipsilateral side just above the buttock. The leg is routinely prepped and draped with the ipsilateral iliac crest exposed as well as the leg down to the level of the knee.

A pelvic tracker is attached to the ipsilateral iliac crest and a femoral tracker fixed to the lateral femoral condyle. It is imperative that the trackers are placed in positions that are able to maintain good line of sight with the camera throughout the entire procedure. This applies especially to the femoral tracker as the leg will be flexed and externally rotated at various times in the operation (Fig. 13.2). Our recommended setup is to have the assistant standing on the ipsilateral side and the navigation unit and camera approximately 2 m away on the opposite side of the patient. The femoral tracker should be angled anteriorly, enabling it to be visible to the camera for the maximal amount of the procedure.

The first generation of trackers, apart from being large and cumbersome, were fixed to bone by threaded Steinmann pin-type devices. These usually required a 3–5 cm incision for direct application to the underlying bone. Especially at the level of the distal femur, this was seen to result in significant patient discomfort which may interfere with an otherwise rapid rehabilitation. Our current tracker design involves the use of small light-weight components fixed to the underlying bone percutaneously (Fig. 13.3). The percutaneous tripod base is applied in the position of maximal stability and then the tracker is attached by a universal elbow construct to allow optimum placement for the camera.

The anterior incision is a longitudinal incision beginning proximally at the level of the tip of the greater

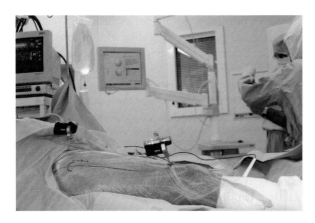

▣ Fig. 13.2. The patient is prepped and draped with pelvic and femoral trackers applied prior to the double-incision approach

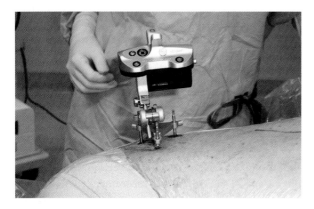

▣ Fig. 13.3. Percutaneous tracker fixation enables minimal rigid fixation with minimal soft-tissue damage

trochanter and extending distally for approximately 6 cm. The fascia is split at the same level and with careful blunt dissection a finger can be passed over vastus lateralis and gluteus medius and below rectus femoris directly onto the femoral neck. Specialized minimally invasive retractors and a fiberoptic light source are of great advantage at this stage in providing retraction and visibility.

At this stage, before resection of the femoral head, registration of the bony landmarks is performed. The pelvic reference plane is created by digitizing the two anterior superior iliac spines and a point on the pubic symphysis. The anterior superior iliac spines are usually easily palpable, even in the most obese patient as they are closely subcutaneous and under any abdominal adi-

pose fold. The pubic symphysis digitization point may be more difficult in the obese patient due to the thickness of the subcutaneous fat layer directly over the symphysis. It is recommended to palpate inferiorly at the level of the suspensory ligament of the penis to obtain a more accurate point. Digitization of the pelvic reference frame is significantly easier with the patient in a supine position rather than a lateral decubitus position.

The next step involves resection of the femoral neck. This is performed through an anterior H capsulotomy and a 2-cm neck section is removed with the head left located, thus allowing the head to be removed with adequate space using a corkscrew. Through the anterior incision, good visualization of the entire acetabulum can be achieved. Further registration of the acetabular surface, the fovea and the acetabular rim can then be performed to provide additional information for the navigation system. The computer is then able to accurately calculate the diameter of the real acetabular surface, allowing the surgeon to introduce an appropriately sized reamer first up. This decreases the number of times reamers are required to be taken past the skin and soft tissues. The navigation unit also provides valuable real-time information to the surgeon about the depth of reaming with reference to the deepest point of the fovea (approximates to the medial wall).

Insertion of the acetabular shell is fully navigated, giving the surgeon information as to the inclination and version of the shell as well as telling the surgeon when the shell has been fully bottomed out to the depth of the reaming. Our preference is then to insert a non-lipped liner.

At this stage, the femoral reference plane has been registered by identifying the piriform fossa, midpoint of the popliteal fossa and mid-point of the tendo-achilles. The longitudinal axis of the femur is then calculated with a sagittal plane and a coronal plane calculated at right angles to this.

The superior incision (approximately 4 cm in length) is then made in line with the proximal femoral axis. This can be best performed by passing a large pair of dissecting scissors retrograde from the cut surface of the femoral neck through the gluteus medius and gluteal fascia. The skin incision can then be made directly over the palpable scissors. The femur can then be broached to the templated size. The navigated broach will provide information as to the varus/valgus alignment of the broach, the amount of anteversion and the predictive change in leg length and offset if the hip were to be reduced with the broach at that level. The navigation system will then provide the same information to the surgeon for the insertion of the definitive femoral stem. The predictive information is able to decrease the amount of trialing required which may be difficult with double-incision procedures. It is likely with navigation of both the broaching and femoral stem insertion better control of version will be able to be obtained, thus decreasing the incidence of femoral calcar fracture.

The Mini-Posterior Approach

Once again as the operative techniques of the mini-posterior approach have been adequately covered elsewhere in this volume, it will not be covered in detail here, only in combination with navigation. The implants used in our mini-posterior navigated THR are the Trident acetabular component and the Secure-fit femoral stem. All components are currently fully navigated, allowing the software to provide "look ahead" predictive features, which are of benefit in limited approaches. Our unit also performs a cemented Exeter through a mini-posterior approach and will perform this navigated in the next version of the software when the Exeter data is also available in the navigation software.

For the mini-posterior navigated THR the patient is placed in a lateral position with both anterior and posterior supports. We currently leave the posterior support a little loose, allowing the patient to be rolled back slightly following prepping and draping. This allows for easier digitization of the contra-lateral ASIS as this may be difficult to accurately identify if covered by a brace. Other units have employed different techniques to overcome this, including insertion of the tracker and performing the registration process with the patient supine prior to prepping and draping. This technique requires re-prepping of the tracker pin and wound site when the patient has been turned and placed in the lateral decubitus position.

The second difference with the navigated mini-posterior approach is the placement of the distal femoral tracker. As the hip is dislocated into a posterior position with 90° of internal rotation of the femur, the tracker should be angled posterior to the sagittal plane to enable it to remain visible to the camera following internal rotation.

The Future of Navigation with Minimally Invasive Total Hip Arthroplasty

As with many other fields of surgery, the uptake of minimally invasive total hip arthroplasty has been rapid and led by patient demand. It is likely to have already made permanent changes to the ways in which we perform our surgery, the instruments we use and the expectations of our patients.

Already described as the "silver bullet application", the combination of the two new technologies of minimally invasive surgery and navigation are mutually complimentary. Many early publications support the advantages of minimally invasive surgery while others report an increased incidence of complications. The introduction of navigation to the techniques of minimally invasive surgery first and foremost serve to provide increased safety for the procedure. The risks of minimally invasive surgery appear related to loss of visibility of the surgeon's normal landmarks, and inability to adequately visualize the bone-prosthesis interface. Early work with navigation in both the double-incision- and mini-posterior approaches have shown this combination to result in superior surgery with better short-term and more reproducible results.

The future of both navigation and minimally invasive surgery will be directed by appropriately constructed prospective studies aimed at ensuring the safety of emerging surgical techniques and the clinical advantages of these techniques to the patient. We will continue to see as rapid developments in computerized navigation as we have witnessed in all aspects of the computer industry with increased accuracy and decreased size of the hardware components combined with more intuitive and smarter software.

References

1. Murray, D.W., A.J. Carr, C.J. Bulstrode. Which primary total hip replacement? J Bone Joint Surg Br 1995. 77(4): 520–527
2. Ali Khan, M.A., P.H. Brakenbury, I.S. Reynolds. Dislocation following total hip replacement. J Bone Joint Surg Br, 1981. 63-B(2): 214–218
3. Demos, H.A., et al. Instability in primary total hip arthroplasty with the direct lateral approach. Clin Orthop 2001. (393): 168–180
4. Dorr, L.D., Z. Wan. Causes of and treatment protocol for instability of total hip replacement. Clin Orthop 1998. (355): 144–151
5. Grossmann, P., M. Braun, W. Becker. Dislocation following total hip endoprothesis. Association with surgical approach and other factors. Z Orthop Ihre Grenzgeb 1994. 132(6): 521–526

6. Hirakawa, K. et al. Effect of acetabular cup position and orientation in cemented total hip arthroplasty. Clin Orthop 2001.(388): 135–142

7. Kennedy, J.G. et al. Effect of acetabular component orientation on recurrent dislocation, pelvic osteolysis, polyethylene wear, and component migration. J Arthroplasty, 1998. 13(5): 530–534

8. McCollum, D.E., W.J. Gray. Dislocation after total hip arthroplasty. Causes and prevention. Clin Orthop 1990. (261): 159–170

9. DiGioia, A.M. et al. The Otto Aufranc Award. Image guided navigation system to measure intraoperatively acetabular implant alignment. Clin Orthop 1998. (355): 8–22

10. Lewinnek, G.E. et al. Dislocations after total hip-replacement arthroplasties. J Bone Joint Surg Am 1978. 60(2): 217–220

11. Paterno, S.A., P.F. Lachiewicz, S.S. Kelley. The influence of patient-related factors and the position of the acetabular component on the rate of dislocation after total hip replacement. J Bone Joint Surg Am 1997. 79(8): 1202–1210

12. Berger, R.A. Total hip arthroplasty using the minimally invasive two-incision approach. Clin Orthop 2003 (417): 232–241

13. Higuchi, F. et al. Minimally invasive uncemented total hip arthroplasty through an anterolateral approach with a shorter skin incision. J Orthop Sci 2003. 8(6): 812–817

14. Rodrigo, J.J., Juan J. Rodrigo. MD on minimally invasive hip surgery. Orthopedics, 2002. 25(10): 1016, 1028

15. Sherry, E. et al. Minimal invasive surgery for hip replacement: a new technique using the NILNAV hip system. ANZ J Surg, 2003. 73(3): 157–161

16. Waldman, B.J. Advancements in minimally invasive total hip arthroplasty. Orthopedics, 2003. 26 [8 Suppl]: s833–836

17. Wenz, J.F., I. Gurkan, S.R. Jibodh. Mini-incision total hip arthroplasty: a comparative assessment of perioperative outcomes. Orthopedics 2002. 25(10): 1031–1043

18. Digioia, A.M., 3rd et al. Mini-incision technique for total hip arthroplasty with navigation. J Arthroplasty, 2003. 18(2): 123–128

19. Leenders, T. et al. Reduction in variability of acetabular cup abduction using computer assisted surgery: a prospective and randomized study. Comput Aided Surg, 2002. 7(2): 99–106

20. Mielke, R.K. et al. Navigation in knee endoprosthesis implantation–preliminary experiences and prospective comparative study with conventional implantation technique. Z Orthop Ihre Grenzgeb 2001. 139(2): 109–116

21. Sparmann M. et al. Knieendoprothesennavigation mit dem Stryker-System. In: Konermann H.R. (ed) Navigation und Robotic in der Gelenk- und Wirbelsäulenchirurgie. Springer, Berlin Heidelberg New York Tokio. 2003. pp 250–255

22. Jenny J.Y. et al. Navigated implantation of total knee endoprostheses – a comparative study with conventional instrumentation. Z Orthop Ihre Grenzgeb, 2001. 139: 117–119

23. Digioia, A.M. III et al. Comparison of a mechanical acetabular alignment guide with computer placement of the socket. J Arthroplasty, 2002. 17(3): 359–364

24. Schep, N.W. et al. Validation of fluoroscopy-based navigation in the hip region: what you see is what you get? Comput Aided Surg 2002. 7(5): 279–283

25. Zheng, G. et al. A hybrid CT-free navigation system for total hip arthroplasty. Comput Aided Surg, 2002. 7(3): 129–145

13

Image-Free Navigation for TKA – Surgical Technique

G.R. Klein, W.J. Hozack

Introduction

While the goal of total knee arthroplasty is the restoration of a quality of life by eliminating pain and improving function, it is clear to most knee-replacement surgeons that this goal is not always achieved. Sharkey et al. [1] reviewed 203 consecutive total knee revisions and found that greater than one-half of these revisions were performed within 2 years of index arthroplasty and one third of these were due to instability, mal-alignment or mal-position (usually avoidable problems). Similarly, Fehring et al. [2] reported on 440 patients who underwent revision total knee arthroplasty and found that 63% of patients required revision surgery within 5 years of their index arthroplasty, 27% were due to instability. It is quite evident that current instrumentation systems leave room for improvement. Stulberg [3] used navigation to assess the position of knee components implanted with traditional methods and found that only 4 of 20 knees were implanted within 3° of ideal component position in all planes. Conversely, occasionally a surgeon performs an operation in which the patient has a near perfect result. Unfortunately, using traditional techniques there is no tangible information or objective data that allows us to reproduce that result in the next patient.

Navigation systems provide us with the potential to quantify data, to have dynamic intra-operative feedback and to obtain more reproducible results. Errors in component positioning and limb alignment that continue to occur using the conventional mechanical alignment jigs can be minimized through navigation instrumentation [4–8]. Another important attribute of navigation system is its ability to provide instant feedback regarding in vivo kinematics of the joint. Alignment and ligament stability can be assessed with the trials in place to ensure

proper function. Coronal deformity, alignment, rotation, and translation can be measured for any specified degree of flexion. This characteristic of the navigation system provides the unique opportunity to assess in vivo kinematics of the knee during surgery and implement beneficial changes such as refinements in soft-tissue tensioning, rotational adjustment of components, or alterations in component selection. Phillips and Krackow [9] reported on thirty patients undergoing total knee replacement with a computer-assisted surgical system and found that range of motion, alignment and knee scores were equal to or better than patients undergoing standard total knee replacement. Surgeons can now take the "subjective feel" of standard knee arthroplasty and translate it into more "objective data" provided by the navigation system. This creates the potential for more consistent reproducibility of the surgeon's clinical result.

Surgical Technique

The following technique is for the Stryker Knee Navigation System using the Stryker Orthopedics Scorpio Total Knee System. During surgical approach the scrub technician/nurse should be setting up the specialized navigation instruments. During the system setup dialog, the trackers are initialized and the Smart Tools are registered. While a medial parapatellar exposure is used to enter the knee joint, it is done so with the knee in 90° of flexion so as to minimize the total length of the incision. During the procedure, the patella is not everted so as to minimize the soft-tissue trauma to the quadriceps mechanism. Bicortical 4.0 mm anchoring pins, which consist of a self-tapping screw design with anti-rotation and tracker attachment features built-into ensure the trackers remain rigidly fixed throughout the surgical procedure, are affixed to proximal tibia and the distal femur. The trackers are then attached to the anchoring pins.

Registration

Registration of the navigation system includes determining the centers of the femoral head, knee and ankle joints as well as surface mapping of particular bony landmarks of the knee. This procedure allows the navigation system to determine the mechanical axis of the extremity. The determination of the mechanical axis involves direct measurement of specific landmarks except for determining the center of the femoral head, which is a calculated value. No imaging studies are necessary when performing this procedure, again minimizing the overall invasiveness of the procedure to the patient.

The first step of registration involves calculating the center of femoral head. The rotational center of the femoral head is determined using motion analysis. As the leg is gently rotated, the femoral LED location yields a set of data points that lie on a sphere with the femoral head theoretically at its center. Feedback is provided to the surgeon through visualization of the digitized data points on the computer screen, seen as 3D tiny spheres (■ Fig. 14.1).

The distal femur is registered next. The navigation system will guide the surgeon through each component of the femoral registration to pick the medial and lateral epicondyles, center of knee, and anteroposterior axis of knee

(■ Fig. 14.2). After key landmarks are identified, the surgeon will digitize the medial and lateral condyles. This is done by tracing the surface of the bone with the pointer for both of the distal articulating portions of the condyles. It is important to identify the most distal portion of the condyles as this will be the basis for the resection levels.

The proximal tibia is registered next. Using the navigation screen as a guide, the center of tibia and anteroposterior axis of the tibia (i.e. rotation) are selected. The medial (■ Fig. 14.3) and lateral tibial plateaus are then digitized in similar fashion to the femoral condyles. Here it is important to identify the most proximal portions of the articulating surface of the proximal tibia. The last step of the registration process involves the ankle. The medial and lateral malleoli as well as the center of the ankle are identified with the pointer.

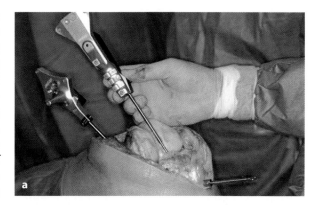

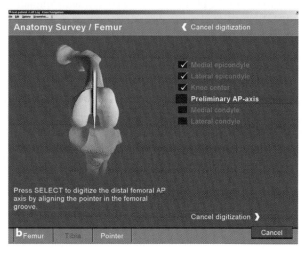

■ **Fig. 14.1.** Navigation system screen shot of digitized points during center of femoral head calculation

■ **Fig. 14.2. a** Surgeon-positioned navigation system pointer indicating the anteroposterior axis of femur. **b** Corresponding navigation-system screen shot

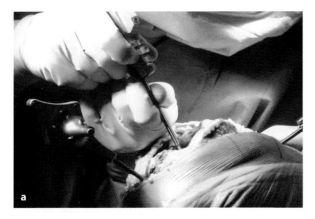

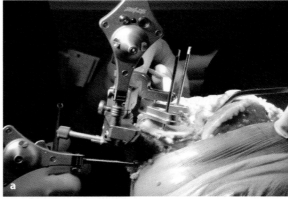

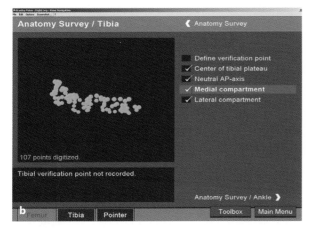

■ **Fig. 14.3. a** Digitization of medial tibial plateau using the Navigation system pointer. **b** Corresponding navigation-system screen shot

■ **Fig. 14.4. a** Navigated tibial cutting guide in place. **b** Corresponding navigation system screen shot. The surgeon has the ability to set the amount of tibial resection, posterior slope and varus/valgus orientation. Note that there is neither an extra-medullary nor an intra-medullary guide on the tibia

Initial Kinematics

After the registration is performed, the initial kinematics of the pathological knee is performed. Data such as maximal extension, flexion and alignment is recorded in table form by the navigation unit. Soft-tissue releases are performed based on this initial pre-operative data. Initial kinematic curves, which give an indication of the initial balance of the knee, are then assessed. This process involves bringing the knee through a range of motion while exerting sequentially a varus and then a valgus stress. It is important to note that the noise (i.e. widening of band) in the curves indicates either bone deficiency or soft-tissue laxity. The absolute values of the curves reflect the distance of the digitized femoral epicondyles to the transverse axis of the tibial plateau.

Overall, the initial registration and kinematic measurements take less than 5 min of time.

Navigated Tibial Preparation

It is the authors' preference to approach the tibia first. However, the Stryker software is flexible and allows surgeon preference. Using the navigation-system computer screen, the surgeon is able to micro-manipulate the depth of tibial resection, amount of posterior slope, and varus/valgus orientation of the cut (■ Fig. 14.4). The initial tibial cut is checked with a navigated flat-plate guide and, if needed, modifications to the cut may be made. The rotational alignment of the tibial component (as determined by the initial registration of the anteroposterior axis during the tibial registration) is then set, using navigated instruments, thus completing the preparation of the tibia.

Navigated Femoral Preparation

Navigated femoral preparation occurs in two steps. First, the sagittal and coronal alignment of the distal cut as well as the depth of distal cut is performed, and then the rotational alignment is set. During the first step (■ Fig. 14.5), we generally cut 10 mm of distal femur (11–12 mm with a large flexion contracture) and prefer to orient the varus/valgus position to 0° and the flexion/extension position to 0° with respect to the mechanical axis of the limb. After the initial distal femoral preparation is performed, the surgeon should check the cut using the navigated flat plate, with modifications being made as necessary.

Navigated anterior referencing instrumentation is used to set the rotational alignment of the femoral component (a posterior referencing software package is available if preferred). The navigation system gives the option to set rotation in reference to the pre-registered Whiteside's line or epicondylar axis. We prefer to set rotation to 0° in reference to the epicondylar axis which in most cases corresponds to Whiteside's line within a few degrees (■ Fig. 14.6).

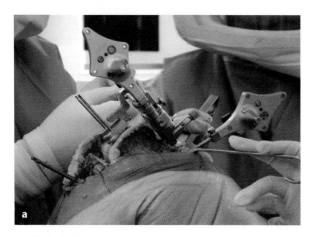

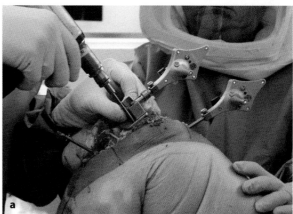

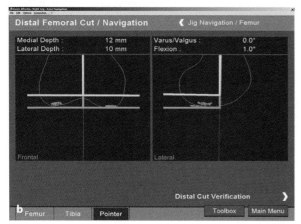

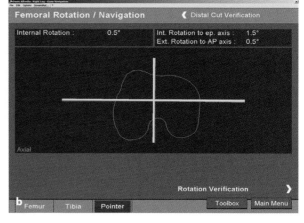

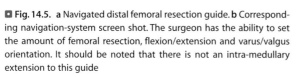

■ **Fig. 14.5.** **a** Navigated distal femoral resection guide. **b** Corresponding navigation-system screen shot. The surgeon has the ability to set the amount of femoral resection, flexion/extension and varus/valgus orientation. It should be noted that there is not an intra-medullary extension to this guide

■ **Fig. 14.6.** **a** Navigated anterior skim-cut instrumentation. **b** Corresponding navigation-system screen shot. Note rotation is indicated in reference to the epicondylar axis as well as Whiteside's line

The remainder of the femoral preparation does not involve the use of navigation. Trial components are now placed and patellar resurfacing, if desired, may be performed at this time.

Final Kinematics

At this point, data, such as maximal extension, flexion and alignment, is re-assessed by the navigation unit (◘ Fig. 14.7). With the trials in place, new kinematic curves are created, which give an indication of the soft-tissue balance of the replaced knee. The goal during the soft-tissue balancing stage is to achieve relatively horizontal, smooth parallel curves for both the medial and lateral compartments throughout the entire range of motion. In general, the wider the curves the more instability is present. If the curves show a poorly balanced knee, soft-tissue- or bony corrections may be made at this point and a new kinematic curve may be generated to evaluate if the changes helped to balance the knee (◘ Fig. 14.8). Based on the information obtained from the navigation software, the surgeon can implement changes in selection of the knee components with beneficial effects in knee kinematics and function.

Navigation and Minimal Invasiveness

At several levels, computer-assisted total knee replacement as described above is already minimally invasive in nature. The Stryker system requires no special radiographic techniques, thereby minimizing radiation exposure for the patient. Exposing the knee in flexion minimizes the total length of the incision. Performing the surgery without everting the patella minimizes the trauma to the quadriceps mechanism. Strict standardization of surgical technique and sequence of steps has lead to an imperceptible change in the total operative

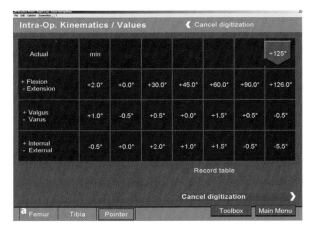

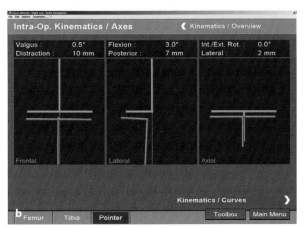

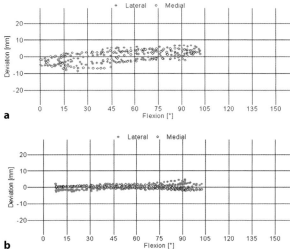

◘ **Fig. 14.7. a** Range of motion analysis after implantation of trial components. **b** Alignment analysis after implantation of trial components

◘ **Fig. 14.8. a** Pre-operative kinematic curve. Note the "noise" or widening of the curves in reference to the blue–blue distance and the red–red distance indicating a poorly balanced or deformed knee. **b** Post-operative kinematic curve. Note the significantly decreased widening of the curve indicating a well-balanced knee

time (and tourniquet time). Review of the most recently performed knee replacements (20 knees), the total surgical time averaged 57 min (range 46 to 63 min). However there is an initial learning-curve period. In the senior authors' experience, the average operative time was 61 min (range 51–84 min) based on the tourniquet times (skin incision to application of dressings) for the first 30 surgeries. However, when critically analyzed, the operative time for the first five knees performed with the navigation system averaged 70 min and the remaining 32 knees averaged 60 min. This result was statistically different (p=0.02).

An important minimally invasive benefit of navigation is the lower chance of emboli related to the use of dedicated extra-medullary instrumentation. During "classic" total knee replacement with intra-medullary instrumentation, numerous studies have documented the release of fat-embolic particles to the lungs and brains of patients. Using trans-esophageal ultrasound, multiple studies have shown the persistence of echogenic material when intra-medullary alignment was used [10, 11]. These studies have attributed the intra-medullary rod as the cause of the fat embolus [12–15]. These particles may lead to pulmonary compromise such as fat embolism or adult respiratory distress syndrome and neurologic changes related to fat in the cerebral circulation [16]. Morawa et al. [17] compared patients undergoing total knee arthroplasty with intra-medullary and extra-medullary instrumentation and found that the risk of embolic events was substantially reduced with the extra-medullary instrumentation. True to the minimally invasive terminology, navigation eliminates a serious risk factor – the use of intra-medullary alignment rods – and thus may decrease the risks of embolic events to the patient. This may result in less pulmonary effects as well and less postoperative mental status changes.

Navigation also has the potential to expand the realm of minimally invasive arthroplasty. Questions about visualization and component orientation can now be overcome by using navigation. In smaller incision surgery, specific landmarks and orientations may be hard to visualize; however, navigation has the ability to solve these problems. Newer and smaller instrumentation is currently being used in preliminary clinical evaluations to couple the fascinating worlds of computer-assisted surgery and minimally invasive surgery.

References

1. Sharkey PF, Hozack WJ, Rothman RH, Shastri S, Jacoby SM (2002) Insall Award paper. Why are total knee arthroplasties failing today? Clin Orthop 404: 7–13
2. Fehring TK, Odum S, Griffin WL, Mason JB, Nadaud M (2001) Early failures in total knee arthroplasty. Clin Orthop 392: 315–318
3. Stulberg SD (2003) How accurate is current TKR instrumentation? Clin Orthop 416: 177–184
4. Bellemans J, Banks S, Victor J, Vandenneucker H, Moemans A (2002) Fluoroscopic analysis of the kinematics of deep flexion in total knee arthroplasty. Influence of posterior condylar offset. J Bone Joint Surg Br 84: 50–53
5. Sparmann M, Wolke B, Czupalla H, Banzer D, Zink A (2003) Positioning of total knee arthroplasty with and without navigation support. A prospective, randomised study. J Bone Joint Surg Br 85: 830–835
6. Mielke RK, Clemens U, Jens JH, Kershally S (2001) [Navigation in knee endoprothesis implantation–preliminary experiences and prospective comparative study with conventional implantation technique]. Z Orthop Ihre Grenzgeb 139: 109–116
7. Hart R, Janecek M, Chaker A, Bucek P (2003) Total knee arthroplasty implanted with and without kinematic navigation. Int Orthop 27: 366–369
8. Krackow KA, Phillips MJ, Bayers-Thering M, Serpe L, Mihalko WM (2003) Computer-assisted total knee arthroplasty: navigation in TKA. Orthopedics 26: 1017–1023
9. Phillips MJ, Krackow, K.A., Bayers-Thering, M. (2002) Computer-assisted total knee replacements: Results of the first thirty cases using the Stryker Navigation System (TM). In: Second Annual Meeting of the International Society for Computer-Assisted Orthopaedic Surgery
10. Parmet JL, Berman AT, Horrow JC, Harding S, Rosenberg H (1993) Thromboembolism coincident with tourniquet deflation during total knee arthroplasty. Lancet 341: 1057–1058
11. Berman AT, Parmet JL, Harding SP, Israelite CL, Chandrasekaran K, Horrow JC, Singer R, Rosenberg H (1998) Emboli observed with use of transesophageal echocardiography immediately after tourniquet release during total knee arthroplasty with cement. J Bone Joint Surg Am 80: 389–396
12. Fahmy NR, Chandler HP, Danylchuk K, Matta EB, Sunder N, Siliski JM (1990) Blood-gas and circulatory changes during total knee replacement. Role of the intramedullary alignment rod. J Bone Joint Surg Am 72: 19–26
13. Monto RR, Garcia J, Callaghan JJ (1990) Fatal fat embolism following total condylar knee arthroplasty. J Arthroplasty 5: 291–299
14. Caillouette JT, Anzel SH (1990) Fat embolism syndrome following the intramedullary alignment guide in total knee arthroplasty. Clin Orthop 251: 198–199
15. Dorr LD, Merkel C, Mellman MF, Klein I (1989) Fat emboli in bilateral total knee arthroplasty. Predictive factors for neurologic manifestations. Clin Orthop 248: 112–118; discussion 118–119
16. Jacobson DM, Terrence CF, Reinmuth OM (1986) The neurologic manifestations of fat embolism. Neurology 36: 847–851
17. Morawa LG, Manley MT, Edidin AA, Reilly DT (1996) Transesophageal echocardiographic monitored events during total knee arthroplasty. Clin Orthop 331: 192–198

14

Image-Free Navigation for Total Knee Arthroplasty

K. Buehler

Introduction

Image-free navigation for total knee arthroplasty is a technology that is in its infancy of development. Like an infant, it has much potential to influence the future if developed and integrated properly with its environment – the operating room. Image-free navigation is based on an open platform computer-based knee-alignment system developed by Stryker Orthopedics, Mahwah, New Jersey. The system is image free, meaning no pre-operative CT scan or fluoroscopy is needed. The current software module (Navigation 2.0) allows for intra-operative assistance for alignment of the leg, instruments, resection planes, trial and prosthetic implants. The Stryker system also provides surgeons an assessment of the patient's joint kinematics before and after prosthetic implantation.

The hardware consists of a mobile workstation containing laptop PC, flat-screen monitor, and infra-red camera system (◘ Fig. 15.1). Instruments and the navigation system communicate via light-emitting diodes (LEDs), thus eliminating the need for cords coming off the sterile field. The surgeon is able to control the system with a pointer which operates like a wireless computer mouse. No specially trained operating-room staff or technicians are necessary to run the system. Setup time takes approximately 3 min to activate the computer and enter patient demographic information.

The benefits of image-free navigation to the surgeon are substantial and unique. The virtual visualization of instrument depth and position prior to osseous cuts helps prevent errors that can be difficult to correct. The continual intra-operative evaluation of alignment at every step in the procedure provides more confidence in the surgical accuracy. The quantitative kinematic data allows an abundance of data for research purposes and forms an automatic registry to track patient outcomes. Image-free navigation of knee arthroplasty should be seen as an important tool for the surgeon that computerizes a previously completely mechanical procedure. It does not replace the eye of the surgeon, but rather enhances it.

Current mechanical instruments and techniques used for knee arthroplasty generally produce good results, but substantial numbers of implants are maligned, have poor soft-tissue balance, markedly abnormal kinematics, or poor patella tracking [1–4]. As recognized in the 2003 National Institute of Health consensus conference on knee arthroplasty, "proper alignment of the prosthesis appears to be critical in minimizing long-term wear, risk of osteolysis, and loosening of

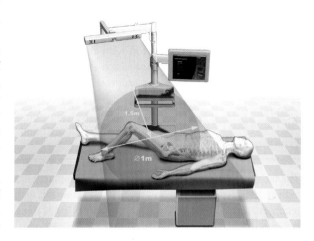

◘ **Fig. 15.1.** The Stryker image-free knee-navigation hardware consists of a mobile workstation containing a laptop PC, flat-screen monitor, and infra-red camera

the prosthesis." Joint-line mal-position, usually secondary to femoral component mis-orientation is also known to have an important effect on range of motion with changes as little as 2.5 mm reducing flexion [5]. Clearly, opportunity exists through use of image-free navigation and other techniques to improve results of knee arthroplasty.

Objectives

The primary objective of any knee arthroplasty technique is to distribute contact stress across the artificial joint as symmetrically as possible [6] while maintaining good knee function. This is thought to occur in most circumstances when implants are placed neutral to the mechanical axis, the collateral ligaments are balanced, and flexion/extension gaps are equal. Ideal rotational and sagittal plane alignment of implants are not well defined and vary depending on prosthetic design. Determining appropriate parameters for rotational and sagittal alignment for knee implants is an area deserving further investigation.

Similarly, what constitutes good knee function following knee arthroplasty is yet to be defined. The work of Dennis and Komistek have focused attention on prosthetic knee kinematics. They have demonstrated that over 60% of some series of patients have abnormal kinematics, such as reverse screw home and paradoxical femoral translation after knee replacement [3]. Currently, the working assumption is that knee kinematics after arthroplasty should attempt to replicate normal knee function. Image-free navigation techniques provide intra-operative information with regards to both knee kinematics and alignment which enables the surgeon to more consistently and accurately achieve their objectives.

Technique

The technique we currently use for knee arthroplasty is a hybrid using methods from traditional balanced gap technique introduced by Insall in the late 1970s [7] and measured resection technique popularized by Hungerford and Krackow in the mid 1980s [8]. Our measured tension technique is dependent on a balancing/tensioning device (❑ Fig. 15.2) which allows measurement of the

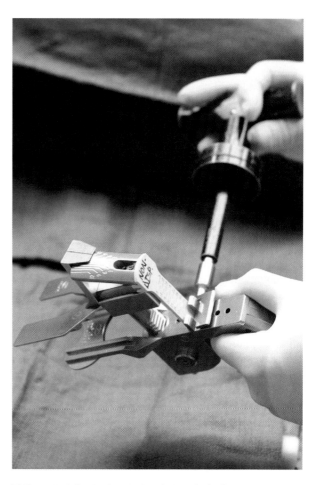

❑ **Fig. 15.2.** Balancing/tensioning device which allows measurement of the flexion/extension gaps in millimeters and collateral ligaments balance in degrees under calibrated tension

flexion/extension gaps in millimeters and collateral ligaments balance in degrees under calibrated tension. Navigation allows fine adjustments in osseous alignment and soft-tissue balance at multiple points throughout the procedure.

Surgical Approach and Navigation Initialization

An anterior medial incision is made with the knee in 60° of flexion. A mid-vastus approach is made to the knee with patella being dislocated laterally but not everted. The combination of the mid-vastus approach [9] and lack of patella eversion through the procedure allows

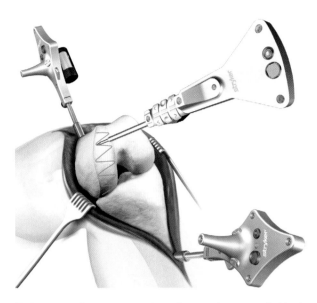

Fig. 15.3. A digitizing pointer is used to enter key anatomical landmarks around the knee

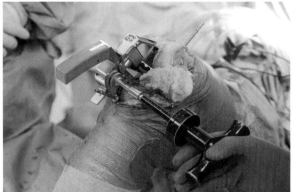

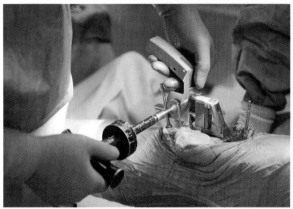

Fig. 15.4. After the tibial resection is made perpendicular to the mechanical axis, a horizontal base is formed for which measurements of flexion/extension gaps and collateral ligament tension can be made with the balancing/tensioning device

quicker patient recovery of quadriceps function. Anchoring pins for the LED navigation trackers are placed in the anterior medial distal femur approximately 3 cm above the joint line and in the anterior medial proximal tibia at the level of the pes tendons insertion. These anchoring pins are placed through the standard total knee incision – no separate incisions are needed. The hip center is determined by a motion analysis program which generates the exact rotational center of the hip through motion of the hip in a spherical pattern. The digitizing pointer is then used to enter key anatomical landmarks (**•** Fig. 15.3) – epicondylyar axis, Whiteside's line, the femoral and tibial centers, rotational axis of the tibia, the malleoli and center of the ankle. Surface mapping of the femur and tibia provides a digital map of the knee identifying defects in the joint surface. This completes the initialization and data-entry portion of image-free navigation and takes on average 7 min to perform.

Data Analysis, Jig Navigation and Tension Measurements

Sophisticated intra-operative data analysis is possible, using the processing capabilities of the knee-navigation software. Initial knee-kinematics axis screen

allows the surgeon to visual the patient's deformity in live time throughout a range of motion. Initial kinematic values are collected in table and graphical form, aiding the surgeon in important decisions with regard to appropriate soft-tissue release and osseous resection levels.

We next proceed with proximal tibia resection instead of the more typical femoral first methods. The advantage of tibia first technique is that with the resection made perpendicular to the mechanical axis a horizontal base is formed for which measurements of flexion/extension gaps and collateral ligament tension can be made (**•** Fig. 15.4). Imbalance of gap tension at this point will influence femoral resection levels. For example, if the extension gap is larger than the flexion gaps, a less aggressive distal femoral resection is performed. Jig navigation is performed before any osseous resection by attaching the LED tracker to the cutting jig. Fine adjustments are then made in jig position to perfectly place it. Frequently, typical intra-medullary alignment instruments need to be adjusted 2–4° in both sagittal and coronal planes to achieve correct alignment.

Similarly, typical intra-medullary instruments are then used to align the distal femur osteotomy with refinement of jig position done with navigation. Femoral rotation and anterior/posterior position are then set, also using a navigated sizing instrument, which accommodates fine changes in rotational and anterior/posterior positioning. This allows the surgeon to make slight changes in femoral component placement to help achieve excellent soft-tissue balance. After every osseous resection, a plane probe is placed flush on the cut surface to verify the cut accuracy (◘ Fig. 15.5). An osseous file is used if necessary to make fine (0.5–1°) corrections.

The balancing/tensioning device is used once again after all osseous resections are completed to measure flexion/extension and collateral gap tension. Further soft-tissue releases are performed to balance the knee as needed.

Kinematic Analysis and Implant Placement

After gaps and collateral ligaments are balanced, trial implants are placed. Similar to the initial kinematic data obtained prior to osseous resections, kinematic values and curves with trial implants are available (◘ Fig. 15.6). The kinematic curves are particularly useful in evaluating the magnitude of soft-tissue laxity in the medial and lateral compartments. Ideally, the curves should be relatively smooth and parallel throughout a full range of motion. The kinematic data is also helpful in measuring any residual flexion contractures. It can be especially difficult to visualize residual knee flexion contractures accurately in obese patients without navigation.

Final implants are placed using normal cement technique. Fine corrections in femoral alignment can be made at this step. We have observed up to 3° of variability in alignment in standard placement of cemented femoral implants. This occurs due to the creation of asymmetric cement mantles on the medial and lateral distal femur either from the cement application or

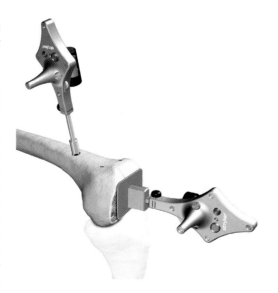

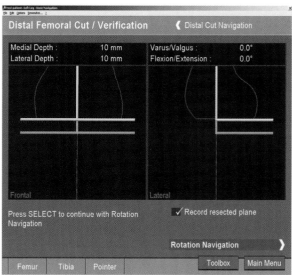

◘ **Fig. 15.5.** After every osseous resection, a plane probe can be placed flush on the cut surface to verify the cut accuracy

uneven pressure on the implant during insertion. We now standardly navigate the cemented femoral implant placement to avoid introducing unwanted changes in the alignment.

Overall image-free knee-navigation technique allows very fine and accurate soft-tissue- and osseous adjustments through nearly every crucial step of the procedure. The ability to perform such incremental adjustments combined with immediate and quantifiable

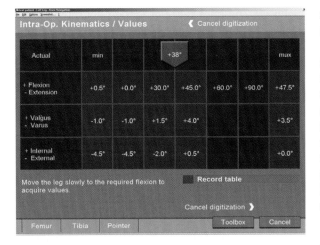

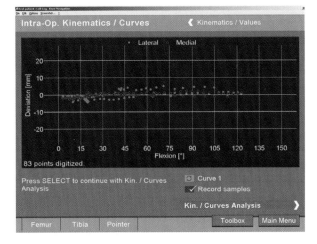

Fig. 15.6. Kinematic values and curves with trial implants are in place. The kinematic curves are particularly useful in evaluating the magnitude of soft-tissue laxity in the medial and lateral compartments

intra-operative data on alignment, gap tension, and kinematics allows surgeons to more consistently attain their surgical goals.

Risks of Image-Free Navigation

The primary risk of image-free navigation is for the surgeon to lose perspective on the value of the system. It is a very sophisticated tool, which, if used correctly, will markedly improve accuracy. It is not a robot that can think independently and take away responsibility from the surgeon for very important intra-operative decision

making. Knee navigation enhances the surgeons perspective, but should never replace it.

Further risks of navigation are standard, such as injury to neurovascular structures during placement of tracker screws and periprosthetic fractures. Over-pentration of the anterior to posterior femoral tracking screw is of particular concern, due to close proximity of femoral artery. Theoretically, the screw holes from the trackers could create stress risers resulting in a periprosthetic fracture especially if multiple drill holes were needed to place the tracking screw. Currently, there have been no reported cases of such periprosthetic fractures associated with knee navigation.

Lessons Learned from Knee Navigation

Important lessons have been learned from our use of knee navigation in over 300 consecutive cases. Knee navigation has clearly brought to our attention common steps in the surgical procedure which can introduce substantial error. Some errors have been recognized in the past but their etiology have been better defined with navigation and still other errors are previously not described.

Intra-Medullary Femoral Alignment

Intra-medullary alignment of the femoral is very inconsistent and highly dependent on the placement of the entry hole into the femur. Enlarging the entry hole as typically recommended, does not alleviate the errors in most cases. It is especially problematic with patients who have vacuous femoral canals. Most commonly intra-medullary femoral alignment introduces errors towards producing excessive flexion and valgus cuts.

Pinning of Cutting Guides

Typical technique used in pinning cutting guides frequently introduce alignment errors. Each time a pin is placed through any cutting guide, there is the potential to shift its position, thus we now place as few pins through guides as possible. Pins are placed with power-pin drivers instead of a mallet. We have found less movement of guides using this method. The design of the cutting guides are also crucial to preventing error. Guides which capture a significant length of the pin before contacting bone are much less likely to shift with pinning. Beware of cutting guides which capture only the tip of the pin – they tend to introduce much error.

Common Surgeon Judgment Errors

We have identified several steps in the surgical procedure of knee replacement where surgeons commonly misjudge alignment. One is to excessively internally rotate the tibial implant. This is most apparent in a varus knee with medial soft-tissue release. In this situation, the tibia in flexion is externally rotating on the intact lateral soft-tissue structures making visualization of rotational alignment difficult. We have found that Incavo's recommendation to use the mid-portion of the patella tendon to rotationally orient the tibial component to be most accurate [10]. Another common judgment error is to overestimate tibial slope using extra-medullary tibial alignment jigs. A final difficult alignment perspective for surgeons is evaluating flexion contractures especially in obese patients. The tendency is to underestimate the amount of flexion.

Early Results

Published results of image-free navigation have recently become available. Sparmann et al. have demonstrated significant improvement in implant alignment and a lower rate of need for knee manipulation in those patients who had a total knee arthroplasty with navigation compared to those without. Significant differences between the two groups in favor of navigation was apparent in overall mechanical limb alignment, frontal and sagittal femoral alignment, and frontal tibial alignment [11]. Similar results have been demonstrated by Stulberg [12].

Our experience in over 300 navigated total knee arthroplasty cases is consistent with the findings of Sparmann and Stulberg. Comparison by an independent reviewer of 100 of our patients with knee arthroplasty performed with and without navigation has shown significant improvements of mechanical alignment, femoral frontal and sagittal alignment, frontal tibial

alignment, and knee range of motion. Tourniquet time averaged 87 min with navigation compared to 78 min without. The learning curve based on length of tourniquet time was approximately twenty cases [13].

Further investigation is needed comparing patellar tracking, rotational alignment of implants, knee scores, post-operative kinematics of patients, and implant survival with knee arthroplasty performed with and without navigation.

Future Perspectives

The early experience of knee navigation has proved that accuracy of implant alignment can be enhanced without increased risk of complication. This has occurred despite the recent introduction of the technology and the still evolving techniques for use of navigation. It is reasonable to expect that as this innovative technology is used more widely, new surgical techniques will develop along with additional instruments which will interface with the navigation system.

In early stages of development are instruments which will completely eliminate all intra-medullary and extra-medullary based cutting guides. This will decrease the number of steps in the operative procedure and thus surgical time. Further electronic integration of surgical instruments, such as saws, drills, and tensioning devices with the knee-navigation system, will be possible.

The continued transition of knee arthroplasty from a mechanical to a fully computerized instrument system will stimulate the development of new techniques, instruments, and speed the innovation cycle for knee-replacement design. When this occurs, knee navigation, now a technology in its infancy, will have quickly reached adolescences fully ready to demonstrate its potential.

References

1. Teter KE, Bregman D, Colwell CW (1995) Accuracy of intra-medullary versus extramedullary tibial alignment cutting systems in total knee arthroplasty. Clin Orthop 321: 106–110
2. Griffen FM, Insall JN, Scuderi GR (2000) Accuracy of soft tissue balancing in total knee arthroplasty. J Arthroplasty 15(8): 970–973
3. Dennis DA, Komistek RD, Mahfouz MR, Haas BD, Stiehl JB (2003) Multicenter determination of in vivo kinematics after total knee arthroplasty. Clin Orthop 416: 37–57

4. Berger RA, Crossett LS, Jacobs JJ, Rubash HE (1998) Malrotation causing patellofemoral complications after total knee arthroplasty. Clin Orthop 356: 144–53

5. Garg A, Walker (1990) Prediction of total knee motion using a three-dimensional computer-graphics model. J Biomech 23(1): 45–58

6. Insall JN, Scott WN (2001) Surgery of the Knee. Churchill Livingstone, Philadelphia

7. Insall JN (1981) Technique of total knee replacement. Instr Course Lect 30: 324–29

8. Hungerford DS, Krackow KA (1985) Total joint arthroplasty of the knee. Clin Orthop 192: 23–33

9. White RE, Allman JK, Trauger JA, Dales BH (1999) Clinical comparison of the midvastus and medial parapatellar surgical approaches. Clin Orthop 367: 117–22

10. Incavo SJ, Coughlin KM, Pappas C, Beynnon BD (2003) Anatomic rotational relationships of the proximal tibia, distal femur, and patella. J Arthroplasty 18: 643–48

11. Sparmann M, Wolke B, Czupalla H, Banzer D, Zink A (2003) Positioning of total knee arthroplasty with and without navigation support. J Bone Joint Surg Br 85(6): 830–835

12. Stulberg S (2003) How accurate is current TKR instrumentation? Clin Orthop 416: 177–184

13. Anderson K, Markel D, Buehler K (2004) Unpublished data

Computer-Assisted Minimally Invasive Total Knee Arthroplasty

S.K. Chauhan

Introduction

Total knee arthroplasty has become one of the most successful procedures in orthopedic practice since its introduction in the early 1970s [1, 2]. Since its development, it has undergone many refinements, leading to good 10–15 year follow-up studies [3–5]. Correct component alignment and soft-tissue balancing have been cited as two of the most important components of successful knee-arthroplasty surgery [6, 7]. Alignment of the components is dependent on many factors including accurate pre-operative planning, normal bone morphology to which standardized instruments are applied and accurate placement of these instruments with the surgeons skill. Incorrect alignment caused by a variation of any of these factors can lead to abnormal wear [8, 9], premature mechanical loosening of the components [10, 11], and patellofemoral problems [12, 13].

Since the inception of total knee arthroplasty, many refinements in technique and instrumentation have been made. However, the majority of surgeries performed today, throughout the world, still involve the use of a large incision, intra-medullary instrumentation and fixed mechanical guides, whose aim is to produce consistent resections in the coronal, sagittal and axial planes in differing patient anatomy.

The orthopedic community is now faced with two new advancements in the field of knee arthroplasty surgery. The first is the introduction of surgeon-controlled computer-navigation systems, and the second is the increasing use of minimally invasive surgery.

Computer-navigation systems, which are widely used in mainland Europe and Australia, are now gaining popularity in the U.K. and North America. Their aim is to provide more accurate component implantation through digital mapping of standard anatomical landmarks and kinematic analysis. Surgical navigation systems can be divided into three groups: those where the information is collected pre-operatively (CT or MRI), those that use intra-operative imaging and, finally, those systems that build up a working model from the surgeon directly mapping out parts of the patient's knee prior to starting surgery, as has already been described in a previous chapter.

A number of studies [14–16] have now shown that there is improved alignment of both the limb and the components, when this technology is used. Further advantages, including reduced blood loss and reduction of fat embolism, have been suggested as most systems are now combined with extra-medullary instrumentation.

The resurgence of unicondylar knee arthroplasty in the 1990s has been due to many factors. One has been the more rapid recovery of patients following surgery when it is combined with a minimally invasive approach. A number of authors [17–19] have now used conventional instrumentation to successfully perform total knee-arthroplasty surgery, through reduced incision sizes. All have used miniature versions of standard IM instrumentation, combined with differing surgical approaches. The results have shown improved pain scores, early ambulation and range of motion, and earlier discharge from hospital. However the positioning of components remains in question with one series [19], showing an average femoral component valgus of 6° in the coronal plane.

With the far superior accuracy of navigation systems, together with their use of extra-medullary instrumentation, it seems a logical progression to try to combine the advantages of navigation systems with minimally invasive incisions to maximize the effects of rapid recovery following surgery with increased longevity of components through more accurate placement of components and reduced wear. The marriage of these two technologies provides further exciting possibility in the use of true quadriceps-sparing lateral approaches, freehand cutting-block placement and in-situ bone cutting where minimal soft-tissue retraction and bone dislocation is performed.

Method

This method describes minimally invasive computer-assisted total knee arthroplasty using:
- either a mini-, mid-vastus or true lateral surgical approach,
- in situ bone-cutting techniques,
- specialist side-cutting instrumentation,
- the Stryker knee navigation system,
- the Scorpio CR knee-replacement system.

In developing a new method for minimally invasive knee-arthroplasty surgery, the ability to place a cutting block in space anywhere around the femoral or tibial surfaces means that there is no longer a need to displace the patella in order to resect the distal femur as the resection can take place in a medial-lateral or lateral-medial direction depending on which approach is used. This essentially leaves the patella in situ whilst the distal cut is made. More importantly, the ability to check the position of the cutting block prior to resection and then to verify the accuracy of resection means that the surgeon can confidently resect from the side and avoid varus or valgus cuts that can occur when using side-cutting techniques. A similar freehand method is used to resect the proximal tibia. The evolution of this technique has led to the development of universal cutting instruments, which result in the same resection blocks being used on the distal femur and proximal tibia. As these blocks are placed into position using a freehand technique, no extra- or intra-medually jigs are needed, which means that the resections are made entirely through captured resection blocks as opposed to the use a partially resected surface of bone to rest the blade on whilst completing the resection. The ability to localize both Whiteside axis and the trans-epicondylar axis results in the correct femoral rotation, being achieved whilst the

kinematic analysis of the deformity prior to resections being made and after trial implantation of components allow accurate soft-tissue balancing to be achieved.

Surgical Technique

The patient is placed supine on a standard operating table. A tourniquet is applied and standard skin preparation and draping is undertaken. The surgeon's usual preference of supports is used; however, closely placed lateral supports may interfere with the initial navigation hip registration. Two distal foot supports are used to allow the knee to be flexed to 45° or 90°, as the surgeon will develop flexion, mid-flexion and extension surgical windows to operate in.

The patient's patella, patella tendon, medial tibial plateau and distal femur are marked out using a surgical marker pen. With the knee flexed, a 10–12 cm incision is marked out medial to the patella and patella tendon. The skin and underlying subcutaneous tissue is then incised to show the underlying knee retinaculum. At the superior end of the wound, the fibers of the vastus medialis muscle (VMO) are seen to insert into the medial side of the patella. A 2-cm stab wound is made in the VMO fibers at the edge of the patella in a 10 or 2 o'clock position, depending on which knee is being operated on. The incision is then continued down along the side of the patella to the inferior aspect of the wound.

Through the medial arthrotomy wound, the fat pad is partly excised together with the anterior horn of the medial meniscus. An interval is created on the medial side by releasing the antero-medial knee capsule/retinaculum from the anterior surface of the tibia. This further aids visualization of the medial side of the knee and creates also a pocket for the dedicated cutting blocks to be placed in.

With the knee in mid-flexion/extension, a soft-tissue retractor (e.g. Langenbeck) is placed under the patella tendon close to its insertion into the tibia. A small segment (no more then 1 cm) of the patella tendon can be released from the tibial surface to aid exposure. With the retractor in position, the surgeon can visualize the antero-lateral surface of the tibia and anterior horn of the lateral meniscus. This can be removed under direct vision.

The surgeon's attention is now focused on the superior aspect of the wound. The leg is held in extension and two soft-tissue retractors are placed under the fibers of the VMO and quadriceps expansion. Both retractors are lifted up to visualize the supra-patellar pouch. In the interval below the VMO/quadriceps mechanism, the anterior capsule is visible to the surgeon as a fine white fibrous layer. This is often attached to the undersurface of the VMO/quadriceps mechanism and needs to be dissected free with Meztabaum scissors. Once free, it is divided longitudinally. The fat and synovial tissue over the anterior surface of the distal femur is next removed and finally any plical bands attaching the medial capsular layer to the medial side of the femur are divided to create a free medial gutter.

Once the proximal and distal releases have been performed, the patella can be easily displaced across the lateral side if required. Next, the surgeon's attention is turned to the insertion of the navigation pins. Due to the desire not to tether the quadriceps mechanism, the interval between the IT band and quadriceps mechanism is identified and a percutaneous stab wound made. A tracker pin is inserted in an antero-lateral to postero-medial direction. A further percutaneous stab wound is made over the anterior tibial surface at least 2 cm below the tibial tuberosity. A tibial tracker pin is then inserted.

The center of the femoral head, distal femoral landmarks, proximal tibial landmarks and ankle landmarks are then registered, using the surgical navigation system. Once this information has been registered, the knee can be analyzed from a kinematic viewpoint to assess the varus/valgus of the knee and the degree of flexion contracture. This can be done not only at 0° and 90°, as with traditional tensioning devices, but through a dynamic arc of movement. The deformity can also be gently stressed to assess how much is easily correctable and how much is fixed. With this simple maneuver, the surgeon can build up a picture of possible soft-tissue contractures and the possible remedial solutions.

The distal femoral resection requires the surgeon to position the block in relation to the three axes of freedom, varus/valgus, flexion/extension and distal resection depth, solely by positioning the block in space. The tibial tracker is attached to the resection-plane probe which in turn is placed into the captured slot of the cutting block. The cutting block/tracker construct is then held by the surgeon with a tripod grip. The cutting block/tracker construct is now an active tool whose virtual position can be monitored on the computer-navigation screen (Fig. 16.1).

The surgeon first places the cutting block against the medial surface of the femur. Then, in a similar method to arthroscopy, he watches the navigation screen as he moves the block into the desired position with one hand, leaving the second hand free to hold the pin driver. Depth of resection is achieved by moving the block in a proximal/distal direction. Flexion/extension of the block is achieved by rotating the block in the appropriate flexion/extension direction. Finally, varus/valgus positioning of the cutting block is achieved by tilting the block in a medial or lateral direction relative to the long axis of the femur (Fig. 16.2).

A blunt curved retractor is placed under the patella/patella tendon, with its tip in the lateral gutter of the knee. This retractor acts as a tissue protector rather then a true retractor, as it separates the quads/patella mechanism from the saw blade.

With the knee in mid-flexion, a saw is then used to cut from a medial to lateral direction through the flat surface of the block. The curved portion of the block can be used to cut the medial femoral condyle in an antero-posterior direction (Fig. 16.3). The resected part of the condyle is removed and the resection-plane probe placed on the distal cut surface to verify the depth and accuracy of the cut. This is the recorded on the femoral cut-verification screen.

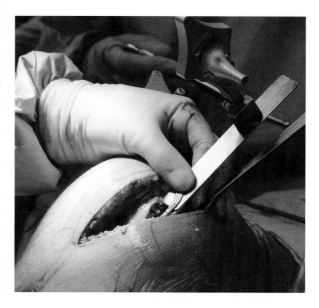

Fig. 16.1. The Universal J Block with attached resection plane probe are seen in the medial mid vastus pocket

The proximal tibial cut is performed with the same cutting block, and a similar freehand technique of cutting-block placement is also used as for the distal femur. The cutting block is first placed into the wound and medial soft-tissue envelope, created during the initial dissection.

The surgeon then orientates the block so that the correct depth, varus/valgus and slope are achieved. The depth is achieved by proximal/distal movement of the block, whilst varus/valgus is achieved by tilting the block in medial/lateral direction about the long axis of the tibia. The desired slope for resection is achieved by tilting the block forward or backward. Once again the block is held with a tripod grip, and the virtual movements of the block can be monitored in real time on the navigation screen.

A retractor is placed under the patella ligament and another placed to protect the MCL. With the knee at 90° of flexion, a saw blade is then introduced into the captured slot and the medial part of the tibial plateau cut through the anterior portion of the cutting block (■ Fig. 16.4). The saw blade is then turned obliquely through the curved portion of the cutting block and the anterior portion of the lateral tibial plateau is cut. Next a curved retractor is placed behind the central tibial plateau, to protect the PCL, and the central and posterior parts of the proximal tibia are cut. Finally, a malleable retractor is inserted between the LCL and lateral tibial plateau, and the posterior-lateral tibial plateau is cut. This latter cut needs to be performed carefully to avoid damage to the LCL.

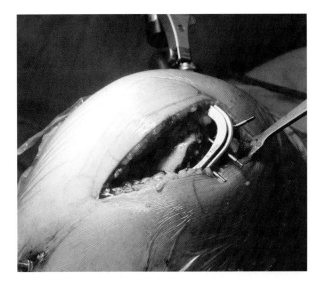

■ **Fig. 16.2.** The Universal J block pinned in situ

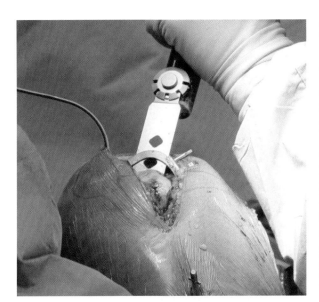

■ **Fig. 16.3.** The Universal J block allows resection in an AP and medial-lateral direction

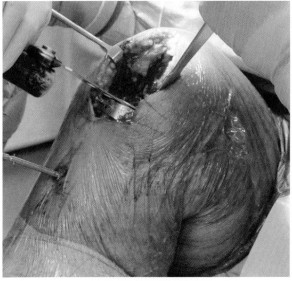

■ **Fig. 16.4.** Proximal tibial resection with the Universal J Block pinned in situ

The knee is then placed into extension, where the previously resected distal femur provides space. An osteotome is used to free the cut proximal plateau, and graspers are the utilized to remove the resected piece of bone. Soft-tissue attachment to the resected bone is removed from medial side, then the posterior aspect and finally the lateral side. The resected piece of bone is then removed and the resection level checked with navigation.

During the resection of both distal femur and proximal tibia, the tibio- femoral articulation has not been dislocated, and, as such, true in-situ cutting has occurred.

During the initial anatomical landmark navigation registration, the lateral epicondyle was approximated. With the distal femur resected, the rotational landmarks of the femur are remapped, using a special referencing guide shown below. This guide is based on the 90° relationship between Whitside's AP axis and the transepicondylar axis (◘ Fig. 16.5).

An anterior skim guide is then used to produce an anterior skim cut, which has the correct rotational alignment, as calculated by the navigation system. A miniature 4-in-1 resection block is then used to finish the femoral cuts (◘ Fig. 16.6).

The tibial baseplate is then inserted and the correct rotation achieved with the navigation unit (◘ Fig. 16.7).

The trial femur is the inserted together with a trial poly insert, and the kinematics of the knee are assessed again. A direct comparison can then be made with the pre-surgery kinematic data, and appropriate changes to

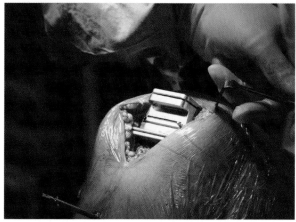

◘ **Fig. 16.6.** The 4 in 1 cutting block placed on the distal femur

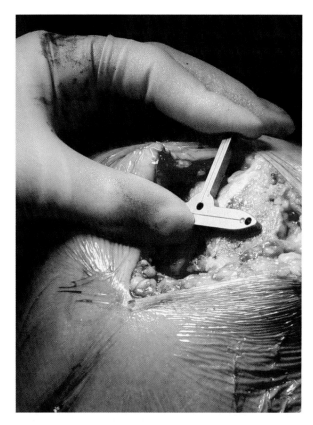

◘ **Fig. 16.5.** The femoral rotational guide placed on the distal femur

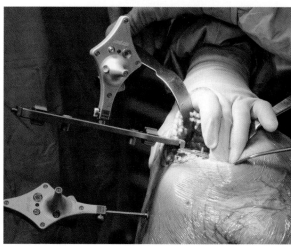

◘ **Fig. 16.7.** Tibial baseplate rotation and sizing

the size of the tibial insert or soft-tissue releases can be performed with instant bio-feedback.

Once the surgeon is satisfied with the limb alignment and soft-tissue balance, the real components can be cemented into place (◘ Figs. 16.8, 16.9).

By utilizing the flexion, mid-flexion and extension windows, the components can be inserted safely and any excess cement can be removed.

The wound is then closed in a standard fashion (◘ Figs. 16.10, 16.11).

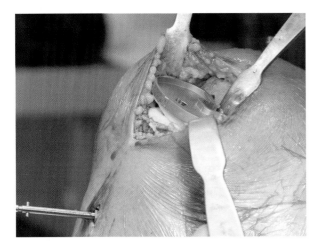

◘ Fig. 16.8. Tibial baseplate insertion

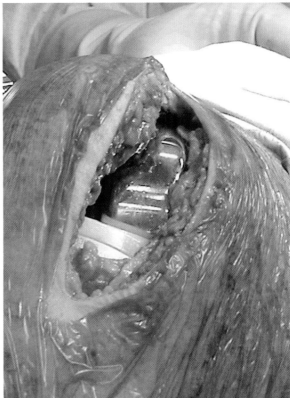

◘ Fig. 16.10. Total Knee Arthroplasty in situ

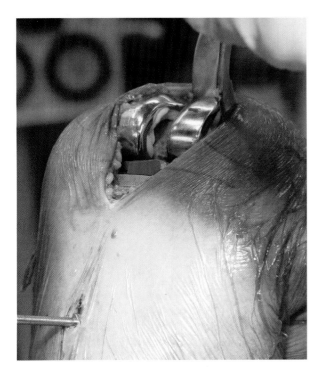

◘ Fig. 16.9. Femoral component insertion

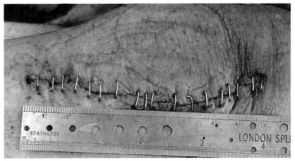

◘ Fig. 16.11. Ten centimetre incision size

Anesthesia and Pain Relief

All patients have spinal anesthesia, the effects of which wear off within 4 h of surgery. Once the patients have sensations in the sole of the foot, they are allowed to mobilize freely. Their pain relief consists of either a PCA pump or a combination of opiods and NSAIDs

Results

One of the most important aspects of minimally invasive surgery, is not to sacrifice shorter term gains in recovery of function for poor component positioning, which ulti-

mately may lead to a higher number of revision procedures later. We therefore watched the first 22 patients who underwent this new procedure looking at the radiological alignment of components, blood loss, length of stay, time to straight leg raise/90° of flexion and surgery times.

On long-leg Maquet views, the majority of patients had a standing femoral-tibial angle of within 3° of neutral, as shown in ◘ Fig. 16.12.

The mean position of the femoral component was 1.5° valgus, whilst the mean position of the tibial component was 0.5° varus. The distribution of position of both components is shown in ◘ Figs. 16.13 and 16.14, where 90° indicates neutral and increasing values indicate a valgus position.

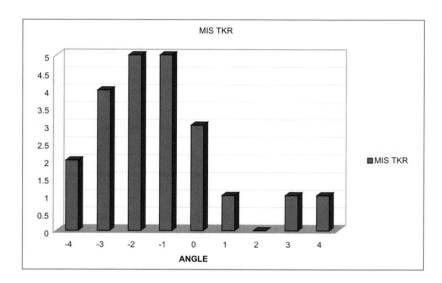

◘ **Fig. 16.12.** Long-leg Maquet angles for computer-assisted MIS TKR. Negative values indicate valgus and positive values indicate varus

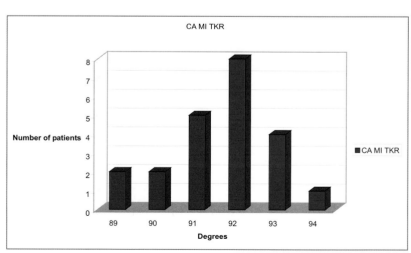

◘ **Fig. 16.13.** Femoral component position on standing Maquet views

The length of patient stay in the MIS group was compared to a similar group of open computer-assisted knee replacements and their distribution is shown in ◘ Fig. 16.15. The mean length of stay for the MIS group was 3.25 days whilst it was 6.04 days for the open computer-navigated group.

Surgical OR time ranged from 180 min at the start of the learning curve to 100 min for the last cases. Patients achieved straight leg raise from 1–9 h after surgery and the majority took 3–12 h to take their first steps with a walking frame.

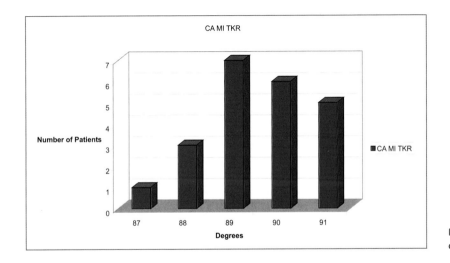

◘ **Fig. 16.14.** Tibial component position on standing Maquet views

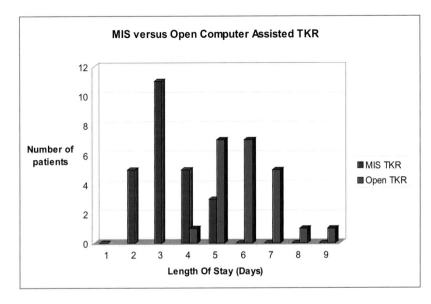

◘ **Fig. 16.15.** Lengths of stay in MIS and open computer-assisted surgery

16

Conclusions

Computer-assisted minimally invasive total knee arthroplasty has, in its infancy, produced a dramatic leap forward in both surgical technique and patient recovery. The ability to cut accurately from the side, leave the joint in situ to avoid repetitive joint dislocation and produce minimal trauma to the entire soft-tissue envelope of the knee – not just the quadriceps mechanism –, is clearly producing dramatic results as shown in our short early series.

All minimally invasive surgery, including computer-assisted techniques, is technically demanding and surgeons must realize the limitations both in terms of their own surgical ability and patient selection. The technique, whilst rewarding, is technically demanding. Some previous use of computer navigation during open arthroplasty surgery is certainly an advantage, as is the progressive down-sizing of the surgical incision. Many manufacturers provide cadaveric courses, which are highly commended. In this era of patient-led decisions, the question is which patients are suitable for such a minimally invasive procedure. Clearly any patient who would be a candidate for total knee-arthroplasty surgery under normal circumstances may be a candidate for an MIS TKR. In those patients who have a varus or neutral deformity, a mid-vastus procedure is applicable, whilst in those with a valgus deformity, a lateral approach is more applicable. Clearly having a universal approach with the same instrumentation has advantages in dealing with the diversity of patients in clinical practice. In obese patients, MIS surgery can be performed more easily than in heavy-muscled male patients. Significant bone loss on either tibial or femoral sides requiring bone wedges or significant flexion contractures is a contraindication to an MIS procedure.

Whilst the aims of all minimally invasive surgery techniques is to reduce soft-tissue trauma, post-operative pain and hospital stays, it is clear that this must not be at the cost of poor surgical positioning of components that will ultimately lead to early failures and revisions.

▼

The potential for surgical inaccuracies when operating through small incisions is a reality, and errors can be frequent as the surgeon's normal visual landmarks are not always clearly visible. This may lead to an excessive amount of retraction on a small wound, which may be more detrimental than performing the surgery through a normal incision. The use of computer navigation has provided many advantages as well as challenges. The use of entirely extra-medullary devices means that the medullary canal of either the femur or the tibia is not violated, reducing the risk of cognitive impairment from fat embolism. The lack of need for an intra-medullary rod also reduces the pressure on the patella and the need to forcibly displace it laterally when inserting such a device. The accuracy that computer navigation gives to the surgeon, both in positioning cutting blocks and verifying resection levels, is unsurpassed and has been proven in many studies to exceed the accuracy of current instrumentation. The ability of these systems to provide instant bio-feedback when performing soft-tissue releases provides the perfect platform to produce a well-balanced knee arthroplasty.

The combination of computer navigation with minimally invasive surgery has provided surgeons with an exciting opportunity. Despite navigation technology still being in its infancy, it has already far surpassed conventional instrumentation and is used in many operating rooms around the world. The future of this technology will be in the development of less invasive tracker attachments, more advanced software developments which map out gap kinematics even more accurately, smart polyethylene inserts which will give the surgeon instant load readings with different sizes of inserts, and a reduction in financial cost. The future of joint replacements as a whole may be the development of specific MIS implants with installed sensors, so the surgeon can monitor a patient's knee for any number of variables. Whilst to many surgeons some of these ideas may seem fanciful, many manufacturers aim to make them real within the next two years.

References

1   Insall J, Ranawat CS, Scott WN, Walker P: Total condylar knee replacement: Preliminary report. Clin Orthop 120:149–154, 1976

2. Insall J, Tria AJ, Scott WN: The total condylar knee prosthesis: The first five years. Clin Orthop 145: 68–77, 1979

3. Stern SH, Insall JN. Posterior stabilised prosthesis: results after follow-up of 9–12 years. J Bone Joint Surg Am 74-A: 980–986, 1992

4. Vince KG, Insall JN, Kelly MA. The total condylar prosthesis: 10 to 12 year results of a cemented knee replacement. J Bone Joint Surg Br 3: 17–25, 1989

5. Ranawat CS, Flynn Jr WF, Saddler S, Hansraj KK, Maynard MJ: Long-term results of the total condylar knee arthroplasty: A 15 year survivorship study. Clin Orthop 286: 96–102, 1993.

6. Freeman MA, Todd RC, Bamert P, Day WH: ICLH arthroplasty of the knee: 1968–1977. J Bone Joint Surg Br 60: 339–344, 1978

7. Insall JN, Scott WN, Ranawat CS: The total condylar prosthesis. A report of two hundred and twenty cases. J Bone Joint Surg Am 61: 173–180, 1979

8. Laskin RS: Total condylar knee replacement in patients who have rheumatoid arthritis. A ten-year follow up study. J Bone Joint Surg Am 72: 529–535, 1990

9. Wasiliewski RC, Galante JO, Leighty R, Natarajan RN, Rosenberg AG: Wear patterns on retrieved polyethylene inserts and their relationship to technical considerations during total knee arthroplasty. Clin Orthop 229: 31–43, 1994

10. Jeffery RS, Morris RW, Denham RA: Coronal alignment after total knee replacement. J Bone Joint Surg Br 73: 709–714, 1991

11. Tew M, Waugh W: Tibiofemoral alignment and the results of knee replacement. J Bone Joint Surg Br 67: 551–556, 1985

12. Figgie HE, Goldberg VM, Heiple KG, Moller HS, Gordon NH: The influence of tibial patellofemoral location on function of the knee in patients with posterior stabilized condylar knee prosthesis. J Bone Joint Surg Am 68: 1035–1040, 1986

13. Figgie HE 3rd, Goldberg VM, Figgie MP, Inglis AE, Kelly M, Sobel M: The effect of alignment of the implant on fractures of the patella after condylar total knee arthroplasty. J Bone Joint Surg 71A: 1031–1039, 1989

14. Chauhan S, Clark GW, Breidahl W, Sikorski JM: Computer-assisted knee arthroplasty versus conventional jig based technique. J Bone Joint Surg 86-B: 366–371, 2004

15. Sparmann M, Wolke B, Czupalla H, Banzer D, Zink A: Positioning of total knee arthroplasty with and without navigation support. J Bone Joint Surg 85-B: 830–835, 2003

16. Krachow KA et al.: Computer assisted orthopaedic surgery – 3rd Annual Meeting of CAOS (International Proceedings), June 18–21, 2003. Steinkopff, Darmstadt

17. Bonutti P, Mont M: Minimum 2 year follow up of MIS TKA. AAOS 2004

18. Tria AJ, Coon TM: Minimal incision total knee arthroplasty-early experience. Clin Orthop 416: 185–190, 2003

19. Laskin RS: New techniques and concepts in total knee replacement. Clin Orthop 416: 151–153, 2003

CAOS as an Adjunct to MIS – the Ideal Partnership in Performing Unicompartmental Knee Arthroplasty

A.J. Cossey, A.J. Spriggins

Introduction

Unicompartmental knee arthroplasty (UKA) has been part of the orthopedic surgeon's armamentarium for the treatment of unicompartmental osteoarthritis for the past thirty years. Its basic premise is that one can resurface only those portions of the knee that are severely involved with degenerate change, whilst allowing relatively normal articular surfaces to remain in situ. This allows for improved restoration of the biomechanics of the knee, leaving the uninvolved compartments and ligaments to function normally. These factors have enabled UKA surgery to develop over the years to become a valuable alternative to total knee replacement and high tibial osteotomy. Many advantages over total knee replacement and high tibial osteotomy in the treatment of isolated medial compartmental osteoarthritis have been advocated, including decreased soft-tissue disturbance, improved physiological gait, preservation of bone stock, decreased blood loss, quicker operation time, and a decrease in hospitalization for the patient [1, 2].

The recent orthopedic literature has reported excellent mid- to long-term results in both fixed and mobile bearing UKAs, performed for medial compartment disease [3–10]. Outstanding survivorship of 95% and 98% have been reported by Carr et al. [11] and Svard et al. [2]. With such positive clinical results, the potential for more orthopedic surgeons to perform UKA surgery is inevitable. However, many factors are associated with successful UKA surgery, including appropriate patient selection, good implant design and meticulous surgical technique [12–16]. Strict patient selection is crucial in order to achieve successful results. Patients with significant patello-femoral symptoms, dysfunctional anterior cruciate ligaments, fixed flexion greater than 10° and poor correction of leg alignment in the coronal axis are poor candidates for UKA surgery.

UKA surgery is technically demanding and less forgiving than other forms of arthroplasty surgery. In particular, poor surgical technique can result in poor soft-tissue balance, component mal-position and incorrect alignment in the coronal tibio-femoral axis. One of the most important predictors of success in UKA surgery is the accuracy with which the components are implanted. Accurate alignment in the coronal plane is important in relation to the survivorship of the prosthesis. In particular, if a varus deformity is over-corrected at the time of surgery, this will lead to excessive loads on the unresurfaced compartments of the knee, leading to disease progression, anterior cruciate ligament dysfunction and ultimately early failure of the prosthesis [17–21]. Biomechanical computer-stimulated models show that over-correction causes increased stress patterns in the lateral compartment allowing a kinematic conflict to develop [22]. Survivorship analysis in many studies shows disease progression to account for as many as 10% of revision procedures [1, 7, 8, 23, 24]. Other studies have shown that at the time of revision as many as 57% of patients show lateral compartment disease progression [25–27]. Over-correction also leads abnormal stresses on the bearing surface of the implant which lead to premature failure of the prosthesis [4]. These studies highlight the importance of achieving the correct intra-operative leg alignment to promote the long-term survivorship of the implant.

Minimally invasive surgery (MIS) is the accepted gold standard in performing UKAs. The advantages of performing small para-patellar incisions include less disruption to the soft-tissue sleeve, a decrease in blood loss and a quicker rehabilitation program. However, this comes at the expense of overall exposure to the knee joint and the anatomical landmarks needed for achieving correct, reproducible component positioning. Improvements in instru-mentation have tried to address the problems associated with the limited exposure but are still far from the ideal in achieving consistently reproducible accurate component position. Is computer-assisted orthopedic surgery (CAOS) the way forward in achieving the surgical aims in UKA?

CAOS enables the orthopedic surgeon to have a high-er degree of intra-operative control in performing accu-rate surgery and can be achieved through small incisions. Its aim is to provide excellent intra-operative feedback so that errors resulting from mal-alignment or poor bone cuts can be addressed immediately and rectified. This has the potential to decrease morbidity, improve functional outcome, improve patient satisfaction and decrease revi-sion rates. It has the potential to have a significant impact in achieving correct component position in minimally in-vasive UKA surgery. The potential for accurate and repro-ducible leg alignment this system theoretically achieves will improve the biomechanical forces within both the re-placed compartment and that of the unresurfaced com-partment. This will lead to less disease progression and, hopefully, an improved environment for the implant to function with the ultimate goal being an improvement in long-term survivorship and reduced revision rates.

Surgical Results

A recent study performed at our unit involved thirty con-secutive patients undergoing UKA surgery. Of this group, fifteen had MIS with no CAOS whilst fifteen had MIS with CAOS. Post-operatively, all patients had long-leg weight-bearing radiographs and CT scanograms of the limb to assess alignment (Figs. 17.1, 17.2). Analysis of this data showed that the implants that were aligned with CAOS had no over-correction of the original deformity unlike the group which did not involve CAOS. This was support-ed statistically with a Fisher's exact test of $p<0.05$. This improved accuracy in radiological leg alignment using CAOS was achieved without significant inconvenience and little change to conventional operating techniques.

Surgical Technique

The EIUS unicompartmental knee system (Stryker Howmedica Osteonics) allows CAOS to act as an adjunct in performing UKA surgery. It relies on an "image-free

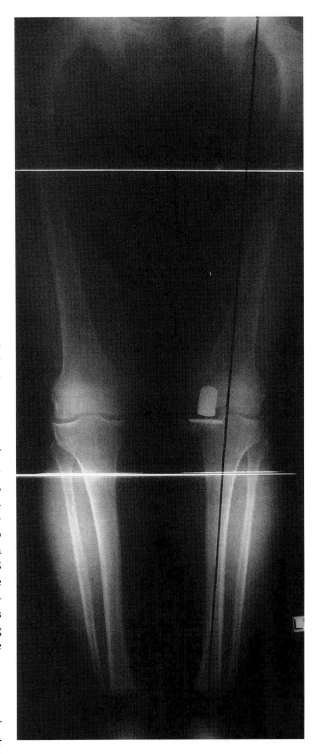

Fig. 17.1. Long-leg weight-bearing radiograph assessing alignment in an EIUS UKA

17

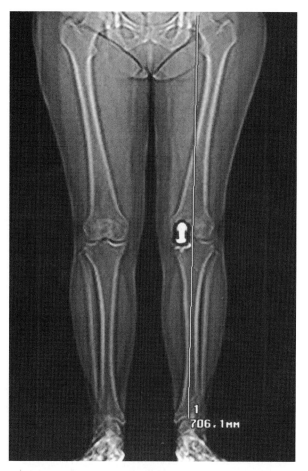

◨ **Fig. 17.2.** CT scanograms assessing leg alignment in an EIUS UKA

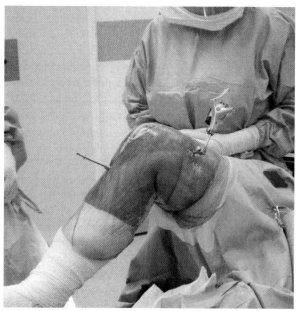

◨ **Fig. 17.3.** Photograph showing pin placement

system" i.e. an anatomical model is embedded in software and upgraded by the process of intra-operative navigation. Six main steps are involved in performing this type of surgery.

- **Pin placement:** Two fixed pins are drilled into position; one on the medial side of the distal femur, the other on the proximal tibia just below the tuberosity (◨ Fig. 17.3). These allow for attachment of infra-red beacons which relay back to the computer allowing anatomical and kinematic data to be collected.
- **Registration of anatomical landmarks:** This involves a pre-determined sequence in which the surgeon identifies key anatomical landmarks using an infrared pointer (◨ Fig. 17.4). These landmarks are logged onto the computer. There are fourteen land-

marks including center of rotation of femoral head, landmarks relating to the distal femur, landmarks relating to the proximal tibia and landmarks relating to the ankle. Accuracy is fundamental.

- **Kinematic analysis:** Data is collected and recorded on the computer relating to the coronal and sagittal axis prior to surgery, i.e. any fixed flexion deformity or varus-valgus leg mal-alignment present.
- **Cutting block set-up and performance of cuts:** The cutting blocks for both tibia and femur are computer-navigated into position (◨ Figs. 17.5, 17.6). Leg alignment and thickness of cuts are verified (◨ Figs. 17.7, 17.8). Varus mal-alignment is never over-corrected. Cuts generated are checked and if the surgeon is not satisfied these are repeated until acceptable.
- **Analysis of alignment and kinematics following insertion of trial prosthesis:** Analysis in real-time allows assessment of the position and performance of the prosthesis. Leg alignment is assessed allowing no over-correction of varus deformities.
- **Final analysis of alignment and kinematics following definitive insertion of prosthesis:** The definitive prosthesis is assessed and data stored on computer in relation to its alignment and kinematic performance.

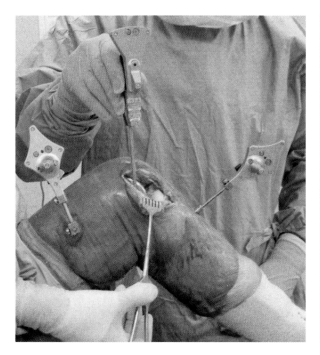

■ **Fig. 17.4.** Photograph showing the use of the mobile beacon to register anatomical landmarks

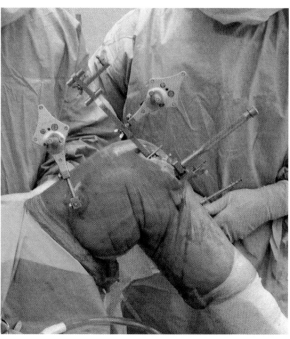

■ **Fig. 17.6.** Photograph showing instrument set-up to achieve femoral cut. The cutting block is computer-navigated into position in order to achieve correct rotation and cut depth

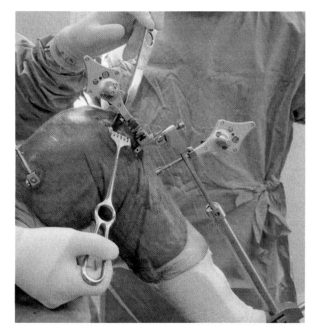

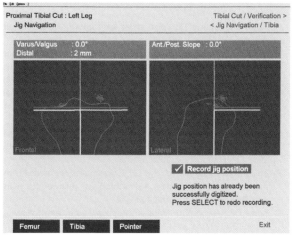

■ **Fig. 17.7.** Visual display of tibial cut verification. Data analyzed enables the correct alignment and depth of cut to be achieved

■ **Fig. 17.5.** Photograph showing instrument set-up to achieve tibial cut. The cutting block is computer-navigated into the correct position with continuous feedback from the visual display unit

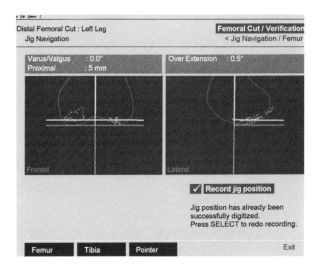

■ **Fig. 17.8.** Visual display of femoral cut verification. Data analyzed enables the correct orientation of the prosthesis to be achieved

References

1. Murray DW, Goodfellow JW, O'Connor JJ. The Oxford medial unicompartmental arthroplasty. JBJS 1998; 80B: 983–989
2. Svard UCG, Price AJ. Oxford medial unicompartmental knee arthroplasty: a survival analysis of an independent series. JBJS 2001; 83B: 191–194
3. Capra SW, Fehring TK. Unicondylar arthroplasty. A survivorship analysis. JOA 1992; 7: 247–251
4. Weale AE, Newman JH. Unicompartmental knee arthroplasty and high tibial osteotomy for osteoarthritis of the knee. A comparative study with 12 to 17 year follow-up. Clin Orthop 1994; 302: 134–137
5. Carter P, Sanouiller JL, Grelsamer PR. Unicompartmental knee arthroplasty surgery. 10 year minimum follow-up. JOA 1996; 11: 782–788
6. Heck DA, Marmor L, Gibson A. Unicompartmental knee arthroplasty. A multicentre investigation with long term follow-up evaluation. Clin Orthop 1993; 286: 154–159
7. Ansari S, Newman JH, Ackroyd CE. St Georg sled for medial compartment knee replacement. 461 arthroplasty followed for years. Acta Orthop Scand 1997; 68: 430–434
8. Tabor OB. Unicompartmental arthroplasty: long term follow-up study. JOA 1998; 13: 373–379
9. Squire MW, Callaghan JJ, Geoty DD, Sullivan PM, Johnston RC. Unicompartmental knee arthroplasty. A minimum 15 year follow-up. Clin Orthop 1999; 367: 61–72
10. Robertson O, Knutson K, Lewold S, Liogren L. The routine of surgical management reduces failure after unicompartmental knee arthroplasty. JBJS 2001; 83B: 45–49
11. Carr A, Keyes G, Miller R, O'Connor J, Goodfellow J. Medial unicompartmental knee arthroplasty. A survival study of the Oxford meniscal knee. Clin Orth 1998; 295: 205–213
12. Marmor L. Unicompartmental and total knee arthroplasty. Clin Orthop 1985; 192: 75–81
13. Andriacchi TP, Galante JO, Fermier RW. The influence of total knee replacement design on walking and stair climbing. JBJS (Am) 1982; 64A: 1328–1335
14. Newman JH, Ackroyd CE, Shan NA. Unicompartmental or total knee replacement: 5 year results of a prospective randomised trial. JBJS 1998; 80B: 862–865
15. Broughton NS, Newman JH, Baily RAJ. Unicompartmental replacement. A high tibial osteotomy for osteoarthritis of the knee. A comparative study after 10 years. JBJS 1986; 68B: 447–451
16. Chestnut WJ. Pre-operative diagnosis protocol to predict unicompartmental knee arthroplasty. Proceedings of the knee society. Anakeim, California. March 10, 1991
17. Weale AE, Murray DW, Crawford R. Does arthritis progress after medial compartment knee replacement. JBJS 1999; 81B: 783–789
18. Dieppe P. Towards a better understanding of osteoarthritis of the knee joint. The Knee 2000; 7: 135–137
19. Weale AE, Murray DW, Baines J, Newman JH. Radiological changes 5 years after unicompartmental knee replacement. JBJS 2000; 82B: 996–1000
20. Deshmuckh RV, Scott R. Unicompartmental knee replacement long term results. Clin Orthop 2001; 392: 272–278
21. Ackroyd CE, Whitehouse SL, Joslin CC, Newman JH.
    The ten year survivorship. A comparative study of the medial St Georg sled and Kinematic total knee arthroplasty. JBJS 2002; 86B: 532–538
22. Barratt D. Over correction causes kinematic conflict in a biomechanical computer simulated model. Intelligent Orthopaedic seminar; Depuy AOA Oct. 2003
23. Scott RD, Cobb AG, McQueary FG, Thornhill TS. Unicompartmental knee arthroplasty: eight to twelve years follow-up evaluation and survivorship analysis. Clin Orthop 1991; 271: 96–100
24. Barrett WP, Scott RD. Revision of failed unicondylar knee arthroplasty. JBJS 1987; 69A: 1328–1335
25. Chakrabarty G, Newman J H, Ackroyd CE. Revision of unicompartmental arthroplasty. Clinical and technical considerations. JOA 1998; 13: 191–196
26. Gill T, Schemitsch E, Brick GW. Revision total knee arthroplasty after total knee arthroplasty or high tibial Osteotomy. Clin Orthop 1995; 321: 10–18
27. Dauwe D, Bellemans J, Ulrus M, Victor J, Farby G. A comparararive study of intramedullary tibial alignment systems. Orthop Int 1996; 4: 21–84

Freehand Navigation For Bone Shaping

P.S. Walker, C.S. Wei, R.E. Forman

Introduction

This chapter describes a method for carrying out knee-replacement surgery where the bone cuts are made freehand, guided by feedback from a computer screen or other means, as opposed to the standard surgical techniques using jigs and fixtures. The potential advantages of freehand navigation are speed, simplicity and accuracy, together with no increase in the cost per procedure. There are numerous total and unicondylar knee systems, each with its own technique, frequently more than one for a particular design. However, there are many similarities between the techniques, the common element being a set of jigs and fixtures which are sequentially positioned on the bones in order to guide the cuts. The goal is to achieve an accurate fit of the components on to the bones, and an accurate overall limb alignment. While experience has shown that the components seldom fit exactly on to the bones, the size of the gaps and irregularities have not been quantified to our knowledge. When cement is used, small gaps may not be important, but that is not the case for uncemented components. Overall alignment has been measured in a number of studies. In a large case study, only 75% of the cases achieved a knee valgus angle of 4–10°, measured from radiographs [5]. When a navigation system was used to measure alignments, it was found that there was a greater spread of results using jigs and fixtures compared with navigation [9]. Several degrees error can result from the use of current intra-medullary rods [7]. The recent introduction of minimally-invasive techniques for total and uni knees [8, 11] similarly increased the range of error compared with standard incisions [2]. Nevertheless, the popularity of reduced incisions has continued to grow due to its advantages, but in contrast, navigation has not become widely used in the USA up to this time, probably because of cost and time. Knee replacement using standard techniques has had successful results as measured by survivorship, but many of the failures or unsatisfactory results that have occurred have been due to mis-alignment and instability, the latter due to incorrect ligament balancing. Alignment and balancing can both be improved using navigation techniques. Hence it can be proposed that, if knee replacements are to be performed more and more using smaller incisions, there needs to be a parallel improvement in the surgical technique with regard to alignment and fit. This chapter aims to show that freehand navigation, being a simplified version of present navigation methods, may be one step in this direction.

Accuracy of Freehand Cutting

Freehand bone cutting is not new, for even now with the availability of accurate instrumentation, some surgeons carry out some of the cuts freehand for the sake of convenience. For carrying out freehand bone sculpting using navigation, the Precision Freehand Sculptor was developed using a burr and the computer screen as a guide [10]. The system has recently been applied to a Repicci uni knee. We experimented with such a system where a burr was used to prepare the surface of foam plastic tibias as if for preparation of a unicondylar component. RMS accuracies of the cut surface of better than 1 mm were achieved [4]. Due to the shape of the burr, the surface was characterized by numerous ripples, although an alternate tool could reduce that effect.

To test the accuracy of freehand cutting using a reciprocating saw, rectangular foam blocks the size of an upper tibia were mounted and the task of the surgeon was to resect 10 mm from the top using metal bars mounted at each side of the block, the surfaces at the 10 mm level, as visual guides. After cutting, the frontal and sagittal angles of the cut surface were measured (■ Fig. 18.1). With the blocks mounted horizontally and the surgeon seated, mean frontal and sagittal errors were 0.6 and 1.2°, respectively. The use of an armrest which gave the surgeon's arm freedom to move in a horizontal plane, gave similar results. When the blocks were mounted at 45° and the surgeon standing, more closely simulating surgery, mean errors were 0.4 and 1.1°. A rigid arm rest gave 0.4 and 0.6° mean errors. As a control, a fixture with a slot, pinned accurately to the block, gave mean errors of 0.3–0.5°. Standard deviations were 0.3–0.5° throughout. This study suggested that freehand bone cutting could produce acceptable accuracy. Future studies will determine whether computer assistance, as described below, can further improve the accuracy.

Freehand-Navigation System

The systems available today use optical navigation for the positioning of cutting jigs through which the bone cuts are made. The placement of the jigs is determined by digitizing various landmarks on the bones to determine the reference axes. In some systems, the mechanical axis of the femur is determined by a kinematic method where the leg is rotated and the center of the hip is thus calculated. Non-image systems rely on the points digitized at surgery and are concerned primarily with alignments. At the other extreme, CT scanning has been used to obtain a 3-D rendering of the patient-specific bone. This has more versatility in that component fit and the extent of the bone cuts can be visualized. An approximation of bone shapes has been achieved at the time of the procedure using fluoroscopy, or by using morphing where a 3-D bone shape stored in the computer is morphed to the patient's bone shape using points digitized at surgery. A freehand-navigation system would use many of the features described above, the main difference being that rather than using the navigation system to position the cutting jigs, through which the bone cuts are made with a saw, the bone cuts are made freehand with the surgeon looking at the computer screen which shows the required planes of cut [12]. The cutting tool and the bone are rendered in real-time so that the surgeon can follow the cuts as they proceed (■ Fig. 18.2).

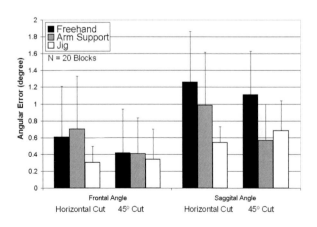

■ **Fig. 18.1.** The angular errors, and standard deviations, for the freehand cutting of a 10 mm thick layer from the top of a rectangular block the size of an upper tibia, using only simple visual guides at each side of the block

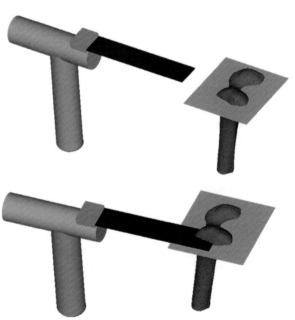

■ **Fig. 18.2.** A typical computer rendering showing the position of the saw and bone together with the required cutting plane in preparation for making the cut; and during the progress of the cut through the distal femur

Goals and Criteria

In order for a freehand-navigation system to be viable, it would need to fulfill certain criteria, as follows:

- applicable to both standard incision or minimally-invasive techniques;
- time for surgery must be less than or equal to that for conventional methods;
- technique is simple to perform, especially for the surgeon who carries out less than 20 operations per year;
- uses only cutting instruments (e.g. reciprocating saw, milling burr), but not conventional jigs and fixtures;
- provides a means for accurate alignment, avoiding "outliers" (errors outside of acceptable limits);
- capability to aid the surgeon in ligament balancing;
- must be able to work with all TKR designs and manufacturers, given CAD data of implant components;
- automatically produces an operating report of all data, measurements, alignments, etc. (this data can be used in future outcome studies);
- must reduce the cost of surgery per case.

Components

The system consists of the following hardware and software (see ◘ Fig. 18.2):

- an optical or electromagnetic tracking system to provide the 3D navigation of the cutting tools and bones;
- a digitizer as a registration tool and for defining key points on the bones;
- an intra-medullary rod which projects outwards from the entry point, to define the long axes of the bones
- a computer to perform the necessary calculations of bone shape, component positioning, and tracking of the surgery in real-time;
- a computer screen for providing real-time visualization to the surgeon on the required planes of cutting and the progress of the cutting;
- cutting tools such as a reciprocating saw, and a milling burr (mainly for uni and minimally invasive);
- a knee support for stability and distraction of the knee at any angle of flexion;
- an arm support to steady the surgeons arm and maximize the accuracy of cuts.

Procedural Steps

The following describes the system at this time although there will be variations depending on preferences and experience (◘ Fig. 18.3). The computer has several representative femurs and tibias stored in STL format. The format has the advantage that the images can be recalculated and moved on the computer screen in real-time. At the time of surgery, key landmarks are digitized on the bones, sufficient to define the extremities of the bones for scaling, with other points determining axes and shape [3]. Special intra-medullary rods which project outwards

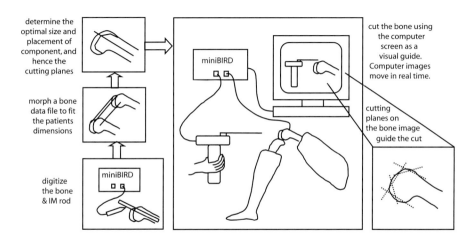

determine the optimal size and placement of component, and hence the cutting planes

miniBIRD

cut the bone using the computer screen as a visual guide. Computer images move in real time.

morph a bone data file to fit the patients dimensions

cutting planes on the bone image guide the cut

digitize the bone & IM rod

miniBIRD

◘ **Fig. 18.3.** A schematic of the freehand-navigation system, showing the initial stage of obtaining the image of the bone, producing an accurate bone model, defining the cutting planes, and making the bone cuts

from the entry point are placed in the bones to define the long axes. Points on the rods are digitized. The computer then selects one of the stored images and morphs it to match the patient being operated on [1]. The computer has CAD models of the implant system being used. For the femoral component for example, the computer will select the most suitable size and its optimal placement. The size selection will be based primarily on the AP dimensions while the positioning will be based on the thickness of the distal cut and the avoidance of notching the anterior cortex. Rotation will be based on the chosen transverse axis whether from the posterior condyles or from the epicondylar line [6]. The required valgus angle will be determined from the intra-medullary rod. The computer will then display the required cutting planes one by one (see ◘ Fig. 18.2). The surgeon will advance the saw to the start of the cut until it is correctly positioned. The saw will be switched on and the cut advanced. The starting point is critical to the subsequent accuracy, because once the cut proceeds, the saw will be largely constrained to follow the same path, which is an advantage. The benefit of having an accurate rendering of the bone shape on the computer screen is that the position of the saw blade relative to the bone boundaries can be visualized, important for the restricted visualization of a minimally-invasive technique. At a suitable stage in the bone preparation, tests will be carried out for ligament balancing along the lines that already exist with some navigation systems [13]. In order to achieve the maximum accuracy using such a freehand technique, an arm support is likely to be a benefit. A design which readily swivels into position is required. Similarly, a leg support where the knee can be flexed at the required angle and held in position, together with the capability of rotation and distraction, will improve stability and accuracy. The screen display shown in ◘ Fig. 18.2 is but one method for providing the required information to the surgeon. Different graphics can be used for the best possible visualization and control, the principle being to align the plane containing the saw blade with the plane of the required cut. A small screen mounted near the knee itself will allow the surgeon to quickly flip from the actual knee to the screen. A display panel mounted directly on the body

of the saw itself is yet another option. The most important factor, which will require extensive experimentation, is to determine how accurately surgeons with different experiences and capabilities can perform the cuts, and how much basic training is required to reach optimum performance. Early tests indicate that freehand navigation is viable and the task now is to systematically develop the system to a practical level.

References

1. Ellis RE, Athwal G, Rudan JF. Image guidance without images: deformable transformations for surgical guidance. International Society for Computer-Assisted Orthopaedic Surgery Conference, Santa Fe, New Mexico, USA, 19–23 June, 2002
2. Fisher DA, Watts M, Davis KE. Implant position in knee surgery. J Arthroplasty 18: 2–8, 2003
3. Incavo SJ, Coughlin KM, Pappas C, Beynnon BD. Anatomic rotational relationships of the proximal tibia, distal femur, and patella. J Arthroplasty 18: 643–648, 2003
4. Lee K, Cruickshank J, Yu H, Walker PS, Wei C-S. Instrument navigation for minimally-invasive knee replacement surgery. Southern Bioengineering Conference, Bethesda, MD, September 2002
5. Mahaluxmivala J, Bankes MJK, Nicolai P, Aldham CH, Allen PW. The effect of surgeon experience in component positioning in 673 press fit condylar posterior cruciate sacrificing total knee arthroplasties. J Arthroplasty 16: 635–640, 2001
6. Matsuda S, Muir H, Nagamine R, Urabe K, Mawatari T, Iwamoto Y. A comparison of rotational landmarks in the distal femur and the tibial shaft. Clinical Orthopaedics 414: 183–188, 2003
7. Novotny J, Gonzalez MH, Amirouche FML, Li YC. Geometrical analysis of potential error in using femoral intramedullary guides in total knee arthroplasty. J Arthroplasty 16: 641–647, 2001
8. Repicci JA. Mini-invasive knee unicompartmental arthroplasty: Bone-sparing technique. Surgical Technology International XI; 1–5, 2002
9. Stulberg SD. How accurate is current TKR instrumentation? Clinical Orthopaedics 416: 177–184, 2003
10. The Precision Freehand Sculptor. Medical Robotics and Computer-Assisted Surgery Laboratory, Carnegie-Mellon University, Pittsburgh, PA. www.mrcas.ri.cmu.edu, 2003
11. Tria AJ, Coon TM. Minimal incision total knee arthroplasty. Clinical Orthopaedics 416: 185–190, 2003
12. Walker PS. Minimally-invasive surgery for total knee. MIS meets CAOS, Pittsburgh, PA, May 31 – June 1, 2003
13. Yagishita K, Muneta T, Ikeda H. Step-by-step measurements of soft-tissue balancing during total knee. Arthroplasty for patients with varus knees. J Arthroplasty, 18: 313–320, 2003

Is There a Place for Robotics in Minimally Invasive TJA?

W.L. Bargar

Introduction

As one who has been involved with robotics in orthopedic surgery since its inception, in my opinion the answer is: yes! We have been taught that the three most important things required for accurate surgery are "exposure, exposure, exposure". Henry's book on "Extensile Exposure" [1] is a classic example. But, with minimally invasive surgery (MIS), there is (by definition) less exposure. This means that many of the usual soft-tissue and bony landmarks are not visible. Thus, to maintain the accuracy required in TJA using minimally or less invasive surgical (LIS) techniques, we need help. That help will come from computer-aided tools such as computer navigation, robotics or other so-called "smart tools". Robotics offers some specific advantages that make it attractive.

Accuracy is the key point.. Using conventional techniques, we currently enjoy a very high success rate in TJA with excellent longevity and a very low complication rate. This is due, in large part, to the accuracy and reproducibility of our technique. There is little question that MIS/LIS techniques offer less peri-operative morbidity and more rapid recovery than conventional open procedures. However, these advantages may be potentially outweighed by a lower success rate due to inaccuracies and human error.

This chapter will compare and contrast navigation and robotic systems. It will emphasize the importance of accurately positioning the components and avoiding human error. Additionally, it will provide a basis for you to evaluate these devices as they become available.

Definitions and Classification

A "robot" is a mechanical manipulator capable of autonomous movement based on a pre-programmed set of instructions. A "navigation system" is a tracking device used to locate and follow an object's position in three-dimensional space.

Surgical robots can be classified as "active", "passive" and "semi-active". An "active" robot manipulates surgical tools that operate on the patient. A "passive" robot manipulates instruments to provide guidance or retraction, but the surgeon is free to use the surgical tool without restriction. A "semi-active robot" restricts the motion of surgical tools along a path or in a specific envelope, but the surgeon provides the motivating force.

Origins of Robotic and Navigation Systems

The first use of a robot in surgery is credited to Kwoh [2] who used it in brain surgery as a passive pointing device in lieu of a stereotactic frame. The first active surgical robot was Robodoc™ (Integrated Surgical Systems, Davis, California, USA) (◘ Fig. 19.1). The chronology of its development is covered in more detail elsewhere [3]·It began in the late 1980s, and the initial application was in primary cementless total hip replacement. Robodoc was approved for sale in the European Union in 1994. It has evolved mainly in Germany to include applications for revision THR, primary TKR and unicompartmental knee replacement. It is not yet approved for sale in the U.S., and is completing its second FDA multicenter study. Caspar™ (URS-Ortho GmbH, Germany, now closed), no longer available, was another active robot developed later in Europe with application in primary THR and TKR. Acrobot™ (The Acrobot Company, Ltd., London, England) is a semi-active robot developed in England by Brian Davies and Justin Cobb [4] with potential applications in orthopedics (TKR), spinal and maxillofacial surgery. Many other robotic devices have been developed for

19

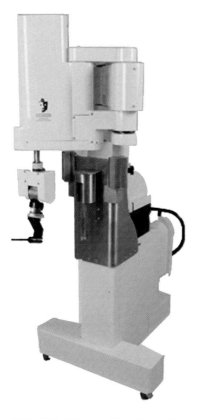

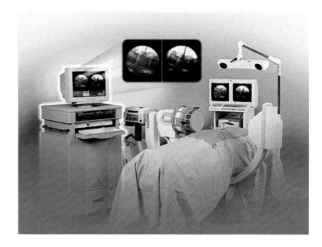

Fig. 19.2. Navigation system. (Reproduce with permission from Medtronic Inc.)

Fig. 19.1. Robodoc. (Reproduce with permission from Integrated Surgical Systems Inc.)

Pre-Operative Planning

While pre-operative planning is important to the success of a TJR, it is rarely performed in more than a cursory fashion by most clinicians probably because they find it of little value. One reason may be that the pre-operative plan is frequently not very accurate. The plan can serve as a general guide, but most surgeons rely more on what they see and feel during the operation, to make the critical decisions on implant size and position. With less invasive techniques, however, accurate pre-operative planning becomes more important.

spine surgery and fracture fixation and are in the pre-clinical application phase.

Navigation systems began as tool-tracking devices used in spine and neurosurgery in the early 1990s [5]. Application in TKR and THR was begun in the late 1990s mainly in Europe. Navigation systems may be attractive because of the rather high cost of robotic systems. Many surgeons will more readily accept freehand use of conventional tools in preference to autonomous mechanical systems. Many navigation systems (■ Fig. 19.2) are commercially available in Europe, and they are slowly being introduced to the U.S. market.

The advent of minimally invasive TJR has generated renewed interest in both navigation and robotic systems. There is an important distinction between these two systems. With navigation systems the surgeon still performs the actual surgery. In active robotic systems, the pre-programmed robot prepares the bone for prosthesis placement.

Conventional pre-operative planning is usually done using radiographs and acetate templates (■ Fig. 19.3). These two-dimensional radiographs are subject to magnification and rotational variations that can introduce large errors. CT scans, on the other hand, can eliminate rotation and magnification errors, and provide the surgeon with three-dimensional information. Robodoc, as well as some navigation systems, use pre-operative imaging with CT scans (■ Fig. 19.4). This can allow more accurate pre-operative planning. The accuracy of the software used to create the image as well as to plan the size and position of the implant is of utmost importance. Unfortunately, information on the accuracy of this part of many systems is not available. If the image in either a robotic or navigation system is not accurate, errors can occur.

In active robotic systems, the robot executes precisely the pre-operative plan. Many surgeons are reluctant to

Chapter 19 · Is There a Place for Robotics in Minimally Invasive TJA?

237 **19**

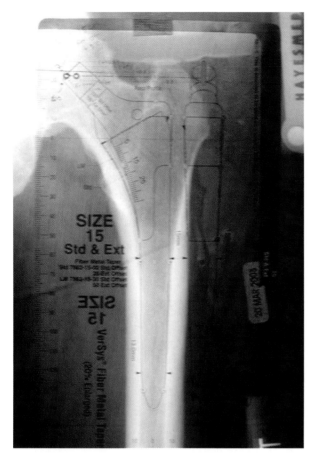

Fig. 19.3. Conventional pre-operative planning with radiograph and acetate template

commit to a pre-operative plan for reasons discussed earlier. They feel this is a major disadvantage of robotic surgery. It is the ability to accurately execute a pre-operative plan, however, which can be considered a major advantage of robotics. Both robotics and navigation systems have as a goal the reduction of human error on the part of the surgeon. Only robotics, however, has the potential to eliminate intra-operative human error.

Some navigation systems offer what they consider the potential advantage of eliminating the need for any pre-operative planning. A phantom bone is used and is scaled using surface point collection. No planning is required as long as the surgeon accepts the goals of the desired implant position and fit that are built into the software. These are the so-called "CT-free" systems [6] most used for total knee replacement.

Registration

Both robotics and navigation require registration of the orientation of the bone(s) to the device's coordinate system. There are two methods by which registration is accomplished: surface point collection/surface mapping and fluoroscopic image matching. Surface point collection requires the surgeon to physically touch a probe to specific bony landmarks or multiple points on a surface of the bone (☐ Fig. 19.5). These points are then mapped onto the CT image and the bone is then registered into the CT coordinate system. Using fluoroscopic image

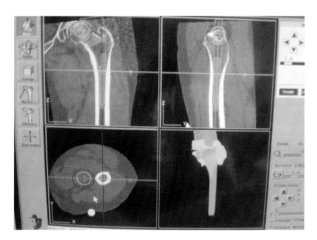

Fig. 19.4. Pre-operative planning screen for Robodoc

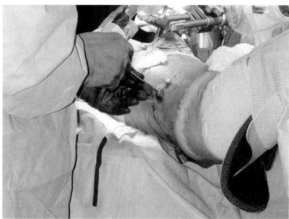

Fig. 19.5. Registration by surface point collection using Robodoc digitizing probe

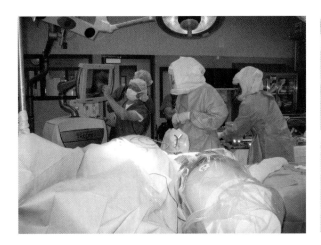

Fig. 19.6. Registration by fluoroscopic image matching

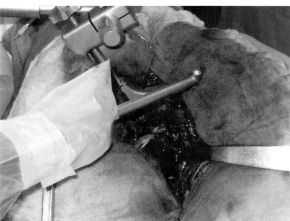

Fig. 19.7. Bone motion monitor for Robodoc system (*left foreground*) attached to femur

matching, points are identified on the image in two views and the position of the bone is then transformed into the fluoroscope's coordinate system (■ Fig. 19.6). Both of these methods can be a potential source of significant error. Studies showing the accuracy of registration techniques are vital for both robotics and navigation systems. Unfortunately these are usually internal studies done by the manufacturer. They are not usually published and therefore have not been subject to peer review.

Bone Tracking

Most surgeons associate this task with navigation. In fact, however, both robotics and navigation systems track the bone position in space. In robotics, the bone is usually held rigidly to avoid unwanted motion during milling. Robodoc uses a mechanical "bone motion monitor" (■ Fig. 19.7) to detect motion. In navigation systems, the bone is allowed to move freely, and metal markers are optically tracked (■ Fig. 19.8). If a bone marker loosens or moves relative to the bone, inaccuracies can occur.

In robotic systems the bone is held tightly in a fixator, so loosening is unlikely. If false movement is detected, the robot stops, re-registration is required, but no surgical error occurs. With navigation systems it is not possible to detect loosening or movement of a marker relative to the bone. If loosening occurs, the surgeon

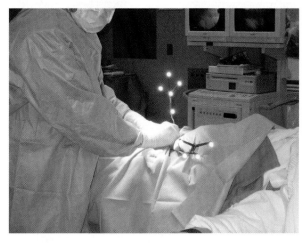

Fig. 19.8. Bone tracking using optical array for navigation system

would not be aware of it, the data on bone position would be inaccurate, and error could result.

Extra Time Required

Both robotics and navigation require extra time in surgery to setup and register the systems. Once the setup and registration are complete, however, the two systems can differ dramatically in the time for surgical execution. For example, Robodoc requires a predictable 12–20 min for milling the femur, depending on the size and

Chapter 19 · Is There a Place for Robotics in Minimally Invasive TJA?

239   **19**

shape of the implant. With navigation, the amount of time needed to complete the surgery depends on how the computer-aided information is presented to the surgeon, and how many choices and actions are required. This can be unpredictable and could take considerably longer. Longer operative times potentially add to the risk of infection and blood loss, factors which may influence a surgeon's willingness to accept this technology.

Clinical Track Record

Robodoc is now a proven technology. Over 10,000 cases have been performed worldwide. A number of Robodoc units are being used in Europe, Japan and Korea. In controlled studies [7], radiographs have shown better accuracy of implant fit, position and alignment. Intra-operative fractures have been virtually eliminated. Laboratory studies [8] have shown that the dimensional accuracy of the implant cavity is nearly 40 times better than freehand broaching techniques. One negative report has been published [9], but the problems encountered in that report can be attributed in part to the type of implant used. In addition, the surgeon apparently did not adequately protect and retract the soft tissues at the time of surgery. These details are the responsibility of the surgeon and are not robot-related errors. The United States multi-center study [7] did not encounter these problems.

Navigation, in contrast, is just beginning to be used clinically. There are few clinical publications showing the efficacy of these systems. With time, their utility and accuracy will be determined. As of now, navigation systems are not in widespread clinical use.

Choice for the Future

While navigation systems are cheaper and more readily acceptable by surgeons than robotic systems, their accuracy is still in question. Robotic systems offer precision. They execute the pre-operative plan, and offer the potential to eliminate human error (although the surgeon must protect soft tissues). In the future, a blend of robotic and navigational technologies may be best. Part of an operation that requires less precision may be more adaptable to navigation (e.g. acetabular cup placement), whereas other parts that require more precision and

pre-operative planning may be more suited to robotics (e.g. femoral stem placement).

Conclusions

Minimally invasive surgical techniques are changing the practice of joint-replacement surgery. The challenge is to maintain the required standard of precision with limited exposure.

The ultimate acceptance of computer-aided surgery techniques in orthopedics depends on the concept of what might be called "clinical utility". This is a term used by the United States Food and Drug Administration, but is not defined. I propose that a new device has "clinical utility" if it can answer at least one of the following questions in the affirmative:

- Does it solve a real problem in orthopedic surgery?
- Does it improve the outcome of patients?
- Does it result in savings without lowering quality?
- Is it worth the investment?

To paraphrase a recent movie: "Clinical utility ... if you prove it, they will come".

References

1. Henry AK. Extensile exposure applied to limb surgery, 1st edn. Edinburgh: Livingstone, pp 53–64, 1950
2. Kwoh YS, Hou J, Jonckheere EA, Hayati S. A robot with improved absolute positioning accuracy for CT guided stereotactic brain surgery. IEEE Trans Biomed Eng 35: 153–160, 1988
3. Paul HA, Bargar WL, Mittelstadt et al. Development of a surgical robot for cementless total hip arthroplasty. Clin Orthop 285: 57–66, 1992
4. Jakopec M, Harris SJ, Baena Fry, Gomes P, Cobb J, Davies BL. The first clinical application of a "hands-on" robotic knee surgery system. Comp Aid Surg 6: 329–339, 2001
5. Nolte LP, Zamorano LJ, Visarius H, Berlemann U, Langlotz F, Arm E, Schwarzenbach O. Clinical evaluation of a system for precision enhancement in spine surgery. Clin Biomech 10: 293–303
6. Stulberg SD, Loan P, Sarin V. Computer-assisted navigation in total knee replacement: results of an initial experience in thirty-five patients. J Bone Joint Surg Am 84-A [Suppl 2]: 90–98, 2002
7. Bargar WL, Bauer A, Borner M. Primary and revision total hip replacement using the Robodoc system. Clin Orthop 354: 82–91, 1998
8. (Internal Data), Integrated Surgical Systems, Davis, CA
9. Honl M, Dierk O, Gauck C, Carrero V, Lampe F, Dries S, Quante M, Schwieger K, Hille E, Morlock MM. Comparison of robotic-assisted and manual implantation of a primary total hip replacement. A prospective study. J Bone Joint Surg Am 85-A: 1470–1478, 2003

How has Computer-Navigation changed TKR?

D. Lucas, T. Bishop, S.K. Chauhan

Introduction

Since the design of the first total condylar knee replacement in 1974, knee arthroplasty surgery has remained one of the most successful procedures in orthopedics. Despite the procedure gaining good 90% long-term follow-up [1–2], there remains a large number (20–40%) of patients who are dissatisfied with the procedure [3–5]. This may be related to patello-femoral pain, medial impingement, instability, increased wear or early failure. A number of studies [6–11] have highlighted the incidence of patello-femoral complications and its relationship to femoral component mal-rotation [12–15]. Polyethylene wear is multifactorial; however, it is accepted that more then 3° of mal-alignment in a coronal plane will lead to differing loading patterns on the tibial polyethylene inserts, and more wear [16, 17]. No thought has yet been given to combinations of mal-alignment, e.g. varus, internal rotation and flexion of the femoral component and in a large series [18] of 212 consecutive TKR revisions, 25% of patients had significant polyethylene wear. Instability of the primary TKR remains a leading cause of revision – with an incidence of 21% in early revisions, whilst overt mal-alignment of the components was present in 11% of revision cases [18].

A number of series have reported on the interval between the index operation and the revision procedure. Fehring et al. [19] showed that 64% of all revision cases where performed within 5 years of the index procedure. Almost 22,000 knee revisions were performed in the USA in 1999 at a cost of $ 262 dollars [20] and the numbers of revisions are rising.

It is clear that the numbers of dissatisfied patients and revisions are rising and the reasons are multifactorial. However, the accuracy of bone resection and implantation together with good soft-tissue balancing clearly play an important role. Since the introduction of standardized knee instrumentation, very little has changed and many implant companies still produce rigid IM/EM rods to which cutting blocks are attached. These instruments are based on normalative anatomical studies which allow some surgeon input in the coronal positioning (varus/valgus) of cutting blocks but even less input in the sagittal positioning (flexion/extension). Many instrument systems still use fixed posterior referencing cutting blocks to determine femoral rotation, which produce mal-rotation by not taking into account posterior condylar wear [21]. Thus a number of errors can be produced which may ultimately lead to premature failure of the total joint inserted. Petersen and Engh [22] reported on post-operative radiography following conventional arthroplasty, 26% (13/50) failed to achieve alignment within 3° of varus or valgus.

Computer-assisted TKR was introduced with the aims of improving component alignment in the coronal, sagittal and axial planes consistently and thus narrowing the "bell curve" of distribution for any individual surgeons results. It logically follows that better kinematics and wear patterns should follow if this is achieved as opposed to a mal-positioned implant. By allowing the surgeon to dynamically assess deformity prior to bone resections, navigation systems allow the surgeon to carefully calculate which soft tissues will ultimately be released, to give the perfectly balanced knee. The ability to immediately assess the effects of any release on kinematics, gives instant biofeedback to the surgeon on which further decisions can be made. One major additional advantage to navigation systems is that the majority now use instrumentation that is entirely extramedullary, thus reducing the risk of fat embolism.

Overview of Computer-Assisted Systems

All navigation systems have a core of components that comprise of a computer, an optical system, mobile trackers (either infra-red or passive reflectors), insertion pins and a working tool that may be hand-held or pedal-operated. In all systems, the computer receives information from an infra-red camera array. The cameras track the signals, which come in from the working area via trackers, which can be active, when they generate the infra-red signal, or passive if they reflect the infra-red radiation, which comes from the source. These trackers can be fixed to the patient and therefore indicate fixed anatomy, or they can be mobile. Mobile beacons can act as pointers or can be attached to specific instruments which the computer can recognize. The progress of an instrument can therefore be followed in its relationship to the anatomy.

Picard [23] first suggested that navigation systems be divided into those that require pre-operative information (CT or MRI scan) to be collected and those where intra-operative information is gathered during surgery. This latter group is further subdivided into two groups of systems. The first is those which use pre-operative imaging, in which usually a fluoroscopic picture is taken and the data transferred directly to the computer through a hard-wire connection. The second is image-free systems, which use an anatomical model embedded in the computer memory, which is upgraded by a process of the surgeon picking anatomical landmarks on the knee during surgery. This itself can be either through geometric mapping or true bone morphing.

Navigation systems require a registration process irrespective of what type of system is being used. The process can take between 7 and 30 min, depending on what system is being used and the experience of the surgeon. Registration requires the surgeon to input key data into the computer using anatomical landmarks in the limb. Thus the center of the femoral head is determined most often by some form of kinematic analysis, whilst the surfaces of the distal femur and proximal tibia can be mapped directly as can key rotation landmarks, which will affect both femoral and tibial rotation. Key-ankle landmarks are mapped directly, thus together with the center of the femoral head, center of distal femur and proximal tibia gives both the anatomical and mechanical axes of the limb. The accuracy of the registration process is fundamental, as although averaging algorithms are used, a poorly performed registration will result in a down-grading of the overall accuracy.

Another feature of importance to surgeons is how "captured" the surgeon is by the system. In closed platform systems the surgeon is often restricted to one particular type of knee arthroplasty with one particular program. More programs increase the surgical freedom to choose between implants but also considerably increases the cost of systems. Closed systems will also often not allow the surgeon to progress unless specific data is acquired – which is often not necessary. Open platform systems allow surgeons to input a key data set of information and then proceed as the surgeon wishes. There is no restriction on choice of component or indeed primary, revision or unicondylar procedure.

Review of Clinical Results

Chauhan et al. [24] produced one of the first randomized controlled trials comparing computer-assisted surgery with conventional surgery using the Stryker knee-navigation system and Duracon prosthesis. This trial is unique in that it is the first to use CT scans to assess all the coronal, axial and sagittal positions of the implanted components. In two equally matched groups of patients, it showed statistically significantly improved position on CT for femoral varus/valgus ($p=0.032$), femoral rotation ($p=0.001$), tibial varus/valgus ($p=0.047$), tibial rotation ($p=0.011$), tibial posterior slope ($p=0.0001$) and femoral tibial mismatch ($p=0.037$). There was further improved alignment on long leg standing Maquet limb alignment ($p=0.004$) and reduced blood loss ($p=0.0001$) in the computer-assisted group but longer OR times ($p=0.0001$) by a mean of 13 min. The trial showed clear improvement in component alignment in the computer-navigated group. The trial also produced one of the first measurements of total cumulative error when looking at component implantation. Here, the deviation from each of 7 CT-based component-alignment parameters was identified for each patient. Each deviation was then added together to give a cumulative error as displayed in ◘ Fig. 20.1.

The literature already suggests that malposition of the component by more than 3° in a single varus/valgus plane may lead to premature failure of the implant [16, 17]. When now looking at the reduction in cumulative error when using computer navigation, the results are significant and the distribution of conventional results

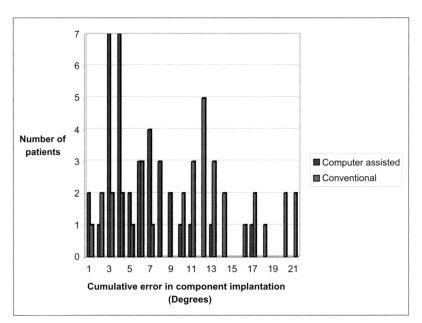

□ Fig. 20.1. A graph showing the cummulative error, in individual patients, of 7 CT alignment variables for Total Knee Arthroplasty based on the Perth CT protocol

may explain accelerated polyethylene wear and failure seen in other series.

Sparman et al. [25] randomized 240 patients into a conventional and computer-assisted group, using the Stryker Knee navigation system and Scorpio prosthesis. This trial used long-leg weight-bearing films to assess coronal alignment, component position in the frontal plane and sagittal plane. The trial showed highly significant difference between the two groups in favor of navigation for all the parameters investigated. Only two out of 120 navigated knees had a post-operative deviation in the mechanical axis of 30, the conventional group 27 cases with 30 or more deviation (22%).

Krachow et al. [26] reported on 90 consecutive computer-assisted Duracon TKRs using the Stryker knee-navigation system and found that 79% of patients reviewed (81 out of 90) had long-leg films within one degree of neutral. The patients also had equal or better ranges of motion; knee and function scores at 1 year follow up. They concluded that the potential gains provided by such a system included faster rehabilitation, improved final range of motion, more complete extension and longer lasting knee replacements.

Clemens et al. [27] reported on a five-center, prospective randomized study between 1999 and 2001. 821 patients were enrolled into the study, 555 patients had navigated procedures and 266 had conventional procedures. The orthopilot navigation system and the SEARCH prosthesis were used in all cases. Implant accuracy was compared in four planes on plain radiographs together with long-leg-standing films to determine mechanical axis which gave 5 axes in total. Results were excellent in 49.6% for all five axes in the navigated group compared with 30.8% in the conventional group.

Stulberg [28] looked at the accuracy of conventional instrumentation using a navigation system. Whilst manual instrumentation allowed accurate frontal limb alignment, there was a tendency to hyperextend and internally rotate the femoral component and place excessive posterior slope on the tibia. Optimal alignment was achieved in only 4 out of 20 consecutive TKRs.

Bathis et al. [29] and Perlick et al. [30] reported a significantly more accurate mechanical axis using CT-based and image-free systems when compared to controls. They also applied navigation to ligament balancing, based upon the work of Katz et al. [31]. A rectangular extension gap was developed with soft-tissue releases; the knee was then moved into flexed position, a spreader tool was then inserted into the space. The navigation system stored this position and recommended the optimal component orientation to achieve a balanced, rectangular flexion gap. Using this concept for femoral component rotation, a balanced flexion and extension gap was achieved in all patients in the navigated group.

Ritschl et al. [32] used the Galileo Navigation and Robotic system to look at ligament balancing and flexion/extension gaps. They found better gap balancing and improved stability in extension and flexion when using a computer-navigation system.

Discussion

Computer-navigation systems, despite there infancy, are clearly here to stay. Whilst the inaccuracies of conventional knee-arthroplasty surgery have been and continue to be documented, navigation systems have now presented the orthopedic surgeon with unrivalled accuracy in producing bone cuts. More importantly, for the first time the surgeon has an advanced biofeedback tool that can be used to his advantage when producing a balanced knee with a combination of accurate bone cuts and soft-tissue releases.

Already there are a number of articles published that show a clear improvement in alignment over the conventional gold-standard techniques. It logically follows that a better aligned and balanced knee should function better and for longer with less likelihood of revision then a poorly implanted component. However, as yet there are no kinematic studies or long-term outcome studies to show this – although the latter is purely a time-dependent phenomenon.

Navigation systems are changing both in terms of hardware and software. No longer are machines the size of large image intensifiers. Many manufacturers have broken machines into smaller components that can be free-standing, incorporated partially into existing OR facilities or integrated completely into an endosuite theater. Software updates arrive once or twice yearly as continuing improvements in our clinical knowledge of knee arthroplasty enables us to fine-tune or even radically change our thought process in performing a TKR. Indeed navigation and the information it has already given us, has led us to challenge a number of long-held beliefs regarding soft-tissue balancing and the ability to accurately determine a resection at a specified angle.

Instrument design is already changing as many manufacturers move to entirely extra-medullary systems. The ability to make universal cutting instruments will make instrument inventories smaller and easier for the OR staff. Many instruments such as IM rods may become obsolete as surgeons minimize the risk of fat embolus. Navigation has not just challenged the accuracy of traditional instrumentation but also challenged the process by which the cutting blocks and cuts have been made [33]. Altered configuration of pin holes in cutting blocks to increase stability of the blocks at the bone interface is a minor example whilst the inadequacies of current saw-blade technology is a more important variable that has been truly highlighted through the use of surgical navigation systems.

The accuracy that computer navigation affords, has led the surgeon to explore other aspects of total knee arthroplasty surgery. One of these is minimally invasive surgery where the accuracy of navigation will have a huge impact and is described in a separate chapter.

Computer-navigation systems will continue to evolve at a rapid pace, much as the general field of computing has done so over the past 20 years and it is not difficult to see how once financial cost issues are resolved, its use will be routine throughout the world within a few years.

References

1. Stern SH, Insall JN. Posterior stabilised prosthesis: results after follow-up of 9–12 years. J Bone Joint Surg [Am] 1992; 74-A: 980–986
2. Vince KG, Insall JN, Kelly MA. The total condylar prosthesis: 10 to 12 year results of a cemented knee replacement. J Bone Joint Surg [Br] 1989; 3: 17–25
3. Aglietti P, Buzzi R, Gaudenzi A. Patellofemoral functional results and complications with posterior stabilised total condylar prosthesis. J Arthroplasty 1988; 3: 17–25
4. Figgie HE, Goldberg VM, Hieple KG, Moller HS, Gordon NH. The influence of tibial-patellofemoral location on the function of the knee in patients with posterior stabilised condylar knee prosthesis. J Bone Joint Surg [Am] 1986; 68-A: 1035–1040
5. Merkow RL, Soudry M, Insall JN. Patellar dislocation following total knee replacement. -J Bone Joint Surg [Am] 1985; 67-A: 1321–1327
6. Aglietti P, Gandenzi A. Patellofemoral functional results and complications with posterior stabilised total knee prosthesis. J Arthroplasty 1988; 3: 17–25
7. Buechell F, Rosa R, Pappas M. A metal-backed rotating bearing patellar prosthesis to lower contact stresses: An eleven year clinical study. Clin Orthop 1989; 248: 34–49
8. Huo M, Sulco T. Complications in primary total knee arthroplasty. Orthop Rev 1990; 19: 781–786
9. Clayton M, Thiripathi R. Patellar complications after total condylar arthroplasty. Clin Orthop 1982; 170: 116–122
10. Insall JN, Binazzi R, Soudry M, Mestriner L. Total knee arthroplasty. Clin Orthop 1985; 192: 13–22

11. Reuben J, McDonald, Woodard P, Hennington L. Factors affecting patella before and after total knee replacement. Trand Orthop Res Soc 1990; 15: 281

12. Berger RA, Crossett LS, Jacobs JJ, Rubash HE. Malrotation causing patellofemoral complications after total knee arthroplasty. Clin Orthop 1998; 356: 144–153

13. Figgie M, Goldberg V, Figgie H. salvage of symptomatic patellofemoral joint following cruciate substituting total knee arthroplasty. Am J Knee Surg 1988; 1: 48–55

14. Figgie M, Goldberg V, Figgie H. the effects of alignment of the implant on fracture of the patella after total knee arthroplasty. J Bone Joint Surg 1989; 71-A: 1031–1039

15. Ranawat C. The patellofemoral joint in total condylar arthroplasty: Pros and Cons based on five to ten year follow-up observations. Clin Orthop 1986; 205: 93–99

16. Jeffrey RS, Morris RW, Denham RA. Coronal alignment after total knee replacement. J Bone Joint Surg 1991; 73-B: 709–714

17. Ritter MA, Faris PM, Keating EM, Meding JB. Postoperative alignment of total knee replacement. Its effect on survival. Clin Orthop 1994; 299: 153–156

18. Sharkey PF, Hozack WJ, Rothman RH, Shastri S, Jacoby SM. Why are total knee arthroplasties failing today? Clin Orthop 2002; 404: 7–13

19. Fehring TK, Odum S, Griffin WL. Revision of failed cementless total knee implants with cement. Clin Orthop 2001; 392: 315–318

20. Ingenix: Data Analyst Group, Columbus, OH, Ingenix 1999

21. Matsuda S, Miura H, Nagamine R, Mawatari T, Tokunga M et al. Anatomical analysis of the femoral condyle in normal and osteoarthritic knees. J Orthop Res 2004; 22: 104–109

22. Petersen TL, Engh G. Radiographic assessment of knee alignment of the femur after total knee arthroplasty. J Arthroplasty 1988; 3: 67–72

23. Picard F, Moody J, Jaramaz B, Digiola AM, Nikou C, LaBarca RS. A classification proposal for computer-assisted knee systems. In: Proceedings. 4th Annual North American Program on Computer-Assisted Orthopaedic Surgery 89–90, Pittsburgh 2000

24. Chauhan S, Scott RG, Breidahl W, Beaver RA. Computer-assisted knee arthroplasty versus conventional jig based technique. J Bone Joint Surg 2004; 86-B: 366–371

25. Sparmann M, Wolke B, Czupalla H, Banzer D, Zink A. Positioning of total knee arthroplasty with and without navigation support. J Bone Joint Surg 2003; 85-B: 830–835

26. Krachow KA, Phillips MJ, Bayers-Thering M. Computer-assisted total knee replacement-Results of the first 90 cases using the stryker navigation system. Computer Assisted Orthopaedic Surgery – 3rd Annual Meeting of CAOS (International Proceedings), June 18–21, 2003

27. Clemens U, Konermann WH, Kohler S, Kiefer H, Jenny JY, Miehlke. Computer-assisted navigation with the Orthopilot system using the search evolution TKA prosthesis. In: Stiehl JB, Konermann WH, Haaker RGA (eds) Navigation and robotics in total joint and spine surgery. Springer; Berlin Heidelberg New York Tokyo 2003

28. Stulberg SD, Adams A, Woods O. At what steps in the performance of TKA do errors occur when manual instrumentation is used? Computer-Assisted Orthopaedic Surgery – 3rd Annual Meeting of CAOS (International Proceedings), June 18–21, 2003

29 Bathis H, Perlick L, Luring C, Kalteis T, Grifka J. CT-basierte und CT-freie Navigation in der Knieenddoprothetik. Unfallchirug 2003; 106: 935–940

30. Perlick L, Bathis H, Luring C, Tingart M, Grifka J. Computer-Assisted Orthopaedic Surgery – 3rd Annual Meeting of CAOS (International Proceedings), June 18–21, 2003

31. Katz MA, Beck TD, Silber JS, Lotke PA. Determining femoral rotational alignment in total knee arthroplasty. J Arthroplasty 2001; 16: 301–305

32. Ritschl P et al. Computer-Assisted Orthopaedic Surgery – 3rd Annual Meeting of CAOS (International Proceedings), June 18–21, 2003

33. Clark G, Chauhan SK, Sikorski JM. The stability of cutting blocks in total knee arthroplasty. Presented at the 62nd Australian Orthopaedic Association, Melbourne, Victoria, October 2002

Part V   Evaluation of MITJA

MIS in Total Hip Arthroplasty: Present Status and Future Direction

C.S. Ranawat, A.S. Ranawat

Introduction

From the time of Sir John Charnley, the pioneer of modern total hip-replacement (THR) surgery, the principles of hip reconstruction have emphasized the reproduction of anatomic geometry to both improve biomechanics and to create the proper myofascial balance. Appropriately performed, THR can reliably and predictably relieve pain, restore function, and improve motion for a period approaching 20 years.

To achieve such a long-term outcome in total hip replacement, proper visualization of the acetabulum and proximal femur was thought to be of paramount importance in order to ensure proper component positioning and to achieve durable fixation. The length of incision was never a consideration. Avoidance of complications was and average hospital stays lasted 1–2 weeks or more.

However, during an era of capitated reimbursements, there was continuing pressure to reduce the length of stay (LOS) in the hospital which demanded earlier recovery of function. The continual strive to speed recovery fostered an "envelope-pushing" mentality using more bone-sparing and abductor-preserving approaches, improved component fixation, aggressive rehabilitation, patient education, improved anesthetic and pain-management techniques and the introduction of clinical pathways. The net result in recent years has been a gradual reduction in average LOS for primary THR to approximately 4 days with the added benefit of improved patient outcomes and lower complication rates than in previous years. Because of this, these improvements have been almost universally accepted by hospitals and surgeons alike.

The trend to push the envelope in THR is a good one encouraging thought-provoking, scientific discussions and new insights. But one must never forget our primary responsibility in medicine: primum non nocere (first, do no harm).

The most recent development that calls this into question has been the introduction of minimally invasive surgery (MIS) to THR. While some patients have demanded speedier recovery, earlier return to work and improved cosmesis, most of the impetus has come from manufacturing companies, hospitals, and some select surgeons eager to capitalize on the market share of a very competitive business, while possibly ignoring the interest and welfare of their patients. Some surgeons have expressed their concern and opinion in opposing this trend, stating that direct marketing of pharmaceutical products, and now, poorly studied orthopedic surgical procedures, like MIS THR, may be unethical. Orthopedic manufacturing companies may have misled the public in the interest of gaining market share and promoting the value of their companies, without scientific evidence to demonstrate the safety, reproducibility, quality of function, and durability of MIS THR.

The purpose of this presentation is to outline how a properly designed study can be carried out to answer the question whether the MIS procedure for total hip replacement, using one or two incisions, is safe, reproducible, functional, and durable. This paper specifically addresses one incision of 10 cm or less, which is used for either posterior or anterolateral exposures, in comparison to a posterior incision of 10–15 cm.

Methods

An appropriately designed scientific study, aimed at investigating MIS in total hip replacement, should be multi-centered, involving 5 to 10 surgeons doing 100 to 300 procedures a year, with a study period of 0 to 5 years. MIS patients should be recruited with proper IRB approval. Informed consent must explicitly delineate the benefits and risks. If possible, patients should be recruited in a randomized manner or at least in two consecutive series of 300 or more patients per surgeon in order to be able to show significant differences between the groups where the incidence of complications may be less than 5%. There should be some uniformity with regards to prosthesis design and fixation. Data collection should be done independently and prospectively using standardized clinical (Harris Hip, HSS, WOMAC) and radiographic evaluations as well as self-administered patient questionnaires at 2 weeks, 4 weeks, 6 weeks, 3 months, and yearly thereafter. The study should address these questions:

- What percentage of patients are concerned about cosmesis and/or the length of incision?
- Is MIS as good as standard total hip replacement in terms of safety, quality, reproducibility and durability?

The following variables should be controlled for:
- Pre-operative patient education
- Patient motivation
- Post-operative pain control
- Rehabilitation protocol

The following parameters should be measured:
- Length of incision
- Time of operation
- Blood loss – based on drop in hemoglobin count
- Intra-operative complications such as mal-position, fracture, nerve palsy, vascular injury, infection, and dislocation
- Difficulty of procedure: learning curve
- Post-operative assessment of pain intensity
- Recovery of activities of daily living
- Return to work
- Normal ambulation (without pain, limp, and support)
- Stair climbing ability
- Return to sporting activities

Discussion

No published studies currently exist that specifically compare MIS total hip replacement to standard total hip replacement using the aforementioned criteria. DiGioia's recently published study, the only properly conducted, prospective, comparative study of mini-incision tech-

nique currently available, concluded that patients in a mini-incision group had significantly faster improvement in their limps and in their ability to climb stairs at 3 months [1]. This accelerated improvement diminished with longer follow-up; by one year, both the standard-incision and mini-incision patients had experienced the same amount of improvement.

Despite the absence of properly conducted, prospective studies comparing MIS to standard total hip-replacement surgery, direct marketing by manufacturers, hospitals, and surgeons has continued unabated lending apparent validation to this technique as a "standard of care."

MIS in total hip replacement does have its place. With the help of special retractors, lighting, reamers and other instruments, a total hip replacement can be done from a posterior or anterolateral exposure, using one or two incisions of 10 cm or less. Many surgeons have championed MIS THR. Those who have performed single-incision MIS total hip-replacement studies, using either posterior or anterolateral exposure, include Dorr, Hartzband, Mahoney, Sculco, Sherry, Waldman, and Wenz [2, 6–9]. Berger, Duwelius, Mears, and Keggi have studied the two-incision MIS technique [2, 4]. According to Berger, Dorr, and Sculco, the recovery of function in a select group of motivated, well-informed patients with properly-controlled pain management have shown early recovery of activities of daily living by 2–3 weeks, such as getting out of bed, walking, and climbing stairs, compared, in their experience, to patients who received standard total hip replacement in the recent past [2, 9].

Yet, the unanswered question remains: Is 2 to 3 weeks of early recovery of hip function with MIS THR worthy of such widespread publicity? Only when the safety, reproducibility, and quality of function of MIS have been documented by qualified investigators, can we say "yes." When the majority of the most serious complications of THR are prevented by proper surgical technique, how can we advertise a less than adequately tested procedure?

RTTS in Total Joint Surgery

We hereby introduce the term RTTS, reduced tissue-trauma surgery, in total joint replacement. In RTTS, a total hip replacement can be performed from a posterior exposure using a properly placed incision of 10–15 cm in the majority of cases. Improved retractors, better lighting and angled reamers developed for MIS THR have made this possible.

After incising the skin, the total joint procedure, whether via MIS or a 10–15 cm incision, is similar in terms of interfering with the gluteus maximus and fascia lata, except the length of the split is lessened by about 30–50% with MIS. Exposure of the external rotators and posterior capsule is similar. The main difference, in MIS is that the quadratus femoris and the insertion of the gluteus maximus are not detached. However, the quadratus is often torn as the leg is internally rotated making it incompetent and more difficult to repair; and not detaching the gluteus-maximus insertion may be responsible for a higher incidence of sciatic nerve palsy as the nerve is compressed under the tense tendon during prolonged internal rotation. Final preparation of the acetabulum and femur is similar in both procedures.

In recent years, pain management in total hip-replacement surgery has been greatly improved. With more effective pain control, pre-operative patient education, and improved post-operative rehabilitation programs, the majority of RTTS patients of all ages at our center have a recovery of function in 4–8 weeks, judged by ambulation without pain, limp, and support, with cemented, hybrid, and non-cemented fixation.

Conclusions

Total hip replacement is indicated to relieve pain, and to restore or improve function and range of motion; in addition, in certain cases, returning patients to sporting activities may be a goal. Safety, reproducibility, quality of function, and durability are the benchmarks for the success of total hip replacement. Compromising these criteria could have a negative impact on total joint surgery. Without appropriately performed studies comparing MIS to the standard incision, MIS total hip replacement cannot be recommended as a standard of care, and must certainly not be promoted or marketed as such. On the other hand, if we can demonstrate safety, quality of function, reproducibility and durability in MIS THR, it will prove to be a definite advance. It will take the next 5–10 years for MIS THR to find its proper place in the management of arthritis of the hip.

References

1. DiGioia AM, Plakseychuk AY, Levison TJ, Jaramaz B: Mini-incision technique for total hip arthroplasty with navigation. J Arthrop 2003; 18: 123–128
2. Berry DJ, Berger RA, Callaghan JJ, Dorr LD, Duwelius PJ, Hartzband, Lieberman JR, Mears DC: Minimally invasive total hip arthroplasty: development, early results, and a critical analysis. The Orthopaedic Forum. Presented at the Annual Meeting of the American Orthopaedic Assocation. JBJS 2003; 85A: 2235–2246
3. Hozack WJ, Ranawat CS, Rothman RH: How to deliver the word? Arthroplasty 2002; 17: 389
4. Light TR, Keggi KI: Anterior approach to hip arthroplasty. Clin Orthop 1980: 255–260
5. Ranawat CS, Ranawat AS: Minimally invasive total joint arthroplasty: where are we going? Editorial. JBJS 2003; 85A: 2070–2071
6. Sherry E, Egan M, Warnke PH, Henderson A, Eslick GD: Minimal invasive surgery for hip replacement: A new technique using the NILNAV Hip System. Anz J Surg 2003; 73: 157–161
7. Waldman BJ: Minimally invasive total hip replacement and perioperative management: Early experience. JAS 2002; 11: 213–217
8. Wenz JF, Gurkan I, Jibodh SR: Mini-incision total hip arthroplasty: a comparative assessment of perioperative outcomes. Orthopedics 2002; 25: 1031–1043
9. Wright J, Crockett H, Sculco T: Mini-incision for total hip arthroplasty. Orthopaedics 2001; 7: 18

Concepts of Clinical Studies

O. Kessler, M. Naughton, M. Kester

Introduction

Over the past few years, there has been considerable interest and much controversy surrounding "minimally invasive" total joint replacement. The advocates say that these methods have a great potential to benefit the patient [1]. Soft-tissue trauma, operative blood loss, post-operative pain, hospitalization time and the need for rehabilitation are theoretically reduced. These reductions may well have a positive economic benefit as well. However, there are surgeons that are concerned that these minimally invasive procedures may introduce new potential problems [1, 2]. In reviewing literature on minimum invasive surgery (MIS) it becomes quickly apparent that there are quite few well-designed studies for hips or knee arthroplasties [3–21]. This is in least in part due to the subjective nature of the clinical variables that MIS is believed to impact. Further, it is quite difficult to conduct a prospective, randomized investigation in this era of the web-educated consumer. Often the surgeon is faced with a self-diagnosed patient who has a stack of pages printed off from various web pages. The content of these web pages are certainly not often subject to peer review, hence the validity of many of the claims is questionable. Hospital Institutional Review Boards now challenged with the added responsibility of the HIPAA (Health Insurance and Portability and Accountability Act – implemented in 2003) patient privacy regulations are careful to assure that patients are highly informed of every aspect of study design and dissemination of information regarding any investigations they are invited to participate in. Although this is clearly the ethical thing to do, such education does inject a potential bias effect that may confound the measured variables. If a patient knows they will get the "standard" incision or a "mini" incision, there is a strong poten-tial that the euphoria from the "mini" or the disappointment from getting the "standard" will bias the subjective variables to be measured. However, other more objective data such as blood loss and operative time may still provide useful information. Certainly, the patient and the evaluators could be blinded in the immediate post-operative phase, but not for the entire 6- to 12-week period in which the benefits of MIS surgery are most likely realized.

A review of the MIS literature reveals a common base of variables being investigated. The common operative variables include blood loss, incision length and complications. The post-operative variables include transfusions, length of stay, discharge disposition, narcotic use, Hip or Knee Society scores, SF12 or 36, complication rate, time to ambulation (use of support, ability to ascend/descend stairs), ability to transfer (bed and/or chair), time to stat rehabilitation (rehab) and number of rehab units required. Readmission, complication rates (such as infections, dislocations, fractures or nerve palsies) and component placement (including any subsequent subsidence) were also generally reported in the post-operative period.

The patient groups and length of follow-up in the literature varied substantially. The majority of studies utilized non-randomized selected and/or non-consecutive series and often the studies would lack an appropriately matched control population. A review of the literature found only one prospective randomized study with a 2-year or greater follow-up [21]. Due to the relative newness of the popularity of the MIS procedures, the follow-up periods in the abstracts and literature vary significantly from 3 months to over 30 years with the vast majority being 2 years or less [19, 20].

Potential benefits of the MIS procedures must be balanced against the associated risks of undertaking a more technically demanding operation. Nevertheless, no surgeon can deny the potential benefits of the reduced soft-tissue trauma. In order to prove the advantages of these methods without marketing, bias objective data has to be generated and evaluated. Unfortunately, there is a paucity of data in existence to aid the surgeon in deciding the viability of the MIS procedures. The goal of this chapter is to present considerations when designing or evaluating MIS clinical studies.

The Importance of Clinical Trials

While laboratory testing and animal studies may provide strong supporting evidence that one product or intervention will produce a desired effect, well-conducted clinical trials are essential to establish that a specific interventional procedure produces the intended clinical outcome. A recent Journal of Bone and Joint Arthroplasty (JBJS) article evaluated the validity of claims made in orthopedic print advertisements and concluded that approximately half the claims were not supported by enough data to be used in a clinical decision-making process. In the article, a well-supported statement was defined as a statement with enough supporting evidence to be used in clinical practice and a high-quality study was defined as a study that could be published in the peer-reviewed literature [22]. In general, the orthopedic literature reports that more higher quality clinical trials are needed to support evidence-based orthopedic practice, and the application of standardized guidelines for the reporting of clinical trials should improve the quality [23, 24]. National agencies, such as US Food and Drug Administration, European Union Medical Device Directives and the UK National Institute for Clinical Excellence offer guidelines for conduct of clinical studies [25–27]. These guidelines set standards for the design, conduct and performance of clinical studies that ensure the accurate reporting of data and protection of the rights, safety, well-being and privacy of the subjects. While pre-market studies that evaluate the safety and effectiveness or clinical performance of a device are obliged to follow these strict study procedures, the guidelines are applicable to the conduct of well-designed post-market studies as well. However, rarely are these stringent guidelines followed outside of pre-market studies. The plan or "protocol" for a well-designed study should include the following: a clear statement of the objective of the study; a method for selection of subjects that provides adequate assurance that the subjects are suitable of the purpose of the study; if randomized, assignment of the subjects to test groups in a way to minimize bias and assure comparability between groups, an explanation of the methods of observation, and a comparison of the results of test and control in such a way to permit quantitative evaluation. The relevance of a study depends essentially on its design, careful implementation and the statistical analysis of the recorded data.

Properly Designed Clinical Trials

Careful monitoring of clinical studies in terms of conformity with rules and specifications of Good Clinical Practice (GCP) therefore should provide a sound basis for study design and protection of study subjects. Adherence to the principles of ethical treatment of clinical research subjects contained in the Declaration of Helsinki, the gold standard for ethical research behavior, insures an appropriate level of conduct [28]. In addition, assurance that specific regional legislation (i.e., US HIPAA patient privacy rules) and local hospital ethical committee regulations are met assures adherence to quality-based principles and methods [29].

Therefore, when designing investigations, they must include approval of the protocol by the hospital ethics committees, such as the Institutional Review Board and, when applicable, governmental agencies. Adherence to GCP guidelines should ensure that strict ethical rules (Declaration of Helsinki and its amendments) in the conduct of clinical trials are observed, that these trials are conducted in accordance with high standards of quality and that authentic, scientifically verifiable and reliable data are the result of such studies.

The first element to consider in the preparation of a sound study protocol is the identification of a clear and concise study objective. This often may be posed as a question. Does my device perform a specific function? Does this surgical intervention offer the specific advantage intended? Answering the question will require the researcher to consider a number of other issues, such as suitable study endpoint or response variable, study design (randomized, cohort, case-control), instruments needed to record study results and acceptable patient population. It is important to select the appropriate patient population for the study, one that is a subset of the general population that is representative of a group of people targeted for the application of the medical device or intervention. Selection of rigorous and unambiguous inclusion and exclusion criteria for the study will uniquely characterize the study population and relate to the intended use of the device. Determination of sample size by a statistician is essential to assure that the research question posed will be able to be answered. Utilization of validated instruments to collect study results not only increases the quality of the study, but also allows comparison to the literature.

Minimal Invasive Total Hip Arthroplasty: Considerations in Designing a Protocol

Pre-Operative

There are multiple variations of surgical approaches to the hip joint and their modifications: the lateral, anterolateral, direct anterior, posterior and posterolateral. In addition to the established conventional approaches with reduced incision length, an anterior-modified Smith Peterson approach can be applied. The typical approaches utilized for MIS THA are subdivided into single- or two-incision techniques. Before starting with any type of MIS approach, the surgeons should be aware of their own learning curve. As always, implementation of any new surgical technique into daily clinical practice should be done in a slow, graduated manner, incorporating cadaver trials and training workshops.

The success of THA depends on several factors, including proper patient selection and education, appropriate implant design, correct surgical technique, proper instrumentation, and effective peri-operative care. A number of studies have suggested that alignment errors outside the safe zone defined by Lewinek [30] are associated with more rapid failure and less satisfactory functional results after THA [31]. The accuracy of implantation is therefore an accepted prognostic factor for the long-term survival of THA.

The primary objective of a clinical investigation of the MIS surgical technique should be to assess the safety and efficacy of the procedure with a dedicated and modified instrumentation. The study protocol should clearly define the parameters unique to the MIS procedure and identify the MIS approach to be evaluated with a detailed surgical

technique for the investigator to follow. Efficacy of the MIS surgical technique should be assessed by short post-operative and long-term data gained from radiographic, clinical and patient outcome assessments and from complication rates. While various options exist for a potential study design, for new techniques, the authors suggest conducting prospective randomized clinical studies in order to demonstrate clinical results that may be directly compared to the standard of care and to keep study bias as small as possible. Blinding the patients to the approach type may minimize the placebo effect. Dependent on the approach, this might not be achievable due to anatomical location (e.g. comparing modified Smith Peterson to conventional antero-lateral). A solution might be to cover all wounds with the same size and identically placed bandages until hospital discharge. By evaluating all patient data by an independent reviewer (blinded when possible), the potential bias can be minimized. Sample-size calculation and primary endpoints of the study need to be defined. Proponents of MIS THA surgery suggest that the procedure has the potential to reduce soft-tissue trauma and thereby reduce operative blood loss, post-operative pain, and hospitalization time, speed the post-operative recovery, and improve the cosmetic appearance of the scar [1]. Therefore, surgical and peri-operative endpoints to evaluate may include intra-operative blood loss (utilizing the method described by Sehat et al. [32]), surgical time, use of pain medication, wound complications, length of hospital stay, day of first ambulation, and walking distance on the day of discharge.

Prior to study initiation, the investigator determines the sample-size calculations and defines the hypothesis and the tests for the statistical calculations. A description of the patient population is identified and incorporated into the inclusion/exclusion criteria. The statistical plan defines tests to be used that will depend on the variability of study results. In case of a non-normal distribution (big differences between median and mean), non-parametric tests have to be used (Wilcoxon rank-sum, Wilcoxon signed-rank test, ANOVA [Kruskal-Wallis test]). With normal distribution, parametric tests will be applied (Student's t test, paired t test, analysis of variance).

Once approval is obtained from the appropriate authorities, the study enrollment may begin. The investigator is responsible for evaluating each patient against inclusion and exclusion criteria and to make sure that the patient meets the study-enrollment requirements. It is not recommended to include patients with characteristics that could influence the outcome independent from any surgical influence. However, since it is generally agreed that MIS THA surgery is not appropriate for every patient, it is extremely important to carefully select the patient population to be included in the study.

Clinical Variables

Patients should be excluded that
- either have or are suspected of having an infection,
- are planning to become pregnant,
- have systemic or metabolic diseases affecting bones,
- are mentally incompetent or non-compliant,
- have significant other joint involvement or other significant co-morbidities, or
- will not sign an informed consent.

Patients should be assessed pre-operatively, intra-operatively and post-operatively according to the study protocol, and appropriate data should be recorded both in their hospital notes and case report forms. Since it is hypothesized that the major benefits of MIS will occur in the short term, a clinical study should be data-intensive in that period in order to assure study end-points associated with early clinical success may be properly evaluated. Follow-up visits may be at 6 and 12 weeks or at 6 and 24 weeks post-operatively. For the first 6 weeks, it may be useful to have the patient answer questions over the phone, via e-mail on a weekly or bi-weekly basis. A patient diary may also be used (see appendix). For the long-term arm of the study, the evaluation should include additional visits at 1, 2, and 5 years after surgery to monitor any effects due to the new surgical technique. As described before, if possible, an independent and blinded examiner should do all follow-up examinations.

The researchers are faced with a plethora of choices of which variables to collect. The challenge is to collect the minimum number of variables necessary to prove the study hypothesis. Initially, the pre-operative variables to be collected must be decided upon, which generally includes basic demographic data (date of visit, patient's study number, patient's initials, date of birth, weight, height, gender, primary diagnosis, affected hip and date of informed consent signature). Since the investigator wants to gain information about a new surgical technique, operative clinical variables associated with the MIS surgical procedure as compared to the standard

incision procedure such as instrumentation used, time to perform surgery, length of incision, blood loss and muscle incision as well as type and size of implants, and method of implant fixation should be recorded. Post-operative evaluation of factors which could be significant changed by the new technique need to be measured. For example, as the MIS surgical intervention could have an influence on the adductor muscles, a Trendelenburg test should be recorded [33]. Additionally, clinical scores may be used. Depending on the objective to prove, the investigator must choose tests designed to answer the hypothesis of the investigation. Since major claimed advantages of MIS are faster rehabilitation and less pain, it makes sense to apply validated tests designed to capture these variables. Patient self-administered questionnaires such as the WOMAC, SF-12 or SF-36 would be preferable in order to minimize potential bias. Also the Harris hip score, or its equivalent, would be additional options [34–40]. A common disadvantage of all the scores is that they may not capture the important variables of the MIS technique. Additional questions posed to the patients in the peri-operative time frame may be necessary to capture information relevant to the MIS surgical technique. Careful recording of this information in well-controlled randomized trials may provide useful data-collection instruments for future studies.

Assessment of Clinical Variables

Intra-Operative

What constitutes MIS should be clearly defined in the study protocol and patients randomized to either group verified by intra-operative variables that confirm that the patient received the appropriate intervention. For example, if the minimally invasive surgical technique is defined as 10 cm to be measured at the time of incision and before closure and the patient's incision is measured as 15 cm at the start of the procedure, then the reason for the deviation from the protocol must be explained and the patient's data analyzed separately. Incision length should be measured with a ruler with the length defined as the widest visible distance from one to the other side of the incision. This should be done at the time of incision and again at the end of the surgical intervention. The minimal desired incision should still be large enough that the surgeon can visualize the circumference of the acetabular rim. In any case, the minimal possible incision length is determined by the half circumference of the cup. Therefore, the report of incision length should be related to the cup size. We would recommend to use a ratio L= C/S where C represents the incision length and S the half circumference of the cup (S = p×r). Even with modified instrumentation, the surgeon should avoid any excessive abrasion against the surrounding skin and soft tissue. In spite of a small incision, it is still possible to induce a large amount of soft-tissue trauma to underlying structures. For example in a two-incision procedure, it may be beneficial to template the cup size pre-operatively to provide a preliminary indication of the skin incision needed to get the implant inserted. Patients requiring an incision larger than the minimal incision size should not be included in a randomized trial. This information should be reflected in the inclusion and exclusion criteria.

The condition of the wound must be carefully monitored in the post-operative period. The authors suggest paying close attention to the wound condition in general (no frazzled edges, no surrounding hematoma) after closing the skin and the following days after surgery. For the assessment of blood loss, it is recommended to compare the estimation of the surgeon and the anesthesiologist. However, these estimates should be correlated to objective values like hemoglobin, hematocrit and the intravenous fluids including the amount of transfusions. For monitoring soft-tissue trauma, the muscle enzymes creatinine kinase, myoglobulin concentration could provide useful markers. As stated previously, surgical time, the type and size of implant, fixation techniques and adverse events have to be recorded. A major focus should be put on the narcotic medication and instantaneous pain-management regime. For this reason, the authors recommend to describe the narcotic usage by equi-analgesic equivalency to morphine (mg EEM) [41]. Patients with spinal anesthetics should be excluded because the EEM cannot be calculated for the intra-operative analysis.

Prior to Discharge

While the patients are in hospital, specific clinical parameters should be measured on a daily basis. Due to budget reasons in European hospitals, most patients will not be discharged before the 5th post-operative day. As opposed to the hospital length of stay, a better variable to measure would be the required medical stay. Therefore, in a multi-center study it is important to carefully review the clinical parameters to be measured with all the study sites and obtain consensus that the parameters are in fact measurable. This will reduce the introduction of bias due to site-specific restrictions. Specific variables to record at the identified intervals may include the post-operative day the patient is able to perform each of the following functions: walk a defined distance (100 meters) on a flat surface, ascend and descend stairs (10 steps), independent transfers to a chair or bed. Independent, daily improvement of walking distance in meters, number of stair steps will also be recorded. Lastly, it is important for the researchers to agree on specific "discharge" criteria that once met would denote that the patient was at the end of their required "medical stay" regardless or not they stayed at the hospital due to some other non-medical reason.

Since the post-operative physical rehabilitation protocol can have an important impact on the outcome, the physical rehabilitation program should be standardized. An example of a typical physical therapy regime is as follows:

- 1st post-operative day: rising from bed, standing, walking on flat surface with two crutches, isometric exercises, active and passive motion, no flexion, adduction and internal rotation; no extension, adduction and external rotation;
- 2nd to 6th post-operative day: continuing of the training of first post-operative day, stair climbing;
- post-operative course: continuing of the training of the first post-operative days.

However, it is understood that these guidelines would be altered in the scenario when the study protocol is such that the patient decides when they are ready to proceed to the next rehabilitation platform.

The wound should be assessed for redness, swelling (measured as the circumference of the fully extended lower limb at 25, 35, 50 cm distances distally to the ASIS) or effusion, and observations documented and recorded as adverse events if necessary. Any operative site-related adverse event should be recorded including but not limited to any signs of neurological disorders, such as nerve palsy or foot drop, dislocation and/or subluxation of components, excessive hip pain with or without the need for medication, hip instability, and limb length discrepancy. If the patient is suspected of having sustained damage of a nerve due to the surgery, an examination by the neurologist should be performed. Systemic medical events, such as urinary retention, and cardiovascular events should be recorded regardless of whether the investigator feels the events are related to the MIS surgery.

Since most conventional tests are too long for frequent administering to the patients, daily diaries while in hospital and weekly thereafter for the first 6 weeks post-operatively could be used. A sample version can be found in the appendix. Careful instruction must be provided to the patient on how to complete the diary. The diary can provide valuable information regarding the dynamics of rehabilitation. Since this is an action to be done by the patients, the bias will be minimized, but compliance is important.

Post-Operative at 6, 12 Weeks and 1,2 and 5 Years

Variables include a conventional clinical examination with measurement of range of motion, Trendelenburg test, leg length discrepancy, WOMAC, and SF-36 score evaluation [39, 40, 41]. Complications need to be recorded. In order to limit the surgeons' bias, patients should be asked for satisfaction (VAS from very dissatisfied to highly satisfied), self assessment of scar (VAS from very dissatisfied to highly satisfied) and measurement of length of scar. The independent reviewer should check whether the scar is dry without any effusions or signs of necrosis. The patient should be asked about the presence of any pain on weight-bearing. If pain exists, the reviewer should ask about the location.

Radiological Analysis

Attainment and maintenance of optimum component placement is essential to long-term success of an implant. Therefore, radiological analysis of anteroposterior and lateral films obtained post-operatively before discharge and at scheduled postoperative office visits should be performed by an independent radiologist, blinded to the surgical technique. The Hip Society recommends a standard method of review for total hip arthroplasty and may provide ease of reference to the literature [42].

Conclusions

It is well known that total hip arthroplasty is considered a very successful procedure that offers patients pain relief and return to function. Minimally invasive surgery for total hip arthroplasty has the potential to offer patients increased satisfaction with shorter recovery time and cosmetic advantage of a smaller scar. However, as with any new procedure, the benefits must be demonstrated clinically. To date, there has been little data to demonstrate unequivocal advantage. We recommend the use of prospective, randomized clinical studies with clearly defined study hypotheses, surgical techniques, and clinical endpoints that will provide surgeons and patients with the information they need to make the appropriate choice.

Appendix: Suggested Clinical Data Collection for MIS Study

Standardized data collection forms (x = complete form)						
Evaluation	Preoperative	Intraoperative	Prior to hospital D/C[a]	Baseline (up to 6 weeks)	3 Months	Yearly
Demographics	x					
Surgical details		x				
Clinical (i.e., Harris hip score)	x			x	x	x
Radiographic A-P and lateral	x		x	x	x	x
Patient outcomes, WOMAC And SF-36	x			x	x	x

[a] Prior to discharge additional information.

Pre-discharge patient activity/medical assessments				
Activity	Day 1	Day 2	Day goal achieved	Day of discharge
Transfer bed to chair			Record date	NA
Walk on flat surface	Record in meters	Record in meters	Date 100 meters	Record meters
Ascend and descend stairs	Number of stairs	Number of stairs	Date 10 steps	Record steps
Ambulatory status (crutches, walker, cane, other)	Record status	Record status	NA	Record status
Discharge disposition (home, rehab, other)	NA	NA	NA	Record status
WOMAC Pain sub score (daily patient diary)[a]			NA	
Medical				
Pain Meds (EEM)[b]	Record	Record	NA	Record

[a] Patient diary to be completed daily in hospital, then weekly until 12 week evaluation. Diary questions utilizing the modified WOMAC [38] should be answered with the same scaling (0 to 10) as the original WOMAC score for the following parameters: ascending stairs, rising from sitting, walking on flat surface, getting in/out of car, putting on socks, rising from bed, sitting.

[b] Equi-analgesic equivalency to morphine.

References

1. Berry DJ, Berger RA, Callaghan JJ et al. (2003) Minimally invasive total hip arthroplasty. Development, early results and a critical analysis. J Bone Joint Surg [Am] 85: 2235–2236

2. Barrack RL (2003) The mini-incision: occasionally desirable, but rarely necessary- in the affirmative. presented at current concepts in Joint Replacement. Orlando, FL, December 2003

3. Argenson JA, Figuera A, Flecher X, Aubaniac JM (2003) A comparative evaluation of minimally invasive open unicompartmental knee arthroplasty. Presented at the annual meeting of the International Society for Technology and Arthroplasty. San Francisco, CA, September 2003

4. Waldman BJ (2003) Advances in minimally invasive total hip arthroplasty. Orthopedics 26 (8 Suppl): s833–836

5. Tria AJ Jr (2003) Advancements in minimally invasive total knee arthroplasty. Orthopedics 26 (8 Suppl): s859–863

6. Berger RA (2003) Total hip arthroplasty using the minimally invasive two-incision approach. Clin Orthop 417: 232–241

7. Romanowski MR, Repicci JA (2002) Minimally invasive unicondylar artholplasty: eight-year follow-up. J Knee Surg 15: 17–22

8. Wenz JF, Gurkan I, Jibodh SH (2002) Mini-incision total hip arthroplasty: a comparative assessment of perioperative outcomes. Orthopedics 25: 1031–1043

9. DiGioia AM 3rd, Plakseychuk AY, Levison TH, Jaramaz B (2003) Mini-incision technique for total hip arthroplasty with navigation. J Arthroplasty 18:123–8

10. Fisher DA, Watts M, Davis KE (2003) Implant position in knee surgery: a comparison of minimally invasive open unicompartmental, and total knee arthroplasty. J Arthroplasty 18 (7 Suppl 1): 2–8

11. Dorr LD (2003) Single-incision minimally invasive total hip arthroplasty. J Bone Joint Surg [Am] 85: 2236–2238

12. Mears DC (2003) Development of a two-incision minimally invasive total hip replacement. J Bone Joint Surg [Am] 85:2238–40

13. Duwelius PJ, Berger RA, Hartzband MA, Mears DC (2003) Two-incision minimally invasive total hip arthroplasty: operative technique and early results from four centers. J Bone Joint Surg [Am] 85: 2240–2242

14. Callaghan JJ (2003) Skeptical perspectives on minimally invasive total hip arthroplasty. J Bone Joint Surg [Am] 85-A: 2242–2243

15. Lieberman JR (2003) Ethics of introduction of new operative procedures and technology. J Bone Joint Surg [Am] 85: 2243–2246

16. Wright JM (2003) Mini Incision for total hip arthroplasty – a prospective controlled investigation with 5-year follow-up. 69th Annual Meeting of the American Academy of Orthopedic Surgeons. New Orleans, LA, March 2003

17. Swanson TV (2003) Advantages of the cementless total hip arthroplasty using mini-incision surgical technique. 69th Annual Meeting of the American Academy of Orthopedic Surgeons. New Orleans, LA, March 2003

18. Sivananthan DKS (2003) MIS for hip replacement using the NIL-NAV hip system. 69th Annual Meeting of the American Academy of Orthopedic Surgeons. New Orleans, LA, March 2003

19. Kennon RE, Keggi JM, Wetmore RS et al. (2003) Total hip arthroplasty thru a mini-incision anterior surgical approach. J Bone Joint Surg [Am] 85: 39–48

20. Sherry E, Egan M, Warnke PH, Henderson A, Eslick GD (2003) Minimal invasive surgery for hip replacement: a new technique using the NILNAV hip system. ANZ J Surg 73: 157–161

21. Chimento GF (2003) Minimally invasive total hp arthroplasty: a prospective randomized study. 69th Annual Meeting of the American Academy of Orthopedic Surgeons. New Orleans, LA, March 2003

22. Bhattacharyya T, Tornetta P 3rd, Healy WL, Einhorn TA (2003) The validity of claims made in orthopaedic print advertisements. J Bone Joint Surg [Am] 85: 1224–1228

23. Bhandari M, Richards RR, Sprague S, Schemitsch EH (2002) The quality of reporting of randomized trials in the Journal of Bone and Joint Surgery from 1988 through 2000. J Bone Joint Surg [Am] 84: 2307–2308

24. Kiter E, Karatosun V, Gunal I (2003) Do orthopaedic journals provide high quality evidence for clinical practice? Arch Orthop Trauma Surg 123: 82–85

25. United States Food and Drug Administration. 21 Code of Federal Regulations: 812 Investigational Device Exemption. Washington

DC, United States Government Printing Office via GPOA Access. April 1, 2002.

26. MEDDEV.2.7.1. European Commission (2003) Guidelines on Medical Devices. Evaluation of Clinical Data: A guide for Manufacturers and notified Bodies. April 2003; Brussel, Belgium.

27. National Institute for Clinical Excellence (2000) Technology Appraisal Guidance -No. 2. Guidance on the Selection of Prostheses for Primary Total Hip Replacement. April 2000; London UK.

28. World Medical Association Declaration of Helsinki (2002) ethical principles for medical research involving human subjects. J Postgrad Med 48: 206–208

29. United States Department of Health and Human Services (2002) 45 Code of Federal Regulations Parts 160 and 164. Standards for the Privacy of Individually Identifiable Health Information. Federal Register: August 14, 2002 (vol 67, no 157).

30. Lewinnek GE, Lewis JL, Tarr R, Compere CL, Zimmerman JR (1978) Dislocations after total hip-replacement arthroplasties. J Bone Joint Surg [Am] 60: 217–220

31. D'Lima DD, Chen PC, Colwell CW Jr (2001) Optimizing acetabular component position to minimize impingement and reduce contact stress. J Bone Joint Surg [Am] 83 (Suppl 2): 87–91

32. Sehat KR, Evans R, Newman JH (2000) How much blood is really lost in total knee arthroplasty? Correct blood loss management should take hidden loss into account. The Knee 7: 151–155

33. Hardcastle P, Nade S (1985) The significance of the Trendelenburg test. J Bone Joint Surg [Br] 67: 741–746

34. Bellamy N, Buchanan WW, Goldsmith CH, Campbell J, Sitt L (1988) Validation study of WOMAC: a health status instrument for measuring clinically-important patient-relevant outcomes following total hip or knee arthroplasty in osteoarthritis. J Orthop Reuth 1: 95–108

35. Ware JE, Sherbourne CD (1992) The MOS 36-item short-form health status survey (SF-36). 1. Conceptional framework and item selection. Med Care 30: 473–483

36. Riddle DL, Lee KT, Stratford PW (2001) Use of SF-36 an SF-12 health status measures: a quantitative comparison for groups versus individual patients. Med Care 39: 867–878

37. Klässbo M, Larsson E, Mannevik E (2003) Hip disability and osteoarthritis outcome score: An extension of the Western Ontario and McMaster Universities Osteoarthritis Index. Scand J Rheumatol 32: 46–51

38. Whitehouse SL, Lingard EA, Katz JN, Learmonth ID (2003) Development and testing of a reduced WOMAC function scale. J Bone Joint Surg [Br] 85: 706–711

39. Harris WH (1969) Traumatic arthritis of the hip after dislocation and acetabular fractures: treatment by mold arthroplasty. J Bone Joint Surg [Am] 51: 737–755

40. Ware JE, Snow KK, Kosinski M et al. (1993) SF-36 health survey, manual and interpretation guide. Boston MA: The Health Institute, New England Medical Center

41. DiPiro JT, Talbert RL, Yee GC et al. (2002) Pharmacotherapy. A pathophysiologic approach. 4th edn. McGraw Hill/Appleton & Lange, Stamford (Rheumatol 2003; 32: 46–51)

42. Johnston RC, Fitzgerald JR, Harris WH et al. (1990) Clinical and radiographic evaluation of total hip replacement. J Bone Joint Surgery [Am] 72: 162–168

22

Scoring Systems for the Comparison of International Data – Hips and Knees

M.J. Dunbar

Introduction

The gold standard for the assessment of outcomes after hip and knee arthroplasty is prosthesis survivorship. However, modern advances in prosthetic design and technique are such that the threshold for joint arthroplasty has moved from salvage operations performed in extreme cases, to an intervention designed to improve the quality of life in patients who might otherwise cope without surgery. Hence, judging the success of the surgery may relate more to subtler improvements in quality of life, including relief of pain and improvement in function. Furthermore, technological innovation has improved the design of prostheses, ensuring survival in situ, barring infection, for at least a decade with relative certainty [19, 29, 47]. Consequently, the homogeneity of current prostheses (with respect to stable and lasting designs) has produced an emerging emphasis on quantifying subtler outcomes after arthroplasty.

Although there is some consensus as to which categories of outcome metrics should be applied to arthroplasty patients, there is no agreement as to which specific metrics are most appropriate. Instead, multitudes of metrics have been put forward in the literature and new metrics continue to be introduced. International researchers are subsequently forced to choose a metric based on its published psychometric properties, or, more alarmingly, based on precedence and extraneous political factors. This practice has led to significant variation in the reporting of outcomes after arthroplasty, particularly between nations. While general trends in outcomes can be contrasted with various outcome metrics, subtler differences in outcomes are lost in the psychometric variability between outcome tools. Ideally, international consensus should determine the most appropriate outcome metrics for wide scale employment. General approaches to standardizing outcome metrics for arthroplasty shall be discussed in this chapter.

Survival Analysis

Arthroplasty Registries

Arthroplasty registries use prosthesis survival as the primary outcome. Survival analysis is a definitive metric that facilitates comparison of outcomes between nations. Currently, several national arthroplasty registries have the potential to compare and contrast survivorship outcomes [14, 19, 41, 46]. However, such comparisons are limited with respect to variation in demographics, including age at time of operation, diagnostic groupings, body mass index, gender, and activity levels. Research efforts should be directed at defining the demographics of each nation/center in detail so that the denominator of the comparative data can be determined. Without this level of research, comparison of outcomes in survivorship between nations/centers is prone to misinterpretation. Furthermore, the specific method of defining survivorship should be standardized [37]. For example, Cox's regression is a particularly useful method as it accounts for other factors such as age and gender, which are known to have an effect on outcomes. If such factors are not considered in outcome analyses, reported differences in survival curves between various prostheses are difficult to interpret, particularly on an international basis.

Arthroplasty registries function best as a surveillance tool for implant failure. As such, favorable and unfavorable trends in the outcomes of certain prostheses can be easily determined and disseminated back to the orthopedic community in a quality-improvement feedback cycle. However, because arthroplasty registries are surveillance tools, there is an inherent lag in the reporting of outcomes, which creates a potential for suboptimal implants or techniques to penetrate into and become part of the clinical norm prior to detection by the registry. A more accurate and predictive form of survivorship analysis would have the advantage of limiting new technology and techniques to fewer patients than is necessary to see trends with arthroplasty registries.

Radiostereometric Analysis

Radiostereometric Analysis (RSA) is a precise outcome tool that has accurate and reliable predictive ability with regard to implant aseptic loosening and, thus, survivorship [26, 48]. At the time of surgery, radio-dense tantalum markers are placed into the host bone and these beads are used to mark the implant. Post-operatively, biplanar simultaneous stereo X-rays of the joint are taken through a calibration cage with known fiducial points. The generated images are then imported into a RSA-software analysis package, and micromotion at the interface of the implant and host bone is calculated in three dimensions. These three vectors are combined into a metric of overall motion – maximum total point motion (MTPM). At six-month intervals, MTPM is plotted on the Y-axis against serial X-ray measures (on the X-axis) (◘ Fig. 23.1). RSA curves follow a typical pattern: the implanted prosthesis either stabilizes with respect to MTPM over time, or it continues to migrate. If the prosthesis stabilizes, revision for aseptic loosening is unlikely. Conversely, if the prosthesis continues to migrate, revision for aseptic loosening is significantly more likely. The power of RSA is such that variation in MTPM patterns can be differentiated accurately as early as one year post-operatively, and as few as 30 to 40 patients need to be exposed to the experimental technology.

It is the author's opinion that RSA is a critical technology for the rational development of minimally invasive surgery (MIS). As new MIS techniques and implants are introduced, earlier concerns over health-quality improvement and cost savings can be effectively addressed. National registries, while useful in overseeing the introduction of new technology, offer outcomes on a near real-time basis, and hence are not predictive. One theoretical concern regarding MIS is that the compromised exposure may lead to sub-optimal fixation and

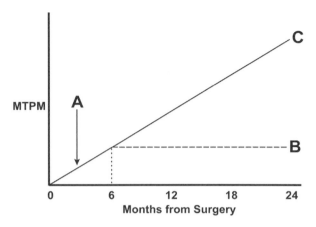

◘ **Fig. 23.1a–c.** A typical RSA curve. Motion is on the Y-axis. **a** All prostheses initially migrate. **b** Some components stabilize and are unlikely to be revised for aseptic loosening. **c** Some components continue to migrate and are more likely to be revised for aseptic loosening. The two curves differentiate early

therefore reduced survivorship. RSA has the potential to predict the long-term survivorship of MIS implants, and, as such, allows for a more realistic determination of the economic model for MIS. What are the savings to the health-care system if hip-replacement patients are sent home on the same day of surgery, only to come to a premature revision? Questions like these can be most definitively answered with RSA.

Limitation of Survivorship Analysis

Arthroplasty registries rely on revision status as the sole endpoint for defining the outcome after arthroplasty. Revision status is a useful measure as it is relatively easy to define and the incidence of revision is definite. While definitive, revision status is a relatively blunt metric and is generally non-representative of the function, degree of pain relief, and overall patient satisfaction after knee arthroplasty. Furthermore, different surgeons have different thresholds for performing revisions and not all patients requiring revision surgery undergo the procedure because of co-existing medical problems, personal wishes etc. [12]. Revision status yields data only on the small minority of operations that fail [1]. The same set of arguments generally holds true for the outcome of continuous migration, as defined by RSA, which essentially acts as a surrogate for revision status. While there is some evidence that subjective outcomes may be correlated with RSA-defined migration patterns, this phenomenon is not widely reported in the literature [20].

The Institute of Medicine defines health-care quality as "the degree to which health services for individuals and populations increase the likelihood of desired health outcomes and are consistent with current professional knowledge" [38]. Previously, the "desired health outcome" of arthroplasty was for a prosthesis that performed in some minimal fashion to alleviate pain and improve function, as long as the prosthesis survived for a period of time without catastrophic complications. Currently, joint arthroplasty is a reproducible, effective and long-lasting procedure [19, 29, 47]. Consequently, comparative analyses of prosthetic models and surgical techniques are increasingly directed toward subjective arthroplasty outcomes.

Subjective Outcomes

Background

In 1947, the World Health Organization defined health as follows: "Health is not only the absence of infirmity and disease but also a state of physical, mental and social well-being." Subsequently, in the surgical realm, the measurement of health moved from simply defining the success of a procedure by its effect on infirmity and disease, to defining what effect the intervention had on physical, mental and social well-being [12]. By this definition, it was no longer adequate to define the outcome of an arthroplasty, for example, by simply stating the prosthesis survival rate. This change in philosophy lead to the development of general health-outcome questionnaires; examples that have been used in arthroplasty research include the 36-Item Short-Form Health Survey (SF-36) [4], the 12-Item Short-Form Health Survey (SF-12) [51], the Nottingham Health Profile (NHP) [23], and the Sickness Impact Profile (SIP) [40]. General health questionnaires focus on patients' perceptions of their own health, including such diverse domains as ability to sleep, energy level, mood, and perception of body pain. These questionnaires are limited neither to specific disease nor patient cohort.

In an effort to avoid the surgeon bias associated with objective outcomes, additional disease-specific questionnaires were introduced to arthroplasty patients. Disease-specific questionnaires attempt to isolate the signal of interest by focusing questions around a particular disease state. In the 1980s, the Lequesne Index of Severity for the Knee (ISK) [33, 34] and the Western Ontario and MacMaster Universities Osteoarthritis Index (WOMAC) [2, 3] were introduced. Site-specific questionnaires attempt to isolate the signal in a similar fashion by focusing questions on a specific region of the body. The Oxford-12 Item Knee and Hip Scores (Oxford-12) were later developed and released in 1998 for use with knee- and hip-arthroplasty patients as site-specific questionnaires [10, 11]. Patient-specific questionnaires, such as the Patient-Specific Index [52], use a novel approach to limit the noise within a questionnaire by asking patients to choose their own goals or objectives prior to an intervention and subsequently requesting that they rate or score how well those objectives have been accomplished. Global- or single-item questionnaires, such as those regarding patient satisfaction, are the most aggressive in their effort to limit noise by asking a single direct question regarding the state or condition of interest [44, 45]. Several authors have suggested that the simultaneous use of general-health- and disease/site-specific questionnaires yields complimentary data [17, 35, 39].

One aspect in the development and assessment of all subjective outcomes that is germane to health-care researchers is the concept of psychometrics. Psychometrics can be defined as "the scientific measurement of mental capacities and processes and of personality " [6]. In other words, psychometrics is the process that allows researchers to apply scientific methodology to the measurement of subjective outcomes. In practical terms, the published psychometric properties of a questionnaire pertain primarily to the validation of the questionnaire (i.e. how well the questionnaire measures what it is supposed to measure). The validation process usually involves three specific elements of questionnaire testing: validity, reliability, and responsiveness. Subjective outcome metrics that are to be applied in a valid fashion for health-outcomes research must meet these three basic criteria.

Validity

In contrast to validation, validity refers more specifically to how well the questionnaire measures the question of interest. The results are usually compared to a gold standard. Unfortunately, there is no gold standard for arthroplasty [28, 31]. Consequently, questionnaires for arthroplasty are usually validated against a postulated effect, or construct, that is an expected outcome of the intervention. Given that postulated constructs typically differ across nations, this practice presents a major limitation in the comparison of international subjective outcomes.

Reliability

Reliability refers to the ability of an outcome metric to remain unchanged when applied on two separate occasions in which no clinical change has occurred [12]. Reliability is the measure of the noise within a metric and can be described by the following equation:

Reliability = Subject Variability/Subject Variability + Measurement Variability

In order for an outcome metric to have acceptable reliability, it must have limited measurement variability.

Responsiveness

Responsiveness is a measure of a questionnaire's ability to detect change when it is applied on separate occasions and a clinically significant change has occurred [12]. There are several methods of determining responsiveness, including the standardized effect size (SES). SES is calculated by subtracting the results of a questionnaire at time two from the results of the same questionnaire at time one and dividing the difference by the standard deviation of the test results from time one. Time one and time two represent a period over which a clinically significant change should have occurred, such as before and after arthroplasty surgery. A SES of 0.2 is considered small, 0.5 as moderate and greater than 0.8 as large [36].

Knee and hip arthroplasty have been shown to have a major impact on health-related quality of life when comparing pre-operative to post-operative status [10, 11, 32, 42, 43]. Dawson et al. have shown a SES of 2.0 for knee arthroplasty when the Oxford-12 Item Knee Score was applied pre- and post-operatively [11]. Such a SES can be considered profound, especially when a SES of 0.8 is considered large. Given the likelihood that such a large signal would mask subtle differences in outcome, an unusually large SES makes pre- and post-operative comparisons of different prosthetic designs or surgical tech-

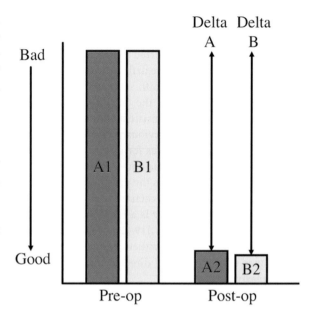

Fig. 23.2a,b. The paradox of arthroplasty outcomes. Patients are randomized pre-operatively (**a**) into two groups. Standard outcome metric is measured on Y-axis. Post-operatively (**b**), because of the large standardized effect size for arthroplasty, the difference in the pre- and post-operative outcome metric is large. Subtle differences in prostheses performance (Delta) are lost in the "noise" of the effect

niques difficult to interpret and potentially irrelevant (Fig. 23.2). Paradoxically, the signal for pre- and post-operative comparisons after hip and knee arthroplasty is so loud (large) that it in effect functions as noise and obscures the subtler signal of interest [12]. Therefore, it may be more relevant to calculate responsiveness using an alternative method and/or to follow arthroplasty patients longitudinally between time two (a defined post-operative period) and time three. In this case, the large signal of the operative intervention would not obscure the subtler signal of interest. This is particularly relevant when comparing international outcomes as the signal will be further degraded by regional variation in demographics, techniques, implants, etc.

Objective Outcomes

A word about surgeon-defined objective outcome metrics is warranted. Initially, as surgeons began to realize a need to formally assess the results of their interventions, they began to derive outcome metrics that incorporated various parameters, including technical procedure-specific outcomes (e.g. alignment, range of motion, etc.) as well as subjective patient-specific factors (e.g. pain). Examples of such assessment tools include the Hospital for Special Surgery Knee Score (HSS) [25], the Knee Society's Clinical and Functional Scoring System (KSS) [24], and the Harris Hip Score (HHS). Unfortunately, and despite their continued popularity, the HSS and KSS scores have never been validated using formal psychometric validation procedures. Moreover, these questionnaires have been found to be exceedingly unreliable [49], leading some authors to conclude that these scoring systems should not be used [30]. The HHS has been validated for use, but it also relies on the objective and potentially biased input of the surgeon [50]. The psychometric robustness of these outcome metrics is limited, and caution should be used in their interpretation, particularly the summary scores that are produced. It is the author's opinion that if these metrics are to be employed, summary scores should be avoided in analyses. Instead, individual sections within each metric should be reported and compared. Finally, given the lack of validated outcomes, these metrics should not be employed when comparing international outcomes.

Sources of Bias when Assessing Outcomes

The assessment of outcomes after hip and knee arthroplasty is subject to bias from several sources. Firstly, patient demographics may influence the results of questionnaire scores. Advanced age (>85 years) has been shown to have an adverse affect on subjective assessments after arthroplasty, as has low socioeconomic status, at least in North America [5, 7]. Gender has also been found to affect the results of health outcome questionnaires, particularly when used in association with hip or knee arthroplasty. Women tend to report greater pain and physical function limitation after hip or knee arthroplasty [27]. Co-morbidity has also been shown to adversely affect the results of knee arthroplasty, as assessed by questionnaire, for both joint-related and medical problems [5, 12, 18]. Charnley was aware of the potential biasing effect of co-morbidity, which was largely the impetus for the Charnley co-morbidity classification proposed for hip arthroplasty [8]. Gender, age, and co-morbidity should be considered when comparing outcomes after hip or knee arthroplasty, particularly international outcomes.

The mode of administration also significantly biases the results of health-outcome questionnaires. When a questionnaire is self-completed by the patient after surgery, as opposed to being administered by the investigator, the resulting questionnaire scores have been shown to be significantly lower (worse) [22, 44]. In addition, non-responders to a self-administered postal survey on quality of life tend to report worse quality of life than responders when followed-up with a telephone survey [21].

Finally, it is inadequate to simply translate a questionnaire into another language [15, 16]. Instead, the translated version needs to be tested for psychometric and cultural equivalence, in order to be deemed valid.

Selecting Appropriate Outcomes

When comparing international results on the introduction of minimally invasive hip and knee arthroplasty, little consensus exists as to which outcomes should be used in order to optimize the comparison. However, it is possible to make some recommendations based on the arguments made above.

As with conventional arthroplasty procedures, all MIS hip and knee arthroplasty procedures should be recorded prospectively into an arthroplasty registry, preferably at the national level. Concomitantly, demographic data, including gender, body habitus, and co-morbidity data, should be recorded. Such data is vital for meaningful international comparisons. Linkages to parallel hospital administrative patient databases could preclude the need to collect this data directly from the surgeon. A significant proportion of MIS hip- and knee-arthroplasty procedures should involve RSA technology in order to assess long-term survivorship at an early stage and limit the exposure of unproven techniques and implants. Without such RSA studies, the true global economics of MIS arthroplasty, which includes the cost of revision as a risk ratio compared to conventional arthroplasty, could not be determined until the survivorship period had been realized.

Surgeon-derived outcome metrics, such as the KSS and HSS knee scores, should generally be avoided as their lack of validation makes international comparisons suspect. The individual components of these scores, however, such as alignment and range of motion, should continue to be collected. Variations in these parameters are significant between nations [9]. Whenever possible, the most accurate form of reproducible measurement should be employed. International standardization would be prudent.

Given that certain outcomes are perception-based (e.g. cosmetic appearance), it is important to collect subjective outcomes for MIS arthroplasty so as to better delineate the patient's perception. There are several categories of subjective outcomes including general health, disease-specific, site-specific, patient-specific and single-item global questionnaires. Unfortunately, there is scant consensus with respect to which outcome measures are most appropriate. Each author advocates his outcome measure over others using, at best, statistical methodology that makes direct comparison of measures difficult to interpret. International consensus is required and should be sought. A general health questionnaire should be incorporated into the assessment process, as it would assist in standardizing comparison between nations. The SF-36 is well validated and has been translated for numerous countries. Site-specific questionnaires, such as the Oxford-12 seem to be better suited for assessing the subjective outcome of arthroplasty than disease-specific questionnaires, although the WOMAC is very popular in North America [13]. Patient-specific indexes may or may not be more appropriate for use in international comparative outcomes; more research needs to be done around this type of outcome metric. Single-item global questionnaires have been shown to be valid and informative for assessing knee arthroplasty outcomes at a national level, and the simplicity of the satisfaction question may transcend cultural differences [44, 45]. When analyzing data from subjective outcomes, demographic variables must be accounted for, especially co-morbidity, if meaningful international comparisons are to be made. Above all, the metrics employed must be validated.

Conclusions

There is currently no consensus as to the type of outcome data that should be collected when comparing international results of MIS arthroplasty. Prosthesis survivorship, as defined by arthroplasty registries and RSA, should be reported. If international comparisons are to be made, it is important to record demographic data as well-defined and accurately measured clinical parameters. Consensus needs to be reached regarding which subjective outcomes should be used, with consideration given to those questionnaires that are best-suited to arthroplasty. Ongoing research is required.

References

1. Apley AG (1990) An assessment of assessment [editorial]. J Bone Joint Surg [Br] 72(6): 957–958
2. Bellamy N, Buchanan WW (1984) Outcome measurement in osteoarthritis clinical trials: the case for standardisation. Clin Rheumatol 3(3): 293–303
3. Bellamy N, Buchanan WW, Goldsmith CH, Campbell J, Stitt LW (1988) Validation study of WOMAC: a health status instrument for measuring clinically important patient relevant outcomes to antirheumatic drug therapy in patients with osteoarthritis of the hip or knee. J Rheumatol 15(12): 1833–1840
4. Brazier JE, Harper R, Jones NM, O'Cathain A, Thomas KJ, Usherwood T, Westlake L (1992) Validating the SF-36 health survey questionnaire: new outcome measure for primary care. BMJ 305(6846): 160–164
5. Brinker MR, Lund PJ, Barrack RL (1997) Demographic biases of scoring instruments for the results of total knee arthroplasty. J Bone Joint Surg Am 79(6): 858–865
6. Brown L (1993) The New Shorter Oxford English Dictionary. New York, Oxford University Press
7. Callahan CM, Drake BG, Heck DA, Dittus RS (1994) Patient outcomes following tricompartmental total knee replacement. A meta-analysis. Jama 271(17): 1349–1357
8. Charnley J (1979) Low friction arthroplasty of the hip. Berlin, Springer
9. Cooke TD, Harrison L, Khan B, Scudamore A, Chaudhary MA (2002) Analysis of limb alignment in the pathogenesis of osteoarthritis: a comparison of Saudi Arabian and Canadian cases. Rheumatol Int 22(4): 160–164
10. Dawson J, Fitzpatrick R, Carr A, Murray D (1996) Questionnaire on the perceptions of patients about total hip replacement. J Bone Joint Surg Br 78(2): 185–190
11. Dawson J, Fitzpatrick R, Murray D, Carr A (1998) Questionnaire on the perceptions of patients about total knee replacement. J Bone Joint Surg Br 80(1): 63–69
12. Dunbar MJ (2001) Subjective outcomes after knee arthroplasty. Acta Orthop Scand Suppl 72(301): 1–63
13. Dunbar MJ, Robertsson O, Ryd L, Lidgren L (2001) Appropriate questionnaires for knee arthroplasty. Results of a survey of 3600 patients from The Swedish Knee Arthroplasty Registry. J Bone Joint Surg Br 83(3): 339–344
14. Espehaug B, Havelin LI, Engesæter LB, Vollset SE, Langeland N (1995) Early revision among 12,179 hip prostheses. A comparison of 10 different brands reported to the Norwegian Arthroplasty Register, 1987–1993. Acta Orthop Scand 66(6): 487–493
15. Guillemin F, Bombardier C, Beaton D (1993) Cross-cultural adaptation of health-related quality of life measures: literature review and proposed guidelines. J Clin Epidemiol 46(12): 1417–1432
16. Guyatt GH (1993) The philosophy of health-related quality of life translation. Qual Life Res 2(6): 461–465
17. Hawker G, Melfi C, Paul J, Green R, Bombardier C (1995) Comparison of a generic (SF-36) and a disease specific (WOMAC) (Western Ontario and McMaster Universities Osteoarthritis Index) instrument in the measurement of outcomes after knee replacement surgery. J Rheumatol 22(6): 1193–1196

18. Hawker G et al. (1998) Health-related quality of life after knee replacement. J Bone Joint Surg Am 80(2): 163–173

19. Herberts P, Malchau H (2000) Long-term registration has improved the quality of hip replacement: a review of the Swedish THR Register comparing 160,000 cases. Acta Orthop Scand 71(2): 111–121

20. Hilding MB, Bäckbro B, Ryd L (1997) Quality of life after knee arthroplasty. A randomized study of 3 designs in 42 patients, compared after 4 years. Acta Orthop Scand 68(2): 156–160

21. Hill A, Roberts J, Ewings P, Gunnell D (1997) Non-response bias in a lifestyle survey. J Public Health Med 19(2): 203–207

22. Hoher J, Bach T, Munster A, Bouillon B, Tiling T (1997) Does the mode of data collection change results in a subjective knee score? Self-administration versus interview. Am J Sports Med 25(5): 642–647

23. Hunt SM, McKenna SP, McEwen J, Backett EM, Williams J, Papp E (1980) A quantitative approach to perceived health status: a validation study. J Epidemiol Community Health 34(4): 281–286

24. Insall JN, Dorr LD, Scott RD, Scott WN (1989) Rationale of the Knee Society clinical rating system. Clin Orthop (248): 13–14

25. Insall JN, Ranawat CS, Aglietti P, Shine J (1976) A comparison of four models of total knee-replacement prostheses. J Bone Joint Surg [Am] 58(6): 754–765

26. Kärrholm J, Herberts P, Hultmark P, Malchau H, Nivbrant B, Thanner J (1997) Radiosterometry of hip prostheses. Review of methodology and clinical results. Clin Orthop (344): 94–110

27. Katz JN, Wright EA, Guadagnoli E, Liang MH, Karlson EW, Cleary PD (1994) Differences between men and women undergoing major orthopedic surgery for degenerative arthritis. Arthritis Rheum 37(5): 687–694

28. Kirshner B, Guyatt G (1985) A methodological framework for assessing health indices. J Chronic Dis 38(1): 27–36

29. Knutson K, Lewold S, Robertsson O, Lidgren L (1994) The Swedish knee arthroplasty register. A nation-wide study of 30,003 knees 1976–1992. Acta Orthop Scand 65(4): 375–386

30. Konig A, Scheidler M, Rader C, Eulert J (1997) The need for a dual rating system total knee arthroplasty. Clin Orthop (345): 161–167

31. Kreibich DN, Vaz M, Bourne RB, Rorabeck CH, Kim P, Hardie R, Kramer J, Kirkley A (1996) What is the best way of assessing outcome after total knee replacement? Clin Orthop (331): 221–225

32. Laupacis A, Bourne R, Rorabeck C, Feeny D, Wong C, Tugwell P, Leslie K, Bullas R (1993) The effect of elective total hip replacement on health-related quality of life. J Bone Joint Surg Am 75(11): 1619–1626

33. Lequesne M (1989) Informational indices. Validation of criteria and tests. Scand J Rheumatol Suppl 80: 17–28

34. Lequesne MG, Mery C, Samson M, Gerard P (1987) Indexes of severity for osteoarthritis of the hip and knee. Validation value in comparison with other assessment tests. Scand J Rheumatol Suppl 65: 85–89

35. Lieberman JR, Dorey F, Shekelle P, Schumacher L, Kilgus DJ, Thomas BJ, Finerman GA (1997) Outcome after total hip arthroplasty. Comparison of a traditional disease-specific and a quality-of-life measurement of outcome. J Arthroplasty 12(6): 639–645

36. Meenan RF, Kazis LE, Anthony JM, Wallin BA (1991) The clinical and health status of patients with recent-onset rheumatoid arthritis. Arthritis Rheum 34(6): 761–765

37. Murray DW, Carr AJ, Bulstrode C (1993) Survival analysis of joint replacements. J Bone Joint Surg Br 75(5): 697–704

38. Palmer RH (1997) Process-based measures of quality: the need for detailed clinical data in large health care databases. Ann Intern Med 127: 733–738

39. Patrick DL, Deyo RA (1989) Generic and disease-specific measures in assessing health status and quality of life. Med Care 27 [3 Suppl]: S217–232

40. Pollard WE, Bobbitt RA, Bergner M, Martin DP, Gilson BS (1976) The Sickness Impact Profile: reliability of a health status measure. Med Care 14(2): 146–155

41. Puolakka TJ, Pajamaki KJ, Halonen PJ, Pulkkinen PO, Paavolainen P, Nevalainen JK (2001) The Finnish Arthroplasty Register: report of the hip register. Acta Orthop Scand 72(5): 433–441

42. Rissanen P, Aro S, Slatis P, Sintonen H, Paavolainen P (1995) Health and quality of life before and after hip or knee arthroplasty. J Arthroplasty 10(2): 169–175

43. Ritter MA, Albohm MJ, Keating EM, Faris PM, Meding JB (1995) Comparative outcomes of total joint arthroplasty. J Arthroplasty 10(6): 737–741

44. Robertsson O, Dunbar M, Pehrsson T, Knutson K, Lidgren L (2000) Patient satisfaction after knee arthroplasty: a report on 27,372 knees operated on between 1981 and 1995 in Sweden. Acta Orthop Scand 71(3): 262–267

45. Robertsson O, Dunbar MJ (2001) Patient satisfaction compared with general health and disease-specific questionnaires in knee arthroplasty patients. J Arthroplasty 16(4): 476–482

46. Robertsson O, Dunbar MJ, Knutson K, Lewold S, Lidgren L (1999) The Swedish Knee Arthroplasty Register. 25 years experience. Bull Hosp Jt Dis 58(3): 133–138

47. Robertsson O, Knutson K, Lewold S, Lidgren L (1999) Knee Arthroplasty for Osteoarthrosis and Rheumatoid Arthritis 1986–1996. Scientific Exhibit SE028, AAOS, Annual Meeting 1999

48. Ryd L (1986) Micromotion in knee arthroplasty. A roentgen stereophotogrammetric analysis of tibial component fixation. Acta Orthop Scand Suppl 220: 1–80

49. Ryd L, Karrholm J, Ahlvin P (1997) Knee scoring systems in gonarthrosis. Evaluation of interobserver variability and the envelope of bias. Score Assessment Group. Acta Orthop Scand 68(1): 41–45

50. Soderman P, Malchau H, Herberts P (2001) Outcome of total hip replacement: a comparison of different measurement methods. Clin Orthop (390): 163–172

51. Ware J Jr, Kosinski M, Keller SD (1996) A 12-Item Short-Form Health Survey: construction of scales and preliminary tests of reliability and validity. Med Care 34(3): 220–233

52. Wright JG, Young NL (1997) The patient-specific index: asking patients what they want. J Bone Joint Surg Am 79(7): 974–983

Part VI Perspectives – The Hip

Is Minimally Invasive Hip Replacement a Winning Concept?

A. Turnbull, A. Leong

To know whether minimally invasive hip surgery will eventually replace standard hip-replacement surgery one would need a crystal ball, but certainly it is a winning idea. Everybody, especially patients, would like surgery to be less painful, have smaller incisions and recover faster from the procedure. This is what minimally invasive hip replacement promises and if it can deliver what it promises it would certainly be a winner.

I consider myself a relatively young orthopedic surgeon, but if I chronicle my age against the changes in surgery that have occurred since I started in medicine I would have to consider myself old. Who would have thought at the time of my training that arthroscopic meniscectomy, arthroscopic anterior cruciate ligament reconstruction, arthroscopic shoulder stabilization, and other endoscopic procedures such as cholecystectomy and appendicectomy would have ever been possible? These procedures have become the accepted standard and have resulted in less patient morbidity and faster recovery. Would any of us now consider having an open meniscectomy? I'm sure the answer is no, but I can remember when arthroscopic surgery was ridiculed as a triumph of technology over good sense just as minimally hip surgery is being ridiculed now. To me it sounds like the same tune just to a different drum.

Even two years ago the concept of minimally invasive hip replacement seemed ridiculous. In fact, I resented the concept as hip replacement remained one of the few bastions of anatomical dissection that is such a delight to most surgeons. Even now, mere discussion of the technique with colleagues seems to arouse the emotion of anger. Standard total hip replacement is one of the great surgical successes of the past one hundred years and who would have thought that something as successful as hip replacement could ever have been challenged as the standard procedure. Most of us would wonder how could we make a procedure that appears to be such a perfect technique even better. It is, however, the testing of such boundaries that leads to improvement and if people did not push the boundaries, we would still be riding horses and traveling in carts.

I first became aware of the technique of minimally invasive hip surgery when I read about it in an orthopedic publication, but I quickly and in an off-handed manner disregarded what I read. It was not until one of my research fellows asked about a research project for his upcoming research year that my interest in the procedure was aroused. At that time the consequences of wear debris and minimally invasive total hip replacements were the controversial topics in joint-replacement surgery and on this basis we decided to research the possibility of minimally invasive total hip arthroplasty.

Dr. Gary Heynan from Auckland in New Zealand was at that time performing the two-incision technique and had accumulated extensive experience using this technique. We traveled to New Zealand to observe the procedure. I was surprised by the remarkably simple concept and astonished to see the rapidity of patient recovery with some patients actually being discharged from hospital the day of surgery. On return to Australia, an ideal patient was chosen and with some trepidation we went ahead with the procedure, using the two-incision technique that we had witnessed in New Zealand. The surgery went surprisingly well with little struggle and the patient has done well. The second case also went smoothly, but with the third and fourth cases we struck difficulty due to poor placement of the proximal incision that resulted in poor alignment of the femoral reamer leading to femoral shaft perforation. As a result of the perforation, the wound required extension to

Chapter 24 · Is Minimally Invasive Hip Replacement a Winning Concept?

267 24

allow better exposure of the proximal femur and insertion a prosthesis that bypassed the femoral perforation. Luckily, the patients' post-operative recovery was uneventful and subsequently they have done well, but this experience gave me severe reservations about the safety of the two-incision technique. I recall also, as I extended the wound for better exposure, my alarm at the amount of damage to the abductors which had been sustained during the preparation of the femur. I could envisage that if this procedure became widely used in the general orthopedic community, we would see a sharp rise in the number of surgical complications. The experience led me to explore other minimally invasive techniques.

One particular orthopedic company in Australia has heavily promoted the use of a two-incision technique and has run cadaver workshops and organized surgeon visits on the technique. Australian orthopedic surgeons initially showed a lot of interest, but it comes as no surprise to me that many surgeons who tried the technique enthusiastically after attending these workshops have subsequently abandoned the procedure and reverted to standard approaches or other minimally invasive techniques.

To those who wish to attempt this technique I would recommend the following. The procedure can be confronting and it is easy to get into difficulties during the surgery so it requires a sense of adventure and a desire to get out of one's comfort zone.

It is essential to attend cases with an experienced surgeon and trial the technique if possible in a cadaver laboratory before proceeding to live cases. Be aware that the learning curve for this procedure is extremely steep. As the procedure is much easier in thin patients I would strongly recommend for the first few cases to select only thin patients.

As the procedure requires the use of image intensification, I have employed the use of a Jackson spinal table. This allows easy access for the image-intensification machine and provides a relatively unobstructed view of the procedure.

The procedure takes longer than with standard techniques so it is important to warn your anesthetist and choose a patient anesthetist.

Special instruments have been designed to perform the procedure and it is essential that you obtain and become familiar with these new instruments. Most companies provide specially designed retractors and these are essential for improved exposure. As the incision is small, it is difficult to illuminate the depths of the wound with a standard operating theatre light and specially designed low-profile light sources are required. As the incision is small and mobilization of the proximal femur difficult through the small incisions modified acetabular reamers are required to minimize damage to the hip muscles. A specially designed acetabular component inserter is also required to allow proper orientation of the acetabular component. As the preparation of the femur is performed through the abductor muscles, special femoral reamers and broaches are required to minimize damage to the abductor muscles during this preparation. As the buttock and the iliac crest make access to the proximal femur, difficult broach handles with a reversed angle are required to avoid these obstacles. With this technique it is difficult to insert all types of prosthesis, so some surgeons may require a change in type of prosthesis that they use. If this were the case, I would strongly recommend that you become familiar with the prosthesis using a standard open procedure before attempting the two-incision technique. At this stage, I do not think that it would be possible to use a cemented femoral component with the two-incision technique. It is almost inevitable that you will strike difficulties at some time using the procedure. If this occurs, a more extensive exposure will become necessary. As the patient is supine, extension of the exposure has to be done through an anterolateral approach. If you are not familiar with this approach, it should be practiced preferably with a cadaver before proceeding with a trial of the technique.

In summary the two-incision technique is possible and can go smoothly with a good result in some cases but I have the following concerns. The procedure is technically challenging and small mistakes can have serious consequences. The lack of exposure and the lack of surgical "feel" increase the risk of component mal-positioning. Mal-positioning increases the risk of dislocation and component loosening. As visualization and surgical feel are compromised, the possibility of incorrect sizing of the components is increased. Insertion of a component that is too small increases the chance of component loosening while insertion a component that is too large increases the risk of femoral shaft fracture. The lack of adequate exposure can cause unnecessary muscle damage and there may be an increased incidence of nerve damage as a result of this.

Even if studies in the future find that the two-incision technique results in shorter hospital stays and faster rehabilitation, I am not convinced that the risks involved with the surgery make the benefits worthwhile.

The fears that I have with the two-incision technique lead me then to explore the mini-posterior approach. As I have always used a modified Hardinge approach for my standard hip replacement changing to a mini-posterior had the two difficulties for me of becoming familiar with the posterior approach and also using a small incision. At first I found it cumbersome and uncomfortable but with perseverance and some work in a cadaver laboratory combined with the development of a purpose designed instrument set the operation has become comfortable and now my standard procedure for uncomplicated total hip replacement even in the more obese patient. For those familiar with the posterior approach and having the retractor instrument set available, I think they will quickly learn the technique and become comfortable with it without much difficulty. I have found certain tricks that have helped to make the procedure less difficult.

Firstly, in positioning the patient in the lateral decubitus position place the contralateral lower limb with the hip extended and the knee flexed. This differs from the standard practice where the contralateral lower limb is normally flexed at the hip and the knee. Having the hip extended allows the upper hip to be more adducted and allows for better exposure of the proximal femur for preparation of the femoral canal and insertion of the femoral component.

Take time to remove the fat and bursal tissue just posterior to the greater trochanter as later in the procedure this will help to identify important landmarks.

Once the hip has been dislocated, remove any remaining capsule and stumps of the external rotator tendons from the area behind the greater trochanter. This gives an excellent view of the femoral neck so that femoral neck-resection angle and length can be better estimated.

I use a spiked curved retractor that I place just anterior and superior to the acetabulum and hammer this into the ilium. This allows excellent retraction of the proximal femur to allow exposure of the acetabulum. A second curved spike retractor is then placed behind the acetabulum at the junction of the ischium and the ilium and this retracts the neurovascular bundle the capsule and the external rotators posteriorly and completes the exposure of the acetabulum.

To expose the proximal femur I use a curved spiked retractor over the greater trochanter underneath the tendons of the gluteus medius and the gluteus minimus and a special curved retractor that is place under the calcar. With these two retractors, excellent exposure of the proximal femur can be achieved and standard femoral preparation then proceeds.

Using this technique, I have found that the mini-posterior approach provides excellent visualization of the acetabulum and the femur. It allows accurate sizing of the femoral and acetabular components and accurate component positioning. Trialing of the components is no more difficult compared to when using a standard posterior approach and I am able to assess stability leg length and offset much more adequately than I can with a two-incision technique. The neurovascular bundle is identified and can be protected adequately. A more accurate assessment of leg length is possible minimizing the possibility of a leg length discrepancy. The approach allows for use of standard components without the necessity to change component types. It allows for either press fit or cement technique. If difficulties are encountered, the surgical approach is easily extended.

I have been using the mini-posterior approach as my standard technique for the last twelve months. The differences in patient outcomes are difficult to quantitate objectively but it is certainly my impression that patients have less pain, mobilise quicker and are happier compared to patients having the standard approach. Patients that have had their other hips replaced not using the mini-incision technique almost universally comment on the relative ease of the second procedure. My physiotherapist who has been working with me for almost thirteen years, has commented without prompting that the patients have less pain and are easy to rehabilitate. Surgeons may not be keen on the technique but the patients are and word travels quickly in the osteoarthritic community. Patients are now beginning to ask about the surgical technique and are starting to demand a less invasive approach. With the increased demand by patients and the encouraging experience that I have had as well as the apparent lack of increased complications I am certain that mini incision hip surgery like other minimally invasive techniques will become the expected norm.

At almost all of the meetings I attend presentations conclude that there is no difference in results at one year comparing patients who have had minimally invasive surgery to those who have had standard hip surgery.

Chapter 24 · Is Minimally Invasive Hip Replacement a Winning Concept?

269   24

This finding is used to conclude that minimally invasive surgery is not good. To me the result is positive for minimally invasive surgery; after all, minimally invasive surgery promises only improvements in the post-operation period hopefully without jeopardizing longer-term results. There is no reason why minimally invasive surgery should improve the results at one year. The results at one year comparing open and arthroscopic ACL reconstruction would show little difference, but who would recommend open reconstruction?

I feel that we have become a little complacent towards hip arthroplasty. One of the other good aspects of this debate has been the reassessment of the procedure that has occurred. New instruments such as retractors, broach handles, component inserters and better light sources for confined spaces have all been positive spin offs of the new procedure. Also, dramatic changes in treatment protocols have occurred. These include better pain-control protocols, faster rehabilitation with earlier weight-bearing and better patient education to facilitate early discharge.

I am confident, however, that surgeons who do not learn and start using minimally invasive techniques will be left behind as surgeons who embrace the procedure will be sought by patients. I am sure, improvements will happen, instruments will improve and prosthetic design may even change to suit the technique, new muscle-sparing approaches will be introduced and the prospect of help from computer-assisted navigation instruments is exciting.

Minimally invasive hip replacement is a winning concept and in fact it has already scored many points. It has stimulated new instrument designs, the development of more rapid rehabilitation programs and the development of better pain-control protocols. It has made us realize that our previous incisions were longer than necessary.

I'm afraid that surgeons who continue to practice hip replacement using standard exposures will be left behind by patients just as those who failed to take up other minimally invasive techniques such as arthroscopic knee surgery were left behind.

References

1. Cameron HU. Mini-incisions: visualization is key. Orthopaedics 2002; 25: 472
2. Cameron HU. Mini-incisions: two for the price of one! Orthopaedics 2002; 25: 473
3. Ramesh M, O'Byrne JM, McCarthy N, Jarvis A, Mahalingham K, Cashman WF. Damage to the superior gluteal nerve after the hardinge approach to the hip. J Bone Joint Surg 1996; 78B: 903–906
4. Kennon RE, Keggi J, Wetmore R, Zatorski L, Keggi K. Total hip arthroplasty using the minimally invasive anterior surgical approach. Yale University School of Medicine Department of Orthopaedics & Rehabilitation (Keggi Orthopaedic Foundation)
5. Wenz JF, Gurkan I, Jibodh SR. Mini-incision total hip arthroplasty: a comparative assessment of perioperative outcomes. Orthopaedics 2002; 25: 1031
6. Tittler MA, Harty LD, Keating ME, Faris PM, Meding JB. A clinical comparison of the anterolateral and posterolateral approaches to the hip. Clin Orthop Rel Res 2001; 385: 95–99

One Universal Approach – or a Split World?

V.E. Krebs, W.K. Barsoum

The evolution and advancements in adult eeconstructive orthopedic surgery over the past 20 years have been tremendous. Total joint arthroplasty has been a major focus of this evolution, and has been recognized as being among the most medically beneficial and cost-effective surgical procedures in the history of modern medicine. The effectiveness of these procedures has been driven by concurrent and multifaceted developments in the basic science of bone and joint biomechanics, material science, manufacturing, surgical techniques and instrumentation, and clinical outcomes measurement. Innovative and forward thinking surgeons have been the catalysts for the process, and these individuals and groups have come from around the globe with very different cultural and educational backgrounds. A certain degree of "ownership" has permeated the process, creating a competitive spirit that has accelerated innovation, sparked creativity, and continually challenged the generalized acceptance of any single procedure, exposure, and/or implant design.

Any complete discussion of the relative advantages and disadvantages of various exposures and the possibility of creating a single universal exposure for hip arthroplasty must first consider what is presently available. Due to the unique anatomy of the hip joint and its relatively deep position within the pelvis, multiple exposures have been described. These exposures take advantage of the various intra-nervous planes that exist around the hip. These planes must be respected to avoid neurovascular injury and maintain hip function. The common approaches presently used for hip replacement include the anterior, anterolateral, trochanteric osteotomy, trochanteric slide, direct lateral and posterolateral.

The trochanteric osteotomy was described and popularized by Charnley, and was the most commonly used approach for total hip replacement during the procedure's early development and widespread acceptance. It is currently used in situations where extensile acetabular and pelvic exposure is required for placement of cages, posterior plating for discontinuity, and can be useful when correcting leg-length discrepancies. Properly done in a controlled fashion, it can also be used to decrease the risk of intra-operative femur fracture when bone stock is poor in patients with osteolysis or osteoporosis. Its historic disadvantages have been related to high re-operation rates for complications such as non-union, migration, bursitis, and fibrous union that occurred with failed trochanteric fixation. The transtrochanteric approach also limits the surgeons' ability to use post-operative irradiation for prophylaxis against heterotopic ossification, as it would further increase the risk of non-union. Despite the excellent pelvic and acetabular exposure, most surgeons would agree that this approach has become antiquated in light of non-osteotomy-approach alternatives that offer equal or better visualization.

The posterolateral approach is one of the most commonly used today. Its wide acceptance is related to the ease and speed of dissection, wide exposure of both the proximal femur and acetabulum, extensibility, application to both primary and revision settings, and rapid recovery of abductor muscle function. This approach spares the abductors and limits the surgical trauma to the major functional muscle groups responsible for gait, balance, and power. This aspect of the approach eliminates the need for weight-bearing precautions and allows for accelerated rehabilitation. The main disadvantage to the posterior approach has been its historically increased incidence of posterior dislocation. With the advent of better soft-tissue repairs and the development of more anatomic femoral and acetabular components this concern has, to a great degree, been eliminated.

The anterolateral, or Watson–Jones, approach was one of the early alternatives to the trochanteric osteotomy and has its principle role in primary total hip replacement. The exposure utilizes a relatively confined plane between the tensor fascia lata and the gluteus medius muscles. The proximity of neurovascular structures limits the ability to extend the exposure proximally, and can limit acetabular access due to the risk of damaging muscle innervation. Common complications with this approach include the risk of abductor avulsion or denervation and post-operative limp. Its advantages include the ability to preserve femoral head and neck blood supply by leaving the quadratus muscle intact posteriorly, requisite for successful femoral head resurfacing arthroplasty. Its other advantage is the very low dislocation rate and excellent joint stability afforded by the retention of the entire posterior capsule and short external rotators.

The trochanteric slide is felt by many to be the next generation of trochanteric osteotomy. This allows for a partial trochanteric osteotomy while maintaining the soft tissue and bony sleeve between the abductor insertion along the greater trochanter and the quadriceps musculature. The osteotomy allows for a complete exposure of the acetabulum while simultaneously allowing for controlled femoral osteotomy and exposure of the femur. Its main advantage over trochanteric osteotomy is that the risk of proximal trochanteric migration is quite low due to the fact that a distal tether is kept intact through the quadriceps. Additionally, the function of the abductor musculature remains physiologic due to the fact that the distal soft-tissue anchor remains intact. This approach is commonly used in the revision situation where either a more extensile exposure of the acetabulum is needed or the removal of the femoral component with or without cement would otherwise be difficult. Drawbacks of the trochanteric slide are a high incidence of chronic secondary trochanteric bursitis that resulting predominantly in response to the prominent and failed hardware essential for reattachment of the osteotomized trochanter. The approach also has the potential for non-union or fibrous union of the osteotomized trochanter fragment that can lead to abductor weakness.

The direct lateral approach is versatile and extendable and therefore commonly used in both primary and revision total hip replacement. Its main advantage is the reduction of posterior instability by maintaining the posterior sleeve of capsule and short external rotators. Although it may be used in complex acetabular revisions, it is difficult to plate posterior column fractures or to use cages with this approach in the hands of surgeons that do not have a significant amount of experience with it. Additionally, there is potential for damage to the superior gluteal neurovascular complex as this is found just 4–5 cm proximal to the tip of the greater trochanter in most patients. Its most common complications are limp and heterotopic ossification. In addition, it is sometimes difficult to gain significant length with the use of this approach due to the limitation in repairing the soft-tissue sleeve. The secondary avulsion of the soft-tissue sleeve may also lead to limp and late instability. On the other hand, this approach does maintain femoral head blood supply to allow for surgical procedures, such as femoral head resurfacing for the management of avascular necrosis by maintaining the posterior structures such as the quadratus muscle and secondarily the femoral head blood supply.

The final approach that should be mentioned in this discussion is the anterior or Smith–Peterson approach. This approach has recently seen some increased interest with the advent of minimally invasive surgical techniques for total hip replacement. This technique utilizes the plane between the sartorius and the tensor fascia lata muscles. This intra-nervous plane is between the femoral nerve and the superior gluteal nerve. The approach is not considered an extensile approach, but may be used for anterior column plating, acetabular osteotomies, simple cup revisions, and femoral head resurfacing. It offers poor visualization of the posterior acetabulum and when used in the minimally invasive surgical setting, a second incision is usually necessary for management of the femur. This approach puts the lateral femoral cutaneous nerve at risk, but for straightforward primary hip replacement it is a reasonable option. Its other main drawback is that it has been frequently recommended that fluoroscopy be utilized at the time hip replacement is being done through this approach. This leads to increased fluoroscopic imaging time for both the patient and the surgical staff. Another drawback that has come to light more recently is the difficulty in assessing and managing intra-operative complications such as intra-operative femoral fractures utilizing this approach.

It is rare in surgery to see so many different surgical approaches for one operation. This fact alone should enlighten us, as orthopedic surgeons, to the fact that one surgical approach is simply not enough for the management of all total hip replacements. Patients with varying pathologies will frequently require different approaches. For example, in the patient with developmental hip dysplasia where a lengthening of the leg may take place, a subtrochanteric osteotomy or trochanteric osteotomy may frequently be necessary. In the patient where a posterior column plate may have been placed for an acetabular fracture, a posterior approach may be more advantageous to facilitate the removal of the old hardware. In the patient with neuromuscular disorders, it is frequently felt that an anterior, antererolateral or direct lateral approach is advantageous due to its historically decreased risk of instability. The key in all of these approaches, as well as in the straightforward primary total hip replacement, is that adequate exposure should allow for correction of the deformity, correction of the deficiency, and proper positioning of the correct implant for the patient. Whether this is done through a posterolateral approach, an anterolateral approach, an anterior approach, a trochanteric osteotomy, a trochanteric slide, or a direct lateral approach is not the point. The point is that the proper patients have their surgery completed through an approach to maximize their postoperative function and minimize their potential for complication. Many factors will play a role in this decision-making, including the surgeon's personal comfort level with different approaches, the patient's primary pathology, the patient's body habitus, the patient's anatomy, the presence of old incisions from previous surgical procedures, and the potential for the need of an extensile approach. Ultimately, it is our responsibility to do what is best for our patients in the best way that we know how. Remember, first do no harm.

References

1. DeWal H, Su E, DiCesare PE. Instability following total hip arthroplasty. Am J Orthop 32(8): 377–382, 2003
2. Kennon RE, Keggi JM, Wetmore RS et al. Total hip arthroplasty through a minimally invasive anterior surgical approach. J Bone Joint Surg Am 85-A [Suppl 4]: 39–48, 2003
3. Masonis JL, Bourne RB. Surgical approach, abductor function, and total hip arthroplasty dislocation. Clin Orthop 405: 46–53, 2002
4. Masterson EL, Masri BA, Duncan CP. Surgical approaches in revision hip replacement. J Am Acad Orthop Surg 6(2): 84–92, 1998
5. Nezry N, Jeanrot C, Vinh TS, Ganz R, Tomeno B, Anract P. Partial anterior trochanteric osteotomy in total hip arthroplasty: surgical technique and preliminary results of 127 cases. J Arthroplasty 18(3): 333–337, 2003
6. Parker MJ, Pervez H. Surgical approaches for inserting hemiarthroplasty of the hip. Cochrane Database Syst Rev (3): CD001707, 2002
7. Weeden SH, Paprosky WG, Bowling JW. The early dislocation rate in primary total hip arthroplasty following the posterior approach with posterior soft-tissue repair. J Arthroplasty 18(6): 709–713, 2003
8. White RE Jr, Forness TJ, Allman JK, Junick DW. Effect of posterior capsular repair on early dislocation in primary total hip replacement. Clin Orthop 393: 163–167, 2001
9. Zimmerma S, Hawkes WG, Hudson JI, Magaziner J, Hebel JR, Towheed T, Gardner J, Provenzano G, Kenzora JE. Outcomes of surgical management of total HIP replacement in patients aged 65 years and older: cemented versus cementless femoral components and lateral or anterolateral versus posterior anatomical approach. J Orthop Res 20(2): 182–191, 2002

What Instruments Do We Need?

M. Nogler, F. Rachbauer, E. Mayr

Introduction

The concept of minimal invasiveness not only implies a reduction in the length of skin incision, as discussed in earlier chapters, but also a reduction in the surgical field, which means there is less working space for the surgeon. At the same time, this task remains unchanged: to implant a prosthetic device whose size and shape are dictated by the joint it has to replace. Significant force must be applied to ream or broach cartilage and bone. The surgeon needs space to maneuver in – to osteotomize, dissect, prepare surfaces and insert implants. Obviously, perfect execution is always important when retracting soft tissue, but it becomes even more paramount within a narrow approach.

When the workspace is limited, the structures at risk of damage remain in closer proximity to the surgical field. Even when retracted out of range, they must still be protected against instruments used for dissection and implantation. Thus, devices that protect the surrounding soft tissue are crucial when minimally invasive approaches are employed.

Retraction and protection involves placing devices into a wound that is already small in circumference. One major task for the engineers and surgeons developing such tools is to design them in such a way that visualization and lighting of the surgical field is impeded as little as possible. Additional lighting should be possible.

To reach anatomical structures, direct axial open approaches have been developed and used for a long time. Firstly, these approaches combine direct access and, secondly, minimize the potential for damage to important soft-tissue structures. In attempting to be minimally invasive, the directness of access is secondary to the minimal invasiveness of the procedure. This will usually result in less indirect access to the whole joint or parts of it. Yet, indirect access means that surgical steps that could previously be performed directly in the axis of the joint now have to be performed indirectly, or outside in the joint axis. This requires tools with angles, curves and offsets as opposed to the straight axial tools used in open approaches. When the axial introduction of alignment guides and jigs is impeded by the periarticular tissue within a narrow surgical space, it is more difficult to align non-axial tools. At the same time, the anatomical landmarks otherwise exposed in open approaches might be hidden from view or are not accessible for palpation.

The use of navigation systems can help the surgeon overcome the problems created by limited access to landmarks, the use of non-axial tools and the inability to align tools within bone. Such systems allow either navigation based on pre-operative images or on intra-operatively acquired anatomical landmarks, thus eliminating the need to visualize or palpate structures directly. Such systems are also able to drive tool position throughout an entire procedure.

In the earlier chapters of this book, different solutions for attempting less invasive total joint replacement have been proposed. Instead of focusing their presentations on either approach or instrumentation, all authors' proposals combine a surgical procedure with a set of sophisticated new tools. The authors of these articles have achieved breakthroughs in their own fields of interest, and are thus aware of how much effort it takes to define one isolated issue and solve even one single problem. Hence, we can hardly address all issues associated with instrument development for minimally invasive approaches. Thus, this chapter will try to do justice to the topic of the instrument-design requirements and highlight some feasible solutions.

Within a structured discussion of the specific mechanical requirements for minimal invasive surgery tools (MIS) we believe the following aspects deserve priority:

- retraction of soft tissue,
- protection of soft tissue,
- lighting,
- indirect instrumentation,
- navigation of instruments and implants.

Retraction of Soft Tissue

Different types of retractors have always been utilized depending on the approach. As a broach-reaching discussion of retractor design issues would exceed the scope of this article, we will specifically focus on some of the more important aspects of retractor design:

- Reduced size: The retraction should be enabled with the lowest possible profile.
- The retractor should be shaped in such a way that it allows early and easy wound exist. The retractor should have a long handle.
- The handle should be long enough to allow assistants to hold it in their hands a good distance away from the surgeon's working area.
- Alternatively, self retaining retractors or frames can be used.

Protection of Soft Tissue

Length and size of the approach are limited by the size of the final implant to be introduced. It is obvious that the length of an incision needed for insertion of a size 64 mm cup has to be longer than when a smaller cup is to be inserted (48 mm in diameter). Skin and muscle can be stretched to some extent, implants can be angulated for implantation. During insertion, it is important that implants are protected against contact with soft tissue and skin, in particular, to prevent contamination as well as injury. Obviously, in the case of reamers, broaches and oscillating saws, it is imperative to protect skin and muscles against potential injury.

Protective Retractors

Defining exact retractor positions is an important task when developing standardized approaches. An optimized retractor shape needs to be developed for each position. One goal for this design is perfect retraction, another one is optimal protection. For the anterior approach to the hip, a retractor set – whether held manually or self-retained – can be arranged so that they form a metal funnel that protects soft tissue against trauma when tools and implants are inserted (■ Figs. 26.1 and 26.2).

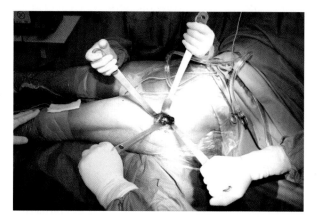

■ **Fig. 26.1.** Special retractors in place demonstrating the above-mentioned principles

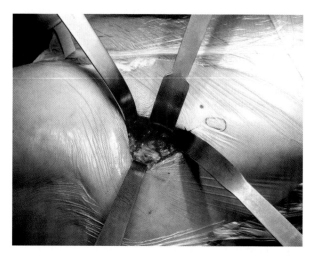

■ **Fig. 26.2.** Retractors form a metal funnel which protects soft tissue

Protection Through Instrument Shape

The success of a minimally invasive approach depends very much on instrument design. Extra protection through instrument design is indeed possible,

- if certain instruments can be eliminated altogether. For example, intra-medullary rods can be avoided if a navigation system is used for jig alignment;
- if instruments are angulated, curved or have an offset. For example, a curved cup-reamer handle prevents pressure on skin, soft tissue and bone. A curved cup inserter can eliminate pressure in a similar manner while preventing misplacement of components;
- if instruments have a low profile. For example, segmented acetabular reamers that are not fully hemispherical allow for easier insertion though narrow spaces. They thereby directly protect the soft tissue and indirectly help prevent the exertion of extensive force on the retractors during insertion;
- if rotating parts are covered. For example, fully covered reamer handles protect skin and soft tissue;
- if instruments are small. For example, small saws with oscillation dips of saw blades only provide soft-tissue protection in total knee arthroplasty.

Protection Through Implant Design

Since MIS access to joint parts is indirect, some angulation might be needed during the introduction of an implant. When femoral components are involved, an angulated instrument might benefit from the following features:

- anatomical form,
- rectangular profile of straight stems,
- cut-off shoulder,
- reduced length.

A protective coating on the surface of the device that can be removed immediately before implantation or after the implant has already been maneuvered through the soft tissue would facilitate insertion while providing protection.

Lighting

Narrow approaches impede lighting more than wide open ones. This may require alternative solutions to the standard OR lights. One alternative could be head-mounted lights. A more sophisticated solution is a system of lighted retractors as shown in ◻ Fig. 26.3. A normal light source can be used to light a broad plastic light via a glass-fiber cable. The light is attached to a retractor.

Indirect Instrumentation

With minimally invasive approaches, direct axial access to all or some parts of the joint might be impeded. Indirect access requires instruments that facilitate maneuvering under such conditions. Solutions to this set of problems include:

- Angulated and curved reamer handles: Angulation and curvature provides offset. As a reamer handle has turning parts, these have to be covered and directed around the angle or curved. This usually involves a loss of momentum.
- Angulated or curved inserters: They follow the same principles as the reamer handles. In addition, fixation of the final cup to the inserter can be an issue. Cups that are screwed to the inserter cannot be unscrewed by simply turning the curved or angulated handle. Collapsible screws might be a solution.

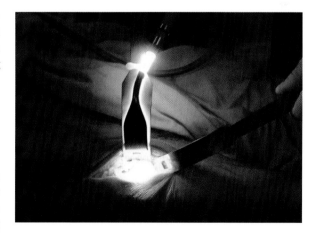

◻ **Fig. 26.3.** A lighted retractor in a minimally invasive approach to the hip

- Broach handles with offsets: anterior, posterior and lateral offset depending on the specific requirements of an approach.
- Low profile jigs for TKA which can be inserted through small incisions.
- Flexible cement-plug introducers allow for bent or angulated insertion.

Navigation

Several articles in this book deal with the application of navigation systems on minimally invasive total joint arthroplasties. We would like to refer the reader to these articles for information on specific systems. We think that there are a few promising solutions already available. However, what are the general principles of navigation support in MIS?

Extension of Our Memory

One guiding principle in orthopedic surgery is the identification and exposure of anatomical landmarks which we need to see or at least feel in order to know where we are and where we need to go. Identification of such landmarks is still necessary in minimally invasive surgery, but exposure to those landmarks will be limited. With poor visibility, palpation becomes more important. Identifying such landmarks might involve changing retractor positions and moving soft tissue – making only one landmark accessible at a time. Navigation alone does not identify anything for us. Using a navigation system still requires showing the system a set of relevant landmarks. Still, with such a system it is easy to identify landmarks one by one and visualize their spatial positions or even relate them to pre-operatively taken pictures of any kind. Without such a device the surgeon must memorize the location and relate them and remember the relation throughout the surgery, or – if not – go back and identify them again.

Visualization

A navigation system offers a virtual picture of the anatomical structures and their relationship after registration. The system can support a surgeon by visualizing invisible anatomic landmarks throughout the surgery in relation to the navigated tool. In a system without images this would/will be an abstract representation of digitized points or surfaces and resulting planes, vectors and axes. Using image-based systems, real images can be overlaid.

Guidance of Non-Axial Tools

It is rather easy to guide a straight tool. Such tools have been used for open approaches for a long time. As described above, the indirect access of minimally invasive approaches is facilitated by tools with curves, angles and offset. While the human brain may have its difficulties aligning a curved cup impactor at a certain anteversion and inclination to a (difficult to remember) palpated frontal pelvis plane – this is an easy task for a computer. If the geometry of an instrument is stored in the system's database, aligning the tool to reference planes is mathematically easy.

Freehand Jig Placement

Jig placement is based on alignment guides, especially in total knee arthroplasty. These are usually extra-medullary or intra-medullarily rods aligned to the femur or tibia axes. A navigation system to which the bone and leg axes have been registered allows the complete omission of such rods A navigated jig can be free-hand-positioned, with the correct alignment visualized on screen (◘ Fig. 26.4).

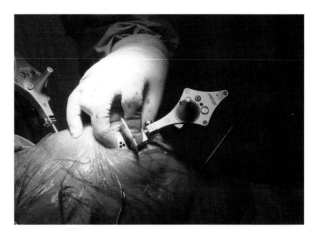

◘ **Fig. 26.4.** Freehand-positioning of a jig in a navigated, minimally invasive TKA

Freehand Cutting

The same is true for the navigation of devices such as a saw. In cases where there is not enough room for jigs, a saw can be equipped with a tracker and navigated to the correct position, orientation and depth (◘ Fig. 26.5).

Functional Navigation

Most navigation systems currently navigate based on anatomic landmarks. Systems that focus on function could be envisioned. Such systems would not require exposure of landmarks but would analyze the function of trial implants as well as the proposed alternative combinations of implant modules and changes in implant position.

Conclusions

We have attempted to structure this chapter looking forward to the future development of instruments that incorporate the different aspects we have identified in our discourses. The anatomic principles for these approaches have always existed while their use in total joint arthroplasty and/or the reduction of incision length are new aspects of established techniques. Minimal invasiveness depends on sophisticated tool designs that empower the surgeon with greater freedom of safe movement despite smaller incisions within narrow surgical fields.

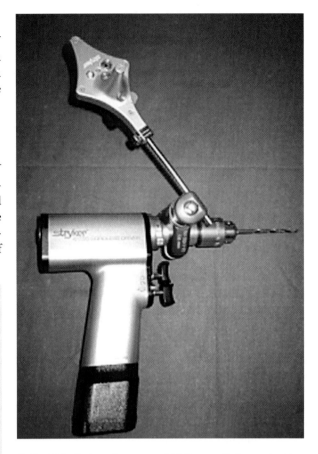

◘ **Fig. 26.5.** Navigated power tool (drill or oscillating saw) with a mounted tracker

Are New Implant Designs Required for MIS?

M. Krismer

Introduction

Several articles in this book discuss the benefits achieved through the use of minimally invasive approaches to hip and knee arthroplasty. These benefits are principally the decreased soft trauma to the skin and the muscles, the potential for earlier mobilization, decreased post-operative pain associated with smaller incisions and less intra- and post-operative blood loss. Although the smaller incisions are thought to be associated with decreased soft-tissue trauma, it is obvious that the maximal potential with regard to soft-tissue trauma could only be achieved through the modification of existing implants and instruments or the development of implants and instruments specific to MIS approaches.

In addition to implant and instrument design, the use of navigated implantation methodologies should assist in decreasing the soft-tissue damage associated with hip and knee arthroplasty through more accurate implant positions and less opportunity for variances. As discussed in several previous chapters dedicated to navigation, the precision afforded through the use of intra-operative navigation for achieving appropriate leg lengths or implant rotation is unprecedented. However, the use of conventional implants has significant potential for complicating the desired outcomes associated with MIS arthroplasty. The implants and instruments should be designed to facilitate, not complicate MIS arthroplasty.

The over-arching goal of arthroplasty is to achieve improved function and decreased pain, both of which depend on the long-term survival of the implant. These goals have been as constant as the surgical communities attempts to improve function and decrease pain. In the early days of the development of arthroplasty, the incision length was dependant on providing satisfactory exposure of the important structures and to permit mobilization of the tissues for implantation of the components. Post-operative restrictions were accepted as inconveniences and some patient complaints were seen in the relation to the initially incredible progress of replacing joints. The surgical community has long attempted to minimize intra-operative trauma and facilitate early mobilization with the goal now focusing on performing arthroplasty with a minimum of pain and restriction, or, in other words, where a return to normal function in the perspective of the patient is reached within days rather than weeks. This is a major change of paradigm, and with this change the question arises whether changes of implants and the instruments used to implant the components are rational.

Examples of Modified Implants

The field of MIS arthroplasty is evolving at a rapid pace and as such the following are examples only and the authors do not claim to be the first to propose them. However, these examples illustrate that solutions can be found where implant changes are made such that the minimally invasive surgical approach with or without navigation is facilitated. There is a dogma that implant changes are made only when improved survival is achieved. The changes are made and the implant placed in our patients, but long-term survival cannot be assessed for a number of years. Although the more recent claim to change implants to reduce intra-operative soft-tissue damage seemed ridiculous just a few short years ago, the surgical community, in the continuous effort to improve patient function is now focused on providing longest possible implant survival when returning to normal function as soon as feasible post-operatively. Within this context, we will discuss changes in implant design.

Offset and Leg Length

Offset and leg length are related parameters which are addressed by different neck angles and different neck lengths of the stem. In the standard open approach, minor differences are of limited importance due to the limits of accuracy in determining leg length. The gross anatomic landmarks used by most surgeons and the intra-operative calculation of the trigonometric values that would help to assess changes in leg length with changes in neck length limit our ability to perfectly match leg lengths. We also do not have a quantitative method to assess muscle- and soft-tissue tension associated with stability of the construct. With the use of intra-operative, computerized navigation, leg length and offset can be determined within the accuracy of a few millimeters (☐ Fig. 27.1). This affords the surgeon the ability to determine intra-operatively whether the intended and

optimal solutions have been achieved. The inability to achieve the desired implant position can often be ascribed to the lack of variation offered by the implant inventory. However, there is also no data to prove that slight deviations from an optimal solution provide any benefit for the patient. Nevertheless, the contrary is not proven as well, and many surgeons empirically know the situation where they must accept lengthening of the leg, because they are not able to restore offset and leg length exactly with the implant under the desired soft-tissue tension and the stability thought necessary to avoid instability and dislocation.

Modular Stems

In a double-incision approach, the femoral stem is implanted directly through the gluteal muscles. A modular stem that incorporates separate pieces of the femoral implant for the diaphyseal and the metaphyseal aspects could assist to further avoid muscle damage. The diaphyseal portion could be inserted through the muscles while the metaphyseal portion could be inserted through the second, anterior approach. For those implants with a hydroxyapatite metaphyseal surface, this two-part implant could assist to keep the biological surface free of soft tissue or other debris that could negatively influence bony ingrowth. Separate diaphyseal and metaphyseal parts of the stem could also be beneficial in a single-incision minimally invasive anterior approach. In a similar fashion, the instruments used to prepare the femoral canal could be constructed of short interconnected lengths rather than a single longer instrument to facilitate turning the corners and avoiding impingement on exterior structures. This modular approach could also be beneficial when a patient's body habitus is such that exterior structures interfere with a straight-line approach to the canal. A straight stem which can be inserted in parts, two or even more when additional femoral component length is required, can be implanted with less soft tissue mobilization and soft tissue trauma (☐ Fig. 27.2).

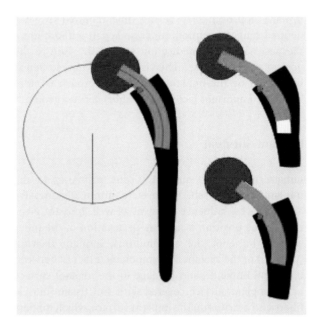

☐ **Fig. 27.1.** An example for a variable modular stem. A bent rod with the exact shape of a segment of a circle can be moved in or out, changing leg length an offset. The position is then fixed by a screw. Long and short heads can be used as well, in order to achieve either more leg length or more offset

Cup Liner with Protection Device

In each MIS approach to the hip, a hydroxyapatite-(HA-) coated acetabular component is inserted through a relatively small operative site with the walls of the incision

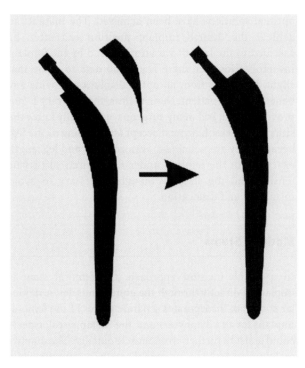

Fig. 27.2. Modular stem for minimally invasive hip arthroplasty, with additional shoulder for rotational stability, which is inserted after stem implantation

containing retractors, muscles and other soft tissues. The trial liners must also be inserted and removed through this incision and the final acetabular insert placed. Moreover, if an angled insert is used, appropriately rotation must be ensured. An acetabular liner with a protection shield would protect the biological coating and could be removed as soon as the liner is in situ, but before press-fit is achieved.

Modifications of Implants: Are they Justified?

The Rule of Incremental Modifications

The history of arthroplasty has demonstrated that modifications in implant design can create important and sometimes disastrous changes in outcome and survival. An incremental modification program is advocated so that the results of a change in any one parameter can be completely and appropriately analyzed before confounding variables confuse the situation. There are enough other variables, such as patient characteristics and activity level, that will confuse the conclusions, so modifying the implants in an incremental fashion will permit a thorough evaluation before moving on to the next modification. To date, surgeons have modified the approach to minimize the surgical incision. Although the outcome studies from these changes are not yet complete nor overwhelmingly positive and convincing, the results are encouraging enough to proceed with implant modifications. The outcomes from modifications in the surgical approach are typically apparent relatively earlier than the outcomes associated with modifications in the implants. Modifications in the implant may also render the MIS arthroplasty components unsuitable for use in traditional approaches. Limitations in available implants may dictate that traditional components will be used for the foreseeable future until rational implant designs can be manufactured and used with a satisfactory chance for long-term success.

Short-Term Outcome Studies

The difference between a traditional and a minimally invasive approach may be the time required to get a defined range of motion, function, a gait without limp, the necessary pain medication and of the pain in the post-operative course. This is perhaps not so much influenced by the implants, and the approach is more likely the important factor in the short-term outcome.

Implant Survival

Long-term implant survival is due primarily to the implant design itself. However, a minimally invasive approach can influence survival as well. Implant position (varus position of a stem, perforation of the inner cortical bone of the acetabulum), implant fixation (press-fit of the acetabular component, exact fit between bone and implant), and damage to the implant surface or an implant surface covered with soft tissue (muscle fibers and detritus on the implant surface, which hinders bony in-growth) can considerably influence survival as well. Implant position can be assessed as a parameter, but the other factors cannot be analyzed independently. Therefore, it cannot be concluded that the long-term outcome of a minimally invasive approach using the same implants will be identical, and when using a new implant design it will remain unclear whether approach or implant contributed to a worse or better outcome.

The Future

Minimally invasive procedures will have a longer learning curve than traditional procedures and need more experience to conduct them safely. Both statements have to be proven, and may in fact turn out to be wrong. More likely, however, after significant trial and error, they will be true, and minimally invasive arthroplasty will be restricted to those surgeons operating on high numbers of patients with the same procedure every year. If the implants are to be specialized, then perhaps so should the surgeons be specialized in MIS arthroplasty. If also the implants are specialized, and if also navigation is used, the procedures will be more complex than tradi-tional arthroplasty. Therefore, we expect that a few procedures will ultimately provide a superior outcome and will need to be conducted in a highly structured manner. Additionally, every modification of an implant or an instrument will need to be appropriately assessed to ensure improved outcomes for our patients.

Conclusions

The advent of MIS arthroplasty dictates the adaptation of existing products or the development of implants and instruments in order to avoid tissue damage, decrease pain, decrease blood loss and facilitate post-operative rehabilitation. The benefits of implants developed specifically for these approaches would also facilitate further minimization of the approach which would supercede any additional costs of new technologies, additional inventories and the inability for implants to be universal to all approaches.

Part VII　Perspectives – The Knee

Is Minimally Invasive Total Knee Arthroplasty a Winning Concept?

P.M. Bonutti

Introduction

Although total knee-arthroplasty (TKA) implants and instruments have continuously evolved, the basic surgical technique and approach has essentially remained unchanged. Current instrumentation and implant design requires extensive soft-tissue disruption for appropriate exposure and implantation. There is an opportunity to evolve the surgical technique for a TKA into something much less invasive, with improved postoperative results.

Minimally invasive surgery (MIS) is relatively new to the orthopedic reconstructive arena. One of its first recognized successes was in unicompartmental knee arthroplasty (UKA), which provided a quicker recovery than seen with the traditional UKA procedure. Even so, one may regard the evolution of MIS to total knee arthroplasty (MIS-TKA) to be unwarranted, given the long and well-established track record of the traditional TKA procedure. MIS presents a unique and more technically demanding procedure, with the learning curve perhaps overshadowing the benefits.

The interest in MIS is greatly patient-driven, highlighted by its benefits of allowing for a quicker recovery with improved function and less scarring. The surgical choice, therefore, needs to be based on what is best for the patient, with the goal of providing them the chance to achieve optimal results.

The Evolution of Minimally Invasive Surgery

Minimally invasive surgery began with the advent of arthroscopic surgery. The arthroscope was used initially as a visualization tool to enhance diagnostic procedures. Over time, these minimally invasive techniques evolved from purely diagnostic procedures to those that were capable of removing tissue and ultimately to actually repairing tissue. Now, MIS developments are going even further toward minimally invasive implantation.

MIS has evolved across the entire surgical spectrum and is in great part patient-driven. In the past several years, hundreds of articles in all surgical fields have been published with regard to MIS developments and results. MIS techniques have been utilized in areas as diverse as pediatric surgery, the treatment of colorectal cancer, and cardiovascular surgery. Only recently has MIS been evaluated for orthopedic reconstructive procedures (◘ Fig. 28.1).

MIS UKA was the first MIS knee arthroplasty procedure introduced. Recently, minimally invasive total hip arthroplasty has also been introduced [1]. The patients for these procedures are highly pre-selected and highly motivated. Short-term benefits have clearly been described, however, there is no documented long-term benefit to date.

Unicondylar Knee Arthroplasty

In the past, unicompartmental knee arthroplasty has had very limited application. Of 228 knees reviewed, Insall identified less than 6% as candidates for UKA [4]. Although using smaller implants, a UKA requires extensive soft-tissue exposure and quadriceps disruption, with instrumentation and a surgical approach that is similar to traditional TKA.

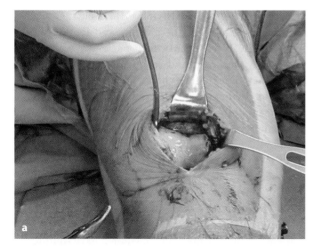

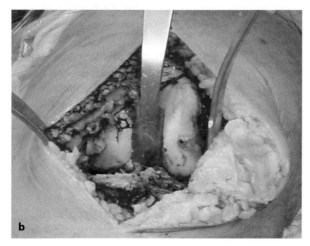

☐ **Fig. 28.1.** **a** Traditional TKA exposure, **b** MIS TKA exposure

Minimally invasive unicompartmental knee arthroplasty (MIS-UKA) was originally popularized because the smaller implant was minimally invasive friendly, this allowed for less hospitalization, a faster recovery, and ultimately a growing patient acceptance. Price performed a study evaluating UKA using minimally invasive techniques and compared them to UKA using a traditional approach with an everted patella [10]. He found that the recovery of an MIS-UKA was two times faster than traditional UKA and three times faster than traditional TKA.

UKA prior to 2002 were less than 2% of the U.S. knee arthroplasty market. In 2003, estimates suggested that

the UKA would grow to between 20% and 30% of the U.S. knee arthroplasty market [8]. This was largely driven by patient demand.

Assessment of Traditional Total Knee Arthroplasty

Traditional total knee arthroplasty has suggested a high degree of satisfaction and long-term survivorship. This data and perspective have been primarily based on surgeons' expectations and evaluations. Orthopedic surgeons evaluate and compare data on the basis of survivorship data, radiographic results and Knee Society scores.

Ryd identified that the knee-scoring systems show "clinical measurements have bias" [11]. Furthermore, he concluded that "Knee Society scores are exceedingly unreliable". A perfect 100 Knee Society functional score suggests a patient can ascend or descend stairs without a rail and can walk 10 blocks without the assistance of a walker or cane. Patients' functional demands, however, are significantly greater.

A recent study by Mont reported that only 35% of patients more than 6 months after TKA, with Knee Society functional scores greater than 90, felt their activities are unlimited [9]. From a subset group of patients, under the age of 60, only 13% felt that they were functionally unrestricted. From the patients' perspective, the majority of TKA results included some level of post-operative functional restriction, especially for the younger and more active patients.

Kelly found that patients under the age of 60 could have a clinically assessed success rate of up to 94% at intermediate term follow-up, concluding that young, active patients can have a high degree of success [5]. He also noted that only 24% of patients felt they could perform all desired activities. He stated "I tell my patients that they may never kneel comfortably, so gardening may be an issue, and descending stairs on occasion".

Additional studies suggest that patients may not be as satisfied with TKA as surgeons would like. A study by Bullens entitled *Patient Satisfaction After Total Knee Arthroplasty* found that "the concerns and priorities of patients and surgeons differ" [3]. Results showed that the surgeons were more satisfied than the patients with the TKA outcomes, something that does not get identified by the Knee Society score.

Independent clinical observation and discussions with patients confirms Bullens' results. Patients do improve and have less pain after TKA, and survivorship of the implant is good at 10 years post-operation. However, patients have significant functional limitations after traditional TKA.

This functional discrepancy may be evident in the revision-arthroplasty market data [6]. The bulk of the revision total hip arthroplasty (THA) market (73%) consists of patients over the age of 65. However, the same data identifies that 62% of revision TKAs are performed on patients under the age of 65. This suggests a high degree of failure in young, active patients and may confirm data suggested by Mont and Kelly.

Traditional TKA – Function

The long-term function of a TKA knee is significantly effected by the trauma that the knee is exposed to during surgery. In the traditional procedure, the knee is exposed (typically via a medial parapatellar approach), the patella gets everted and the tibiofemoral joint is dislocated, with further disruption of the soft tissue to allow for instruments and implantation.

A study by Silva and Schmalzried evaluated patients using isokinetic testing two years after traditional TKA [12]. They found that "isometric extensor peak-torque strength after TKA is reduced by 30.7%". These data strongly suggest that there is permanent damage to the quadriceps mechanism after TKA. This may correlate with significant functional limitation noted by patients.

Mahoney evaluated a simple test of quadriceps strength by asking patients to rise from a 16 inch chair without the use of their arms [7]. At 3 months post-operation only 40% of his traditional TKA could arise from a chair without the use of their arms, and by 6 months post-operation only 64% of his original patients could arise from a chair without using their arms. This simple test identifies how TKA done with an everted patella affects the quadriceps muscle.

Patient Expectations

Patient expectations prior to and after total knee arthroplasty have not been well evaluated. Trousdale performed a study evaluating patients' concerns prior to

undergoing TKA and THA [13]. He evaluated 54 pre-operative concerns of the patients and found that the two greatest concerns for patients undergoing TKA/THA was pain and length of recovery. He also found that "older patients had more modest goals for the function of their joint replacements". Men were concerned about the ability to lift heavy objects, and women were more concerned than men in 19 of 54 questions.

Physical and occupational therapists assess patients with activities of daily living (ADL). ADLs include activities such as squatting, kneeling, and for many patients getting down on the floor or into a bathtub. Functionally, the majority of TKA patients are unable to perform these activities [5]. Further data show that 61% of TKA patients in the U.S. are women. Women have significantly greater functional concern after TKA, which may not be assessed by traditional Knee Society score measurements.

Obesity is becoming a major problem and etiology for TKA. In the U.S., obesity is predicted for over 40% of the population by 2010 [14]. The need and indication for knee arthroplasty in this segment of the population is also growing. With additional weight, additional quadriceps strength is required and further destruction to the quadriceps mechanism, as with traditional TKA, may further incapacitate these patients.

Minimally Invasive Total Knee Arthroplasty

Minimally invasive total knee arthroplasty (MIS-TKA) is being developed to target patient-related issues, such as pain, recovery, and function, both in the short- and long-term post-operative periods. MIS-TKA greatly reduces the trauma to the quadriceps mechanism, thus making less pain, faster recovery and improved function realistic goals. There is also a cosmetic benefit with respect to a reduced length of skin incision, which plays a big role in patient demand for this procedure. Reducing the incision also creates less of a neurologic injury, with less denervation to the skin than with a TKA incision (◘ Fig. 28.2).

The goal of MIS-TKA is to reduce collateral soft-tissue damage while implanting a well-aligned and well-fixed total knee arthroplasty. The criteria for MIS-TKA are variable and include:
- reducing length and optimizing location of incision,
- muscle-sparing approaches – reducing quadriceps trauma,

Chapter 28 · Is Minimally Invasive Total Knee Arthroplasty a Winning Concept?

287

28

- avoiding everting the patella,
- in situ bone cuts,
- in situ implantation
- avoiding intra-medullary canal alignment,
- reducing post-operative pain,

- faster post-operative recovery,
- more rapid hospital discharge; but most importantly,
- enhancing the overall function for the patients.

The goal is to develop surgical principles, approaches, techniques, and instrumentation which are applicable to all patients, not a pre-selected few, and to obtain both short-term as well as long-term benefits. The future will also bring minimally invasive friendly implants.

Surgeons clearly are concerned about MIS-TKA. It is a new technical challenge, with less visualization of the surgical site, an extended time in the operating room, and no increase in surgeon reimbursement. However, the goals of MIS-TKA are to address patient-related issues both in the short term and the long term, and that goal must remain in the foreground of this evolution.

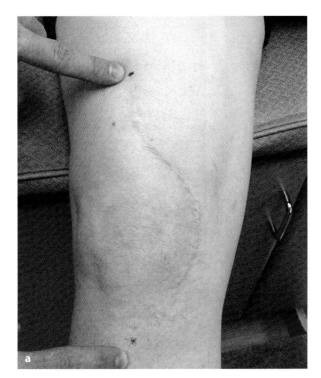

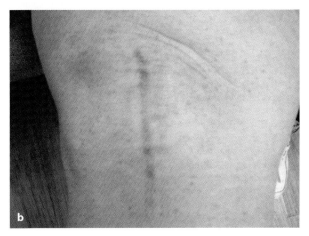

Fig. 28.2. a Traditional TKA incision (11 inches), **b** MIS TKA incision (3.5 inches)

Conclusions

MIS-TKA is a winning concept because the goal is to address the patients needs. Patients with traditional TKA are pleased with the reduction in pain and good long-term survivorship. However, all patients fear pain and the extensive length of recovery after TKA. Cosmetics and skin denervation are minor issues, however, function after traditional TKA clearly can be improved upon. The goals of MIS-TKA are to address patient-related issues, while developing techniques and approaches which allow not only faster recovery, but long-term improved functional results.

As a caveat it is important not to excessively promote potential benefits in advertisement and corporate promotions, but to direct minimally invasive surgery in an evolution based on science. Surgeons do not want to mislead patients, as has been evidenced in the orthopedic corporate advertisements. Bhattacharyya found the majority of orthopedic advertisements were unsupported and arthroplasty advertisements were most misleading [2]. Our goal should be not to mislead the patients, but to direct them in an evolutionary and scientific-based approach to improve short- and long-term recovery, with improved overall function (**Fig. 28.3).

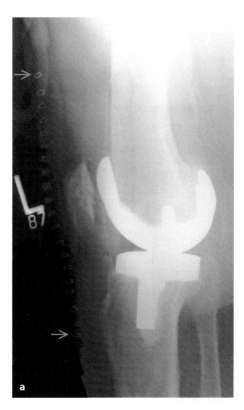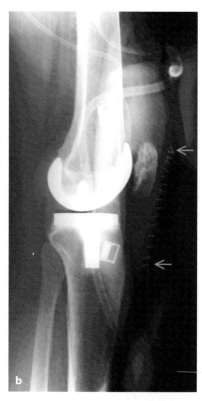

Fig. 28.3. a MINI incision (14 cm),
b MIS TKA incision (8 cm)

References

1. Berger (2003) Symposium: minimally invasive total hip arthroplasty. development, early results, and a critical analysis. JBJS Am 85: 2235–2246

2. Bhattacharyya T et al. (2003) The validity of claims made in orthopaedic print advertisements. JBJS 85: 4–9

3. Bullens PH, van Loon CJ, de Waal Malefijt MC, Laan RF, Veth RP (2001) Patient satisfaction after total knee arthroplasty: a comparison between subjective and objective outcome assessments. J Arthroplasty 16: 740–747

4. Stern SH, Becker MW, Insall J (1993) Unicondylar knee arthroplasty. An evaluation of selection criteria. Clin Orthop 286: 143–148

5. Kelly M (2003) TKA can be an option for the young active patient. Orthopedics Today 23: 43

6. Lipes N (2003) Stryker Howmedica Osteonics; Internet 2003

7. Mahoney OM, McClung CD, dela Rosa MA, Schmalzried TP (2002) The effect of total knee arthroplasty design on extensor mechanism function. J Arthroplasty 17: 416–421

8. Merrill Lynch (2002) Orthopedics Update

9. Mont MA, Stuchin SA, Bonutti PM et al. (2004) Different surgical options for monocompartmental osteoarthritis of the knee: high tibial osteotomy versus unicompartmental knee arthroplasty versus total knee arthroplasty: indications, techniques, results, and controversies. Instructional Course Lectures 53: 265–283

10. Price A et al., Oxford Hip and Knee Group (2001) Rapid recovery after oxford unicompartmental arthroplasty through a short incision. J Arthroplasty 16: 970–976

11. Ryd L, Karrholm J, Ahlvin P (1997) Knee scoring systems in gonarthrosis. Evaluation of interobserver variability and the envelope of bias. Score Assessment Group 68: 41–45

12. Silva M, Schmalzried T et al. (2003) Knee strength after total knee arthroplasty. J Arthroplasty 18: 605–611

13. Trousdale RT, McGrory BJ, Berry DJ, Becker MW, Harmsen WS (1999) Patients' concerns prior to undergoing total hip and total knee arthroplasty. Mayo Clin Proc; 74: 978–982.

14. USA Today (2003) Obesity predicted for 40% of America. Life Section, 7D, Oct. 14

28

Minimally Invasive Total Knee Arthroplasty – What Instruments Do We Need?

P.M. Bonutti

Introduction

Traditional total knee arthroplasty (TKA) relies on significant soft-tissue exposure to obtain access to the knee joint. The exposure is achieved by making extensive release of the quadriceps muscle, fully everting the patella, and dislocating the tibiofemoral joint. Extensive exposure is essential due to the large size of the instrumentation used in a TKA, whether for alignment, sizing, cutting, trialing, or implantation. Although a large incision and exposure may be advantageous in the operating room, it is clearly not advantageous for the patient post-operatively. Cosmetic issues, skin denervation, length of recovery, and function of the quadriceps mechanism are all negatively effected by traditional TKA approach [3].

Minimally invasive TKA (MIS-TKA) was developed specifically to reduce the soft-tissue trauma to the knee while obtaining the same well-fixed, well-aligned implant as achieved during traditional TKA procedures. The expected result is an improvement in the post-operative recovery as well as improvement in long-term function. This reduction in exposure, however, requires new and innovative approaches to instrumentation for access, visualization, alignment, preparation, and implant design for TKA. These changes impact pre-operative planning in addition to anesthesia, patient positioning during surgery, and post-operative pain management.

Current TKA instrumentation and implants must be refined to become more soft-tissue- and MIS-friendly. This evolution enhances the surgeons' ability to implant a MIS-TKA with the same confidence and survivorship as traditional TKA techniques.

Pre-Operative Instruments

Pre-operative planning for MIS is essential. Computer-assisted outcomes provide user-friendly media for collecting, and analyzing data throughout the pre-operative and post-operative periods is essential.

Pre-operative imaging is critical for planning MIS-TKA. Digitized computer software which allows analysis of imaging (X-ray, CT, MRI) provides a clear assessment of patients' deformities, and aids in pre-operative templating and sizing. The surgeon may customize the surgical approach for each patient, determining location and type of incision, exposure needed, with bone removal and soft-tissue releases assessed.

Pre-operative rehabilitation – "prehabilitation" – should be administered prior to MIS-TKA. This introduces the patient to work on range of motion and strengthening pre-operatively to enhance post-operative recovery and function. Computer-linked protocol could improve results and outcomes overall.

Anesthesia – Muscle Relaxation

Optimizing muscle relaxation during MIS-TKA greatly aids in improving access. Although general anesthesia with paralysis can offer the best relaxation, due to safety and post-operative analgesia, regional blocks are often used. Guidance technology with neuro-sensors will assist anesthesiologists in performing regional blocks, and even delivery of medication for relaxation, hemostasis, and analgesia post-operatively.

Expandable catheter designs, continuous pain pump with biodegradable tubing and reservoirs, and extended length pharmaceuticals are helpful for analgesia, relaxation, and hemostasis both systemically and locally. These delivery systems will help intra- and post-operatively.

Patient Position

Traditional TKA is performed with the patient in the supine position with the leg varied between two or three positions, controlled by an assistant. MIS-TKA requires the ability to progressively flex and extend the joint in a controlled fashion to enhance visualization through a small incision. Progressive flexion and extension moves the small incision to the area of the knee worked on, thus optimizing the "mobile skin window". Variable and controlled patient position and an adjustable leg support is essential. A mechanical, pneumatic, or electric leg holder would allow the knee and body to be reproducible and precisely positioned during MIS-TKA surgery. This support may also allow distraction of the joint and controlled adjustable position of the patients body, and would greatly aid in all phases of MIS-TKA surgery. This may reduce the need for surgical assistance and in the long term may be voice-activated.

Similar systems can be used for retraction. Current devices must be downsized and made more soft-tissue-friendly.

A newer approach called the "suspended leg technique", modeled after arthroscopic technique, is being used for MIS-TKA [1]. In this method, the patient's leg is positioned over a padded bolster, hanging over the table, with the surgeon seated. The surgeon controls flexion and extension while being protected with new sterile draping technique that creates a mobile sterile field (□ Fig. 29.1).

Currently, a tourniquet is used to control bleeding. Hyperflexing the patient's knee and hip prior to inflation of the tourniquet relaxes the quadriceps muscle and aids in exposure. To decrease quadriceps tension, it is useful to pre-stretch the quadriceps mechanism by inflating the tourniquet with the hip and quadriceps maximally flexed. This allows greater mobility to the quadriceps mechanism during access.

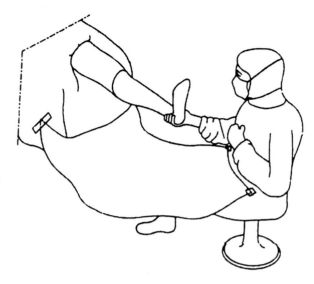

□ **Fig. 29.1.** Suspended leg technique with sterile drape

Surgical Access

Pre-treatment of soft tissue may enhance mobility and define muscle fiber along inter-nervous planes. Balloon expanders could be used to pre-stretch the skin, muscle, or capsule intra-operatively stretching the soft tissue. Expanding cannulas, balloon dissectors, or mechanical tissue expanders may pre-treat the tissue prior to the surgical incision. This would temporarily lengthen tissue, decrease incision length, and reduce soft-tissue trauma, thereby enhancing the ability to position cutting blocks and implants during MIS-TKA (□ Figs. 29.2, 29.3).

Specialized retractors, which are down-sized and soft-tissue-friendly, are required (Hohmann, Goulet, etc.). The future will find disposable, selectively malleable, retractors with built in light sources to allow retraction and visualization. Instruments and implants may be delivered through cannulas which stretch and protect soft tissue.

Retractors, including lighted systems, must be re-designed to be soft-tissue-friendly and procedure-specific. Malleable retractors, such as those made out of heat-deformable polymers, may protect soft tissue, while making bony cuts. These may be pinned directly to the bone for protection, but also may facilitate implantation and cementation.

Chapter 29 · Minimally Invasive Total Knee Arthroplasty – What Instruments Do We Need?

291   29

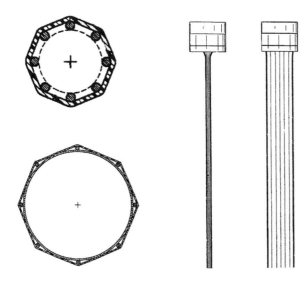

Fig. 29.2. Expanding cannula system

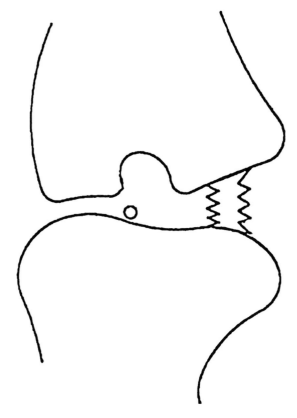

Fig. 29.3. Joint Jack – balloon expand soft tissue and bone

Visualization during TKA requires extensive exposure for direct vision. The "mobile skin window" in MIS-TKA surgery provides access to portions of the joint, but the entire joint cannot be seen all at one time. With direct lateral or medial exposure, visualization of the opposite compartment can be challenging. Additional visual access can be provided via endoscopic assistance, using either straight-line or malleable fiberoptic cameras and light sources. Expanding trocars can stabilize the distal end of the arthroscope and improve visualization.

Additional intra-operative imaging utilizing ultrasound or low radiation fluoroscopy could be linked directly to instrumentation to optimize visualization during access.

Long-term MIS-TKA will be performed without a tourniquet ("bloodless surgery"). Possible features of bloodless surgery may include increasing operating-room barometric pressure, selective cooling of tissue, local sealants, innovative cautery systems and possible use of pressurized fluid, balloons, or a clear gelatin-based operative field.

MIS-TKA Instrument Systems

MIS-TKA requires a whole new platform of surgical instruments. Traditional TKA utilizes large bulky instruments, filling up to eight sterilization trays. The down-sized MIS instruments will be smaller and lighter and require fewer trays. These traditional instruments were not designed to be soft-tissue-friendly. Minimally invasive instruments must be soft-tissue-friendly, down-sized, with rounded smooth edges. These instruments will be significantly less bulky, while allowing pivoting or sliding motions protecting the skin and muscle (◘ Fig. 29.4).

Specific instrumentation and trials will become disposable. Although this may increase cost, ultimately it would decrease the risk for infection and time for re-sterilization, allowing faster operating-room turnover. Transparent disposable retractors, cutting blocks, and/or trials would allow the surgeon to watch tissue and bone, reducing the risk for collateral soft-tissue trauma.

Computer-assisted navigation is a key technology which will be required to maintain the highest accuracy, alignment, bone cuts, and implantation for MIS-TKA. Navigation will replace the need for intra-medullary or extra-medullary alignment devices which add to exposure, quad trauma, and post-operative bleeding. Currently, navigation is not minimally-invasive-friendly. The optical trackers are bulky and require additional incisions, which may increase the risk for infection [2]. Navigation also requires surface mapping, which can be difficult to perform with a minimal incision (◘ Fig. 29.5).

Long-term, down-sized or skin-mounted trackers, and kinematic mapping rather than topical mapping, will make this more navigation MIS friendly and accurate. Freehand cutting jigs positioned through navigation will be a future cornerstone for MIS-TKA surgery. Coupling navigation with ultrasound or other imaging modalities for mapping and alignment may be useful. MIS navigation systems will evolve as MIS-TKA is further miniaturized.

Bone-Preparation Instruments for MIS-TKA

MIS-TKA systems currently use extra-medullary alignment for tibial cuts with cutting guides down-sized to fit underneath soft-tissue and pin fixation to the bone. The bone cuts are made from anteromedial to posterolateral quadrants of the tibial plateau. If desired, an IM rod may be placed down the tibia after the initial skim cut is made, providing IM alignment and clean-up cuts.

Femoral alignment currently is set via intra-medullary rod. Instruments currently used are a down-sized anterior-posterior- or posterior-referencing guide, distal femoral cut, and a 4-in-1 cutting jig, all of which are soft-tissue-friendly and between 30 and 50% smaller than traditional TKA instruments (◘ Fig. 29.6). A sliding cutting block fitting underneath the tissue could prepare each condyle separately. Ultimately, a down-sized distal cutting block which can cut side to side, in situ without dislocating tibiofemoral joint may be optimal.

A composite of pre-operative templating and intra-operative measurement is used to size the knee. Femoral sizers that can be down-sized, may reference the medial or lateral condyles or can be assessed via navigation.

Patellar cutting systems must obtain a flat reproducible cut without everting the patella. The preferred systems are either a milling approach or an oscillating saw. They may also be used to cut the patella in situ, once it is sitting in the femoral groove.

An interferometer can be used to scan the cut surfaces to make sure the bone cuts are smooth and consistent. Currently visualization and direct manual palpa-

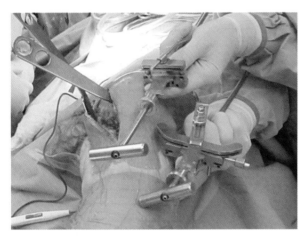

◘ **Fig. 29.4.** MIS down-sized vs. standard instruments

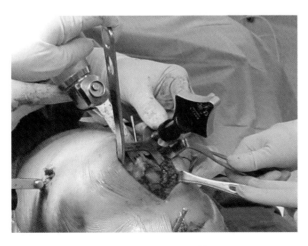

◘ **Fig. 29.5.** MIS computer-navigated cutting blocks

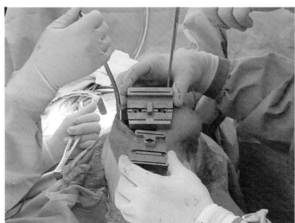

◘ **Fig. 29.6.** Standard vs. down-sized 4-in-1 femoral cutting block

Chapter 29 · Minimally Invasive Total Knee Arthroplasty – What Instruments Do We Need?

293

29

tion is utilized, however, additional feedback could be obtained. Navigation could be linked to the cutting systems interferometer and trials.

Trials for MIS-TKA are metallic and re-usable, however, a disposable or transparent trial may be preferred. Transparency allows visualization of the bone cut and surrounding soft tissue while trialing, thus providing the chance to clearly see where soft tissue invaginates or whether additional releases may be required. Current tibial inserts are mono-block polyethylene spacers, sequentially inserted to assess the appropriate thickness needed for ligament balancing. Alternatively, if these trials were mechanically distractible, expanding by 1 or 2 mm increments during trialing and balancing, one trial could replace the purpose of several. This single distracting spacer would be optimal for minimally invasive techniques. The future may bring trial systems for the femur, tibia, and patella with embedded sensors which would allow force and load readings during surgery. Furthermore, if these "smart" trials were linked to navigation systems, they may provide additional feedback for ligament balancing and range of motion.

Implants

Regardless of any advances made with the instruments, if TKA implants remain unchanged, the continual improvement of MIS-TKA will eventually hit a wall. The current size of total knee implants with the width of the femoral component and length of the tibial keel impact the surgical approach. No matter how small the incision is for preparing the bone surfaces, it must be stretched enough to accommodate for the bulk of the implants.

Modular implants would be helpful. A modular tibial keel assembled on the bony surface is one option. Another is to eliminate the tibial keel or use down-sized lugs or pegs for fixation, although, for long-term success fixation is an issue.

A modular femoral component with two condyles assembled and fixed on the bone surfaces may also make implantation easier. Without modularity, existing monoblock femoral and tibial components can be utilized with this. It must have reduced fixation posts and keels. Femoral components may be decreased in the medial and lateral dimensions with fixation slots rather than lugs.

Bicompartmental knee design may also be a consideration. It is a combination of a medial or lateral uni-

compartmental, with a patellofemoral implant. The modular femoral components may be linked on the bony surface (□ Fig. 29.7).

MIS-TKA surgery will cause renewed interest in cementless fixation. Cemented TKA requires appropriate cement pressurization and cement removal, which requires additional exposure. Cementless fixation with hydroxyapatite, foam metals, BMP, or other enhancements for fixation may ultimately obviate the need for cement and enhance opportunities in MIS-TKA.

If one does use cement for fixation, treating the peripheral tissue and edge of the implant with materials

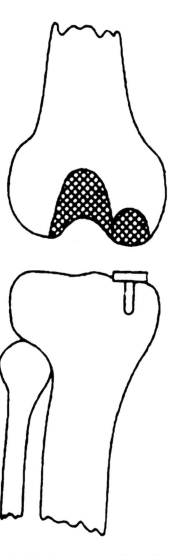

□ **Fig. 29.7.** Bicompartmental knee arthroplasty

to prevent cement bonding and improve cement removal would be helpful.

Post-Operative Instruments

Post-operative instruments include analgesia, drug-delivery systems, methods for achieving post-operative hemostasis, and improved post-operative rehabilitation. When optimized, these aspects of post-operative recovery will allow the patient to take full advantage of the benefits of MIS procedures.

Pain pumps with enhanced distribution utilizing "pulsed pressurization flow" could be utilized rather than either via continuous nerve blocks or locally. Drug eluting implants or biodegradables, delivering local medication to the wound, are on the horizon.

Hemostasis is addressed intra-operatively and post-operatively. Balloons may be placed internally around the knee joint. These may be as simple as tissue expanders to allow direct pressure to the soft tissue to stop bleeding. Once hemostasis is obtained, the balloons are deflated and removed. These can be coupled with drains or pain pumps to improve post-operative hemostasis, as well as to maintain a soft-tissue envelope to improve range of motion.

Improved post-operative rehabilitation is critical to increase overall function. Functional rehabilitation, utilizing new devices, for strengthening and range of motion may be required immediately following surgery. If damage to the quadriceps mechanism can be avoided, faster recovery is possible with early activity. Changing the overall algorithm of post-operative therapy will be required to improve post-operative function, which is essential for best results with MIS-TKA.

Summary – Future of MIS-TKA

The future of MIS-TKA will require a complete change of visualization, access, instrumentation, and implants, as well as pre- and post-operative management. Surgical approaches include medial, lateral, or multi incision, but will involve quad-sparing approaches, in situ bone cuts, and implantation.

Access technologies will include tissue expanders, endoscopic visualization, expanding cannulas, and light-ed malleable retractors. Technologies will be adapted from other minimally invasive surgical fields.

Instrumentation will revolve around MIS-friendly computer navigation, with virtual cutting guides, laser sights on cutting technology, robotics, or haptic assistants, interferometers to scan cut surfaces and smart trials.

Implant technologies will evolve into down-sized implants with reduced fixation keels, modular implants assembled on the bone surface, and bicompartmental designs. Cementless fixation – hydroxyapatite, foam metal, etc. will be utilized. Drug-eluting implants and smart implants with sensors (R.F.I.D.) are on the horizon.

Finally, post-operative hemostasis and pain-delivery systems may be biodegradable, implantable, and controlled by the patient. Pharmaceutical agents to reduce risk of DVT may be replaced by external mechanical devices to mechanically break up blood clots. Rehabilitation may be more self-directed by the patient, but still monitored by smart implants and computers. Patients will be provided with more direct control of their rehabilitation protocol to ensure optimal return of function.

Eventually metallic implants will be replaced by biologic resurfacing, but MIS techniques will still be used to align, position, and implant these biologic resurfacing technologies.

Conclusions

Overall, MIS-TKA is evolving. MIS-TKA addresses the patient's needs of reduced pain, faster recovery, and improved overall function, both in the short- and long-term periods. The orthopedic industry is obligated to continue development of appropriate instrumentation, implants and protocols to optimize access, alignment, bone cuts, implantation, and post-operative function. Patient satisfaction is the ultimate goal, and any available technology should be used or developed to ensure that the best options are available.

References

1. Bonutti P, Neal D, Kester M (2003) Minimal incision total knee arthroplasty using the suspended leg technique. Orthopedics 26: 899–903
2. Sikorski JM, Chauhan S (2003) Computer-assisted orthopaedic surgery: do we need CAOS? JBJS (Br) 85: 319–323
3. Silva M, Schmalzried T et al. (2003) Knee strength after total knee arthroplasty. J Arthroplasty 18: 605–611

Do We Need New Implant Designs?

M. Austin, G. Klein, W.J. Hozack, M. Kester

Introduction

The basic principles of minimally invasive total knee arthroplasty (MIS-TKA) emphasize changes in surgical technique and instrumentation to maximize exposure through a limited incision. These include smaller incisions, modified surgical techniques including no patella eversion [1], no frank joint dislocation, quadriceps-sparing, and also down-sized instrumentation. Many of these ideas have been adapted from the experience with unicompartmental knee replacement. Modifications such as not resurfacing the patella, careful incision placement, and instrumentation-design changes have all helped unicompartmental arthroplasty trend towards minimally invasive and these changes have carried over to MIS-TKA. Furthermore, exact incision planning and placement is paramount to facilitate proper component orientation and fixation through the smallest incision possible. Unicompartmental knee arthroplasty has specific component designs that can accommodate the smaller incisions and reduced exposures. Unicompartmental femoral component designs conducive to implantation in the coronal plane ease insertion of the femoral component, and tibial trays that have smaller keels or pegs do not require significant joint distraction for implantation.

MIS-TKA has adopted all of the above, with the exception of component-design changes. The traditional knee-replacement prosthesis continues to be used with both standard and MIS surgical approaches. The thesis of this chapter is that, perhaps, the time has come to consider modifying the standard total knee-prosthesis design in order to facilitate MIS techniques.

Femoral Component

Incision location is the key to reducing the size of the ultimate incision. Current focus on incisions that are closer to the flexion/extension axis of the knee (near the femoral epicondyles) may reduce soft-tissue tension with knee motion. These incisions may provide adequate visualization but at the same time may reduce post-operative pain and stiffness, and improve cosmesis due to less tension at the wound edges. However, these newer incision locations will require new instrumentation and will pose a significant challenge to device implantation. Implants will have to be conducive to "side-insertion" as opposed to the traditional insertion from the front. This will present a particular challenge for components with pegs and boxes (i.e. posterior-stabilized designs).

The femoral component in traditional total knee arthroplasty tends to occupy the greatest spatial volume. Efforts to reduce this mass effect should involve creating a less bulky component as well as perhaps customizing the prosthesis to the patient's disease. The preponderance of gonarthrosis involves a varus deformity with medial compartment degeneration. The lateral compartment is often not as significantly involved in the disease process. In this common scenario the majority of pathology is found in the medial and patellofemoral compartments. Taking this into consideration, a possible solution would be a modular design that features a lateral compartment that can be later added. This implant could be assembled in situ at the time of primary arthroplasty or added later if the lateral compartment subsequently degenerates. Theoretically, the reverse situation would be applicable should a valgus deformity exist.

Another change in the femoral component may include an implant that can be made more compact during insertion and then expanded, like coronary stents, once inside the knee.

Tibial Component

There are two basic challenges to implantation of the tibial component through a limited incision. The first obstacle is appropriate sizing and placement owing to the restricted visibility. The second and perhaps more important obstacle is component placement without frank joint dislocation. Joint dislocation (tibia forward) further adds to the surgical insult through stretching of the posterior capsular structures [2].

Contemporary total knee tibial component designs have keels that help offset the significant coronal, sagittal, and rotational forces experienced by the tray. The keel presents a challenge in MIS-TKA not only with bony preparation, but also with implantation of the final component. Current parts are designed for implantation in the sagittal plane, which requires frank anterior dislocation of the tibia. This approach is concerning not only because of the resultant trauma to the soft tissues but also because dislocation requires a larger incision to allow for forward translation of the tibia within the soft-tissue envelope. Ideally, MIS-TKA components would have tibial tray designs akin to UKA trays. Design changes might include smaller keels or pegs oriented perhaps in the direction of implantation (for example, from anterior-medial). Clinical results with cemented PCA and MG prostheses show that these less invasive designs have the potential for excellent long-term fixation [3]. It might also be important to selectively replace compartments, in conjunction with the femoral component. Care must be taken with any of these proposed changes not to alter the biomechanical stability of the tibial tray.

Patellar Component

The basic challenge encountered with resurfacing the patella is to avoid eversion, which creates a technical problem if resurfacing is to be performed. The rationale for avoiding patellar eversion is to minimize traumatic stretching of the quadriceps mechanism, which can be significantly weakened after standard TKA [4]. One option is to not resurface the patella. Appropriately selected patients, such as those without anterior knee pain, patellofemoral crepitus, obesity, or other risk factors for anterior knee pain in conjunction with minimal degeneration of the patellofemoral compartment, may function well if the patella is not resurfaced. In patients for whom the patella must be resurfaced, the ideal situation would involve in-situ bone preparation and an implant that can facilitate insertion from the side without patellar eversion and also without compromising biomechanical fixation.

Fixation of Components

Cement fixation of all components continues to be the gold standard for total knee arthroplasty. However, as visualization becomes more challenging with MIS techniques, proper cementation will become increasingly difficult to achieve. Smaller incisions and less available working area will make it more difficult to clean the bone, apply cement, and ultimately implant the components. More worrisome will be the ability to remove excess cement from poorly visualized areas once the components are implanted. The new era of MIS surgery forces us to re-visit the issue of cementless fixation for total knee arthroplasty. While there have been reports of excellent clinical results with cementless TKA, the preponderance of published data suggests that cementless fixation in TKA has less than predictable results [5–10]. Newer fixation substrates, such as titanium foam and tantalum, or fixation augments, such as periapatite or bone morphogenic protein [11–13], may improve bone in-growth potential and eliminate the need for cement.

Conclusions

In order to stay within the tenets of current MIS-TKA and to better address the future direction of MIS (i.e. new incision locations) new implants must be evaluated and developed. It is paramount that these new designs not compromise the ultimate goals of TKA – pain relief and restoration of quality of life. This is dependent to a large degree on accurate component placement and dependable, long-term fixation. Any new designs must not compromise these principles.

References

1. Price AJ et al. Rapid recovery after oxford unicompartmental arthroplasty through a short incision. J Arthroplasty 2001; 16(8): 970–976

2. Brautigan B, Johnson DL. The epidemiology of knee dislocations. Clin Sports Med 2000; 19(3): 287–297

3. Miller CW, Pettygrow R. Long-term clinical and radiographic results of a pegged tibial baseplate in primary total knee arthroplasty. J Arthroplasty 2001; 16(1): 70–75

4. Silva M et al. Knee strength after total knee arthroplasty. J Arthroplasty 2003; 18(5): 605–611

5. Sundfeldt M et al. Long-term results of a cementless prosthesis with a metal-backed patellar component: clinical and radiographic follow-up with histology from retrieved components. J Long-term Effects of Med Implants 2003; 13(4): 342–354

6. Hofmann AA et al. Ten- to fourteen-year follow-up of the cementless Natural Knee system. Clin Orthop 2001; 388: 85–94

7. McCaskie AW et al. Randomized, prospective study comparing cemented and cementless total knee replacement: results of a press-fit condylar knee replacement at five years. J Bone Joint Surg 1998 80-B: 972–975

8. Kim YH, Oh JH, Oh SH. Osteolysis around cementless porous-coated anatomic knee prosthesis. J Bone Joint Surg 1995; 77-B: 236–241

9. Worland RL. Bone cement-porous coated or hydroxyapatite coated prosthesis in total knee arthroplasty-state of the art-future trends. Acta Orthop Belg 1997; 63 [Suppl 1]: 109–113

10. Collins DL et al. Porous-coated anatomic total knee arthroplasty. A prospective analysis comparing cemented and cementless fixation. Clin Orthop 1991; 267: 128–136

11. Akizuki S, Takizawa T, Honiuchi H. Fixation of hydroxyapatite-tricalcium phosphate-coated cementless knee prosthesis. Clinical and radiographic follow-up seven years after surgery. J Bone Joint Surg 2003; 85-B: 1123–1127

12. Hildebrand R et al. What effect does the hydroxyapatite coating have in cementless knee arthroplasty. Orthopade 2003, 32(4): 323–330

13. Bragdon CR et al. The efficacy of BMP-2 to induce bone ingrowth in a total hip model. Clin Orthop 2003; 417: 50–61

Part VIII   Perspectives on MIS and CAOS

Introducing New Surgical Technologies

M.J. Dunbar

Introduction

Modern hip and knee arthroplasty are largely successful procedures that impart profound improvement in quality of life and physical function [7, 15, 16, 22]. Implant survivorship for hip and knee implants at 10-years' post-surgery has been recorded at over 90%, depending on the implant and fixation method [8, 18]. Total hip arthroplasty is considered to be the most cost-effective surgical intervention in all of medicine [12]. Despite such favorable outcomes, innovative and technological improvements for hip and knee arthroplasty persist over a wide range of subjects, including design, fixation, bearing surfaces, and materials. Minimally invasive surgery (MIS) is currently proposed as the next major innovation for hip and knee arthroplasty. How should innovations in surgery be assessed, and what risks are associated with the innovative process? This is the premise of the following chapter.

Historical Perspective

It is useful to consider the evolution of arthroplasty when contemplating the introduction of new technology. Gluck reported on the first endoprosthetic knee arthroplasty, which was made of ivory and employed for severe tuberculosis of the knee [5]. It is important to remember that, at this time, the only alternatives to an interpositional spacer were amputation, arthrodesis, or benign neglect. The following decades saw considerable evolution in surgical materials and techniques until the "modern" derivation of knee arthroplasty, the total condylar knee, was developed [10]. A similar pathway of innovation occurred in the field of hip arthroplasty,

leading to the equivalent modern derivation, the Charnley cemented hip [1]. Given that the alternative to modern arthroplasty yielded, at best, substandard results, the introduction of new technologies by these early pioneers was paradoxically simpler than in modern times. The field of arthroplasty changed immensely, however, as modern hip and knee arthroplasty offered profound improvement in quality of life and function in a reliable and reproducible fashion. Continued improvement in technique and technology have resulted in lower complication rates along with a subsequent need for larger sample sizes to obtain statistical significance in new and more rigorous clinical trials. Consequently, as this trend continues, it will become increasingly difficult for a single author or institution to conduct and complete appropriately powerful studies [6].

Currently, the Scandinavian National Registries demonstrate excellent survivorship of specific prosthesis at 10 years for both hip and knee arthroplasty [8, 18]. The introduction of new technology in the field of arthroplasty no longer serves to impart a profound improvement in outcome, but instead to effect subtle changes aimed at improving outcomes, usually measured as survivorship. Given that the indications for arthroplasty are extending into younger age groups [17], improved survivorship will play a central role in mitigating increasing demand for revision surgery. Unfortunately, small changes in implant technologies introduced to improve outcomes have occasionally resulted in decreased survivorship. Examples are found in the fields of changes to polyethylene, bone cement, surface finish, and overall implant design [2, 9, 14, 19]. Given that excellent results are obtainable with specific implants, and that small changes in implant factors can have deleterious effects, is there a more logical way to introduce new technologies?

Phased Innovation

Gross has previously introduced the concept of the surgical cycle, which illustrates the acceptance of new technique or technology followed in a delayed fashion by the presentation of complications (◘ Fig. 301.1) [6]. After sufficient data on complications is accrued, the surgical community either revises the technique/technology, limits the indications, or abandons the procedure altogether [6]. Gross subsequently calls for a "... more systematised approach to the design, evaluation, implementation and general release of new surgical procedures or implants." In an effort to find a more systemized approach, Gross has adapted the example of how chemotherapeutic agents are introduced in four distinct phases. The four phases are as follows:

Phase 1 – Feasibility Study. A feasibility study aims to determine the balance between toxicity and therapeutic effect of a new agent. The study usually takes the form of a laboratory animal trial. Efficacious human doses are extrapolated from the animal model.

Phase 2 – Efficacy Study. An efficacy study aims to determine if a given dose regime is effective. Generally, relatively small numbers of patients are required for such a study.

Phase 3 – Comparative Trials. Comparative trials incorporate randomized control trials to test the hypothesis that the new agent, tested in Phase 1 and 2, is more effective than current treatment regimes. Larger numbers of patients are needed in this phase.

Phase 4 – Surveillance Study. A surveillance study follows patients who have received the treatment in order to monitor for events unforeseen or unaccounted for in the initial phases.

Borrowing from this four-phase methodology, Gross has proposed that new surgical techniques/technologies be introduced in the following fashion:

Phase 1 – Laboratory Study. Laboratory studies include both animal and biomechanical testing of new implants, bearings, methods of fixation, etc.

Phase 2 – Cohort Study. A rigorously controlled study involving a limited number of patients, for whom the outcome of a new technology is determined using predefined endpoints.

Phase 3 – Randomized Control Trials. Allows for the testing of a new procedure or implant in a larger population by surgeons other than the originators of the new concept.

Phase 4 – Surveillance Study. Like the therapeutic drug trials, the surveillance arm monitors for unforeseen or untested outcomes, especially complications.

The surgical cycle and subsequent proposed phases of innovation were expanded on in an editorial by Malchau, entitled "Introducing New Technology: A Stepwise Algorithm" [13]. Malchau has represented the stepwise introduction of new technology in graphic form, as seen in ◘ Fig. 31.2. Malchau again recommends four steps in the introduction of new technology. These steps are largely synonymous with those proposed by Gross, but are expanded on from the Swedish context. The steps are as follows:

Initial Step – Preclinical Testing. Preclinical testing is largely used by industry to prove that a new device meets basic biometric parameters. The evolution of mechanical testing devices, particularly in the field of

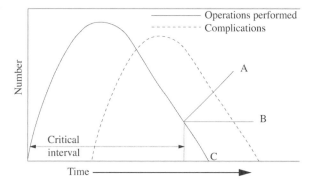

◘ **Fig. 31.1.** Surgical innovation cycle as proposed by Gross. As a new technology is introduced, a lag exists in the onset of complications. At some point the surgical community either A continues with the technology or B modifies the technology. At some point C the procedure is abandoned. (Reprinted with permission from M. Gross)

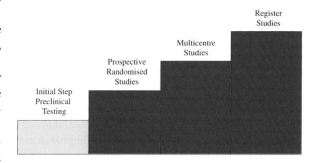

◘ **Fig. 31.2.** Stepwise algorithm for introducing new technology as proposed by Malchau. (Reprinted with permission from H. Malchau)

tribology, has improved the likelihood that such devices will be offered to surgeons for general release. Nevertheless, numerous technologies that have been shown to perform optimally in bench-top studies have gone on to perform sub-optimally in vivo [2, 9, 19]. Some devices have in fact performed poorly, with considerable consequence to the patient and significant incurred costs to the health-care system [4, 14]. This type of outcome clearly demonstrates the need for additional in vivo investigation, or addition steps in the stepwise introduction.

Clinical Step I – Prospective Randomized Studies. Once the new technology has passed the initial step of industry testing, the prosthesis can be released via well-designed prospective randomized trials. Ideally, the new technology should be investigated in a rigorous and precise fashion so as to determine relevant differences in outcome while limiting the exposure of the new technology to as few patients as possible. Radio stereometric analysis (RSA) is an accurate and predictive methodology that accomplishes these goals [11, 20]. RSA studies, however, also limit the exposure of the new technology to only a handful of specialized test centers and surgeons. The results are therefore biased and there is a subsequent need for release of the new technology to a broader audience.

Clinical Step II – Multicenter Studies. Multicenter studies, as the name implies, sees the release of the new technology to multiple centers and surgeons. Study outcomes reflect a broader and more diverse patient base and are therefore more relevant to a general orthopedic audience, and some of the reporting bias seen in clinical step I is reduced. However, the results of multicenter studies are generally in the form of objective and subjective clinical outcomes, such as health-outcome questionnaires, which are less accurate than RSA [3]. Such studies are less powerful and rely on the larger number of patients recruited in the multiple centers to generate statistical significance.

Clinical Step III – Register Studies. The final step in the introduction of new technology is the analysis of a contiguous group of patients using register studies based on large cohorts to reveal early or unusual and potentially clinically catastrophic complications [13]. National registers in Sweden have reported continuing improvement in prosthetic survivorship over the past two decades. Such progress can be attributed to not only the dissemination of clinical findings from the registry to the surgi-

cal community, but also a stepwise approach to technological advancement, especially the use of RSA studies.

Chaotic Innovation

Unfortunately, the introduction of new technology in North America has not followed a stepwise algorithm and could be considered chaotic (◨ Fig. 31.3). The initial step, preclinical testing, is robust in North America. However, instead of incorporating new technologies into prospective randomized studies (clinical step I) prior to general release, they are often made immediately available to a wide surgical community, including those who perform small numbers of arthroplasties per year. There is little emphasis placed on formal study of clinical outcomes. Only a few specialized academic centers conduct prospective randomized studies, which again, introduces a reporting bias in the literature. Unlike the United States and many European countries, national registers are a recent reality in Canada. Finally, the majority of studies published on new technology are retrospective in nature [21], often published after the technology has already changed.

The Introduction of Minimally Invasive Surgery

The introduction of MIS of the hip and knee does not appear to be driven by an effort to improve prosthetic survivorship, the major limitation in arthroplasty outcomes. In fact, MIS has the potential to worsen survivorship and the motives for its introduction should be scrutinized. While cosmetic and length of stay outcomes may be improved with MIS, what has been gained if the

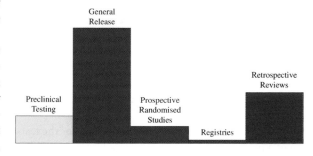

◨ **Fig. 31.3.** Chaotic innovation of new technology as proposed by Dunbar

patient comes to premature revision? Given that the major health benefit imparted by hip and knee arthroplasty may be perturbed with MIS, its introduction should, at the very least, incorporate a logical and rigorous evidence-based methodology, such as the stepwise introduction proposed by Gross and later Malchau. Efforts should be made to prevent the chaotic introduction of this new technology – orthopedic patients deserve better.

Conclusions

Hip and knee arthroplasties are profoundly successful surgical interventions with the major limitation of finite survivorship. Efforts to improve survivorship by introducing new technologies have occasionally resulted in catastrophic outcomes. MIS surgery of the hip and knee, while in some ways an attractive technology, has the potential to adversely affect the outcome of these highly beneficial procedures. When assessing new technologies in surgery, particularly MIS, efforts should be made to avoid the North American paradigm of chaotic innovation. Sound methodologies with proven positive feedback on outcome have been advocated and should be embraced when introducing new surgical technologies.

References

1. Charnley J (1972) The long-term results of low-friction arthroplasty of the hip performed as a primary intervention. J Bone Joint Surg [Br] 54(1): 61–76
2. Chmell MJ, Poss R, Thomas WH, Sledge CB (1996) Early failure of Hylamer acetabular inserts due to eccentric wear. J Arthroplasty 11(3): 351–353
3. Dunbar MJ (2001) Subjective outcomes after knee arthroplasty. Acta Orthop Scand Suppl 72(301): 1–63
4. Furnes A, Lie SA, Havelin LI, Engesaeter LB, Vollset SE (1996) The economic impact of failures in total hip replacement surgery: 28,997 cases from the Norwegian Arthroplasty Register, 1987–1993. Acta Orthop Scand 67(2): 115–121
5. Gluck T (1890) Die Invaginationsmethode der Osteo- und Arthroplastick. Berl Klin Wschr 19: 732
6. Gross M (1993) Innovations in surgery. A proposal for phased clinical trials. J Bone Joint Surg Br 75(3): 351–354
7. Hawker G et al. (1998) Health-related quality of life after knee replacement. J Bone Joint Surg Am 80(2): 163–173
8. Herberts P, Malchau H (2000) Long-term registration has improved the quality of hip replacement: a review of the Swedish THR Register comparing 160,000 cases. Acta Orthop Scand 71(2): 111–121
9. Howie DW, Middleton RG, Costi K (1998) Loosening of matt and polished cemented femoral stems. J Bone Joint Surg Br 80(4): 573–576
10. Insall J, Scott WN, Ranawat CS (1979) The total condylar knee prosthesis. A report of two hundred and twenty cases. J Bone Joint Surg [Am] 61(2): 173–180
11. Kärrholm J, Herberts P, Hultmark P, Malchau H, Nivbrant B, Thanner J (1997) Radiostereometry of hip prostheses. Review of methodology and clinical results. Clin Orthop 344: 94–110
12. Laupacis A, Bourne R, Rorabeck C, Feeny D, Wong C, Tugwell P, Leslie K, Bullas R (1993) The effect of elective total hip replacement on health-related quality of life. J Bone Joint Surg Am 75(11): 1619–1626
13. Malchau H (2000) Introducing new technology: a stepwise algorithm. Spine 25(3): 285
14. Nilsson KG, Dalen T (1998) Inferior performance of Boneloc bone cement in total knee arthroplasty: a prospective randomized study comparing Boneloc with Palacos using radiostereometry (RSA) in 19 patients. Acta Orthop Scand 69(5): 479–483
15. Rissanen P, Aro S, Sintonen H, Slatis P, Paavolainen P (1996) Quality of life and functional ability in hip and knee replacements: a prospective study. Qual Life Res 5(1): 56–64
16. Rissanen P, Aro S, Slatis P, Sintonen H, Paavolainen P (1995) Health and quality of life before and after hip or knee arthroplasty. J Arthroplasty 10(2): 169–175
17. Robertsson O, Dunbar MJ, Knutson K, Lidgren L (2000) Past incidence and future demand for knee arthroplasty in Sweden: a report from the Swedish Knee Arthroplasty Register regarding the effect of past and future population changes on the number of arthroplasties performed. Acta Orthop Scand 71(4): 376–380
18. Robertsson O, Lewold S, Knutson K, Lidgren L (2000) The Swedish Knee Arthroplasty Project. Acta Orthop Scand 71(1): 7–18
19. Roy N, Hossain S, Ayeko C, McGee HM, Elsworth CF, Jacobs LG (2002) 3 M Capital hip arthroplasty: 3–8-year follow-up of 208 primary hip replacements. Acta Orthop Scand 73(4): 400–402
20. Ryd L, Albrektsson BE, Carlsson L, Dansgard F, Herberts P, Lindstrand A, Regner L, Toksvig-Larsen S (1995) Roentgen stereophotogrammetric analysis as a predictor of mechanical loosening of knee prostheses. J Bone Joint Surg Br 77(3): 377–383
21. Ryd L, Dahlberg L (1994) On bias. Acta Orthop Scand 65(5): 499–504
22. Wiklund I, Romanus B (1991) A comparison of quality of life before and after arthroplasty in patients who had arthrosis of the hip joint. J Bone Joint Surg [Am] 73(5): 765–769

Complications of Total Hip and Total Knee Arthroplasty: Lessons Learned

J.A. D'Antonio

Introduction

Over the past four decades, an evolution of peri-operative medical management, surgical technique, implant designs, and rehabilitation protocols have led to improved results with fewer complications. Currently, in the U.S. 200,000 total hip replacements (18% revisions) and 300,000 total knee replacements (8.0% revisions) are performed on a yearly basis. Outcome studies for these total joint replacements looking at health-related quality of life issues have shown a marked increase in overall physical function with a decrease in pain [9, 10, 14, 17, 18, 20, 34, 40]. Total knee arthroplasty (TKA) improves at a slower rate than total hip arthroplasty (THA), but the quality of life outcomes are greatly improved for both. The predictors in general for inferior results include the presence of co-morbidities of a systemic nature, previous hip and/or knee surgery, young age, and low severity of disease pre-operatively [6, 12, 15, 22]. Patients who are most disabled pre-operatively tend to have the best results post-operatively. Additionally, key contributors to the ultimate outcome of THA and TKA include patient expectations, surgeon expertise and experience [1, 2, 23, 25, 27].

As a result of years of adjustments to complications and failures, new innovations and techniques have expanded the indications for THA and TKA to younger and more active patients. A high incidence of infection decades ago has been reduced significantly with the adoption of new surgical approaches, reduced surgical time, peri-operative antibiotics and clean air rooms [1, 2, 32]. Incidence of deep vein thrombosis (DVT) and pulmonary embolism (PE) has been reduced with the use of regional anesthesia, rapid mobilization of patients post-operatively and some form of prophylactic anticoagu-

lant therapy [1–3]. New implant designs with and without cement have decreased wear, improved long-term fixation, biomechanics and functional results [5, 7, 8, 10, 11, 14, 16, 24, 36]. Thirty years ago, the trans-trochanteric approach was the standard by which other surgical approaches were measured. Over the years both anterior and posterior approaches have led to multiple patient benefits, including faster recovery, increased speed of operation, fewer complications and lower overall costs [21, 37]. Because of these and other successful developments, the success of THA and TKA has placed those procedures near the top of all treatment modalities in medicine with regard to cost-benefit ratio to society. With this in mind, it is incumbent upon us when embarking upon new technology and/or new techniques that change must

- provide a proven benefit to the patient,
- have the same or better lasting result,
- have less complications,
- enhance the OR experience for the high- and low-volume surgeon,
- and not increase the cost of total joint arthroplasty.

More now than ever it is imperative that well-constructed prospective and randomized studies be performed to delineate the efficacy and safety of new technology and new approaches.

Peri-Operative Complications

General surgical peri-operative complications can be life-threatening as a result of anesthetic complications, thromboembolic phenomena, myocardial infarction (MI), congestive heart failure or hemorrhage. The overall frequency of serious complications which would include MI, PE, and death has been reported to be anywhere from 0.5–2.0% and is related most often to older age, pre-existing cardiopulmonary disease, surgeon's procedure volume, anesthetic management, and anticoagulant prophylaxis [1, 2, 23, 25]. Specific mortality rates following hip and knee arthroplasty range from 0.2–0.5% within 30 days of surgery and is most often secondary to MI or PE. These mortality rates have been shown to be lower for joint-replacement arthroplasty than for a comparable general population not undergoing surgery.

Venous thrombosis is one of the most common post-operative complications of total joint arthroplasty reported to occur as high as 50% in TKA. However, not all cases of DVT are clinically significant and most do not result in serious events [1, 2, 30]. With appropriate treatment and precautions, with regional anesthesia, and early mobilization, clinically significant DVT is now reported to be between 2% and 4% with the incidence of symptomatic PE being reduced to less than 1% and the rate of fatal PE reduced to 0.1–0.2% after THA and/or TKA. This low incidence of fatal PE has been shown to be a result of chemical prophylaxis of any type including the use of aspirin, and is significantly lower for all forms of prophylaxis when compared to patient populations who have received no form of prophylaxis [1–3].

Deep joint infection has been reported between 0.5% and 12% for both THA and TKA with rates of 0.5% for primary joint arthroplasty in recent years becoming more common [1, 2, 32]. An increased risk of deep peri-prosthetic infection occurs in the multiply operated upon joint, patients on immunosuppressive therapy, those with poor nutrition, those who are obese, patients who abuse alcohol or smoke, those with diabetes mellitus, renal failure, and patients with dental and/or bladder infections. Specific increased risk occurs for patients who suffer with rheumatoid arthritis (1.2%), psoriatic arthritis (5.5%), diabetes mellitus (5.6%), and post-operative urethral instrumentation in males (6.2%). The most commonly occurring organisms are coagulase-positive *Staphylococcus aureus,* causing acute infection following surgery, and *Staphylococcus epidermidis,* causing late infection. The reduction of infection over the years has been directly related to the use of peri-operative antibiotics which achieve a high-tissue concentration at a time of the skin incision. Important additional measures that have reduced the overall infection rate include maintaining a meticulously clean air operating-room environment, surgery performed in less than 2.5 h, antibiotic impregnated cement, and the use of laminar flow and/or body exhaust suits by medical personal.

Dislocation is a painful and troubling complication that occurs in 0.3–10% of primary THAs, 3–20% in revision THAs, and rarely with TKAs [1, 2, 21, 37, 40]. The majority of hip dislocations occur within the first 3 months following surgery, and the risk factors for total hip dislocation include patient, surgeon and prosthetic factors. Patient factors include a history of prior surgery, poor patient compliance, older patients with compromised mental status, patients with neuromuscular problems, a history of alcoholism and the female gender. Surgeon skill and experience is a primary factor in dislocation of the hip [1, 2, 23, 25]. In a prospective randomized study comparing metal-on-polyethylene to alumina ceramics, 723 hips were implanted by 22 surgeons [11]. The overall dislocation rate for these patients was 2.6% in the first 2 years but it varied from 0% for the surgeon who did the most cases (139) to 17% for a surgeon who performed 29 implants. It has been reported that the rate of dislocation in THA reduces dramatically after a surgeon has conducted 30 or more procedures. Surgical technique to minimize the risk requires that the acetabular component be properly positioned consistently, areas of impingement be removed, and soft tissues be adequately repaired. The ideal placement of an acetabular component to maximize the functional range of motion of any design before impingement occurs is approximately 45° (±5°) of abduction and 25° (±5°) of anteversion assuming a femoral anteversion of 15°. Excessive acetabular anteversion, any amount of retroversion, inclination greater than 60° of the acetabular component or excessive femoral mal-position all contribute to instability. Dislocations with TKA are uncommon and related to instability in flexion for both cruciate retaining and cruciate substituting designs. The risk of subluxation is a greater problem for the substituting design where the post-cam mechanism becomes disengaged and subluxed with an unstable flexion gap.

Intra-operative fractures are most commonly seen in cementless reconstruction of the hip and revision THA. For primary THA, femoral fractures with cemented femoral prostheses occur in 0.3–1.8% and for cementless femoral components in 3–18%. [1, 38]. The incidence is significantly higher in the revision setting. Peri-prosthetic femoral fractures secondary to trauma in the immediate post-operative period is estimated at 1% for primary hips and 4% for revision THA. Intra-operative and immediate post-operative fractures of the acetabulum and the knee are less common and are seen more often in the hip with press-fit components and in the knee most often with posterior stabilized and total stabilized designs where condylar fractures can occur. Displaced intra-operative femoral condylar fractures are uncommon but implant and technique are related. In one reported series, 40 out of 532 posterior stabilized TKAs suffered a femoral intercondylar fracture intra-operatively [26]. Five of those fractures were displaced and required re-operation for stabilization. The majority of post-operative fractures reported to occur about the knee can be divided into patellar fractures and supracondylar fractures of the femur [28].

Nerve injuries, although rare, occur in 0.6–3.7% of cases [1, 2]. The incidence for THA increases with a diagnosis of DDH and revision surgery. The sciatic nerve is most often involved, particularly in women, and the femoral nerve secondly most often. Recovery from nerve injury occurs in the majority of patients but sustained permanent damage results in a devastating complication. Nerve injury following THA is most often related to excessive lengthening of the extremity, intraneural hemorrhage, extrusion of methyl methacrylate adjacent to the nerve, constriction with a trochanteric wire or suture, or injury from acetabular screw placement. Nerve damage following TKA is rare but catastrophic when it occurs. Perineal nerve palsy is the most frequent complication seen in TKA and is associated most often with pre-operative severe valgus or flexion deformities.

Bleeding complications into the wound site of joint arthroplasty can occur for several days following surgery and most often as a result of anticoagulant therapy. Significant wound hematomas with or without draining wounds may require discontinuation of aggressive anticoagulant therapy and additional surgery to relieve and drain the blood accumulation. Relatively unique to THA are the complications of heterotopic ossification and leg-length discrepancy. Heterotopic ossification that is clinically significant occurs in 2–10% of patients and has a greater chance of occurring in patients with hypertrophic arthritis, ankylosing spondilitis, diffuse idiopathic skeletal hyperostosis, patients with a history of previous hip surgery and the

male gender [1, 2, 4]. Leg-length discrepancy is a relatively common cause of post-operative dissatisfaction and can lead to an unhappy patient with increased morbidity, the need for revision surgery, and litigation. The average reported leg-length inequality following THA surgery ranges from 2.8–11.6 mm with an ideal target being less than 7 mm of lengthening [1, 2]. Because stability of the total hip takes precedence over attempts to match leg length, pre-surgical understanding between the patient and the orthopedic surgeon regarding these issues is a high priority.

Early (<2 Years Postoperative) and Late Failures

Patient satisfaction rates following THA and TKA are reported to be in the 90–95% range. In addition, the results of these surgical procedures are durable with 10–15 year implant survivorship of greater than 90% [5, 7, 8, 12, 14, 16, 24, 35]. Despite these excellent results, patients do achieve poor results and at times require revision before 2 years as well as suffering later failures beyond the 2-year period. The most common reasons for revision of TKA are infection, loosening, instability, and extensor mechanism complications [6, 15, 19, 27, 39]. Currently, in the U.S., 300,000 TKA are performed each year and 8% are revisions. In a report by Fehring, 64% of patients had revision surgery within 5 years of their index procedure [15]. Looking at mechanisms of failure early and late, Sharkey and group evaluated 212 consecutive total knee revisions in 203 patients [39]. The average time to revision for patients in the early group was 1.1 years and in the late group 7 years. 55.6% of revisions were done less than 2 years after the index operation and the remaining 42.4% greater than 2 years following the index operation. The most prevalent mechanism for failure was poly-wear seen in 25% of all revisions, accounting for 44.4% of all revision in the late failure group. In the early failure group, the most common mode was infection (25.4%) while in the late group infection occurred in 7.8% of patients. Component loosening was a cause of early as well as late revisions with an incidence of 16.9% and 34.4%, respectively. Early loosening was associated with uncemented components as well as surface-cementing of tibial components without cementing the keel. Instability was seen in 21.2% of early and 22.2% of late revisions. Of those knees requiring revision for instability, 37% were cruciate sparing while the remainder were cruciate substituting. Significant stiffness associated with arthrofibrosis was present in 16.9% of patients requiring early and in 12.2% of patients who had late revision surgery. Extensor mechanism failures were responsible for revision surgery because of significant extensor lag (6.6%), AVN of the patella (4.2%) and revision of unsurfaced patella (0.9%). Component mal-alignment and mal-position was present overall in 11.8% of revisions with 11.9% in the early subgroup and 12.2% of the late revision knee subgroup. Peri-prosthetic fractures accounted for 2.8% of all revisions.

Following THA, early failures requiring revision are most often due to infection, recurrent dislocation, peri-prosthetic fracture and leg-length inequality [1, 2, 5, 12, 16, 17, 19, 36, 40]. Late revisions today are most often the result of poly-wear and/or osteolysis, component loosening, and to a lesser degree recurrent dislocation and infection. Revision rates within the first 12 months have been reported in the 1–6.5% range being higher for uncemented than cemented prostheses. Our own experience participating in two different prospective multi-center studies, both of which have been closely monitored with routine follow-up evaluations, are somewhat representative of recent experiences with cementless fixation. In the first study, four surgeons who were a part of the larger multicenter study began implanting implants in 1987 and continued to follow 262 patients beyond 15 years [12]. In that group, the revision rate in the first 2 years was 1.1% (3 hips) and secondary to pain of unknown etiology, deep joint infection, and peri-prosthetic fracture. Revisions that occurred beyond 2 years equaled 44 for a 16,8% revision rate and were a result of two deep joint infections (0.7%), one for pain of unknown etiology (0.37%), one for peri-prosthetic femoral fracture (0.37%), one for recurrent dislocation (0.37%), 12 for wear and/or osteolysis (4.5%) and 26 for loose acetabular components (9.9%). Only one femoral stem was revised for loosening (0.37%). The high rate of socket loosening was a design issue which involved press-fit cups that had no in-growth surface and a high failure rate. The breakdown of socket revisions shows porous in-growth socket failures of 3.5%, threaded HA socket failures at 5.6% and the HA press-fit non-ingrowth socket failures at 10.3%. The second study was a prospective randomized controlled study comparing metal-on-poly to alumina-on-alumina ceramic bearings and involved implantation of 723 hips followed out to 5

years [11]. The failures leading to revisions in less than two years totaled 12 (1.6%): peri-prosthetic fracture accounted for 3 (0.4%); recurrent dislocation for 4 (0.54%); deep joint infection for 2 (0.27%); acetabular loosening for 1 (0.14%); and leg-length discrepancy for 1 (0.14%). Failures leading to revision after 2 years in this study totaled 8 (1.1%): 2 for recurrent dislocations (0.27%); 2 for acetabular loosening (0.27%); 1 for deep joint infection (0.14%); 1 for pain of unknown etiology (0.14%); 1 for trauma (0.14%); and 1 for osteolysis in the poly-control group (0.14%). Approximately 200,000 THA are performed in the UA yearly 18% of which are revisions.

Summary

Based on published clinical and outcome studies, THA and TKA surgery is safe, cost-effective, alleviates pain, and restores function to patients who do not respond to non-surgical treatment. There are few contra-indications to the surgery and overall these operative procedures have been very successful with low risk of complications despite variations in patient health, a variety of prosthetic types implanted, variation in orthopedic surgeon experience and skill, and a variety of surgical facilities with varying volumes of total joint-replacement experience. As we look forward to the rapidly growing new interest in navigation, computer-assisted surgery, and minimally invasive surgery, we must not forget the past and lessons learned. History teaches that while new is not always better, innovation continues to improve our surgical skills and clinical results. However, because of the high success of total joint arthroplasty today, any dramatic shift in technique or design must be critically compared with the result of today's standards. Questions that can only be answered through prospective and randomized studies include:

- Will the new procedure benefit the patient?
- Will the complications be less
- Will long-term fixation be compromised
- Will less experienced surgeons be capable of performing the surgery
- Will the price of new equipment and designs be cost-effective?

Our ultimate goal is long-term success with an absolute minimum of complications.

References

1. AAOS: IMCA Information Series: OA of the Hip: October 2003
2. AAOS: IMCA Information Series: OA of the Knee: September 2002
3. Ansari S, Warwick D, Ackroyd CE et al.: Incidence of fatal pulmonary embolism after 1,390 TKA's without routine prophylactic anticoagulation, except in high-risk cases. J Arthroplasty 12(6): 599–602, 1997
4. Ayers DC, Evarts C, Parkinson JR: The prevention of heterotopic ossification in high-risk patients by low dose radiation therapy after THA. JBJS 68A: 1423–1430, 1986
5. Berry DJ, Harmsen WS, Cabanella ME et al.: 25 year survivorship of 2,000 consecutive primary Charnley THR's: factors affecting survivorship of acetabular and femoral components. JBJS 84A(2): 171–177, 2002
6. Bono JV, McCarthy JC, Turner RH: Complications in THA. In: Pellicci PM (ed): Orthopaedic knowledge update: hip and knee reconstruction 2. American Academy of Orthopaedic Surgeons, Rosemont, IL, pp 155–166, 2000
7. Callaghan JJ, Albright JC, Goetz DD et al.: Charnley THA with cement: minimum twenty-five year follow-up. JBJS 82A: 487–497, 2000
8. Callaghan JJ, Dennis DA, Paprosky WG et al.: Long-term results in TKA. In: Pellicci PM (ed): Orthopaedic knowledge update: hip and knee reconstruction 2. American Academy of Orthopaedic Surgeons, Rosemont, IL, 303–316, 1995
9. Callaghan CM, Drake BG, Heck DA et al.: Patient outcomes following tricompartmental TKR: a meta-analysis. JAMA 271(17): 1349–1357, 1994
10. Chang RW, Pellissier JM, Hazen GB: A cost-effective analysis of THA for osteoarthritis of the hip. JAMA 275(11): 858–865, 1996
11. D'Antonio JA, Capello WN, Manley MT et al.: New experience with alumina-on-alumina ceramic bearings for THA. J Arthroplasty 17(4): 390–397, 2002
12. D'Antonio JA, Capello WN, Manley MT et al.: Hydroxylapatite femoral stems for THA: 10–13 year follow-up. CORR 393: 101–111, 2001
13. D'Antonio JA: TKA: Looks good, feels bad. Sem Arthroplasty 14(4): 215–221, 2003
14. Diduch DR, Insall JN, Scott WN et al.: TKR in young, active patients: long-term follow-up and functional outcome. JBJS 79A(4): 575–582, 1997
15. Fehrin TK, Odum S, Friffin WL et al.: Early failures in TKA. Clin Orthop 392: 315–318, 2001
16. Garellick G, Malachau H, Herberts P: Survival of hip replacements: A comparison of a randomized trial and a registry. Clin Orthop 375: 157–167, 2000
17. Garellick G, Malchau H, Herberts P et al.: Life expectancy and cost utility after THR. Clin Orthop 346: 141–151, 1998
18. Hawker G, Wright J, Coyte P et al.: Health-related quality of life after TKR. JBJS 80A(2): 163–173, 1998
19. Heck DA, Partridge CM, Reuben JD et al.: Prosthetic component failures in hip arthroplasty surgery. J Arthroplasty 10(5): 575–580, 1995
20. Heck DA, Robinson RL, Partridge CM et al.: Patient outcomes after knee replacement. Clin Orthop 356: 93–110, 1998
21. Hedlundh U, Hybbinette CH, Fredin H: Influence of surgical approach on dislocations after Charnley hip arthroplasty. J Arthroplasty 10(5): 609–614, 1995
22. Jorn LP, Johnsson R, Toksgiv-Larsen S: Patient satisfaction, function and return to work after knee arthroplasty. Acta Orthop Scand 70(4): 343–347, 1999
23. Katz JN, Losina E, Barrett J et al.: Association between hospital and surgeon procedure volume and outcomes of THR in the US Medicare Population. JBJS 83A(11): 1622–1629, 2001
24. Knutson K, Lewold S, Robertsson O et al.: The Swedish knee arthroplasty register: a nationwide study of 30,003 knees. Acta Orthop Scand 65(4): 375–386, 1992
25. Lavernia CJ, Guzman JF: Relationship of surgical volume to short-term mortality, morbidity, and hospital charges in arthroplasty. J Arthroplasty 10(2): 133–140, 1995
26. Lombardi AV, Mallory TH, Waterman RA et al.: Intercondylar distal femoral fracture: an unreported complication of post-stabilized TKA. J Arthroplasty 10: 643–650, 1995
27. Mahomed NN, Liang MH, Cook EF et al.: The importance of patient expectations in predicting functional outcomes after total joint arthroplasty. J Rheum 29(6): 1273–1279, 2002
28. Malkani AL, Karandikar N: Complications following TKA: The prevention and management of early loosening. Semin Arthroplasty 14(4): 203–214, 2003
29. Parvizi J, Johnson BG, Rowland C et al.: 30-day mortality after elective THA. JBJS 83A(10): 1524–1528, 2001
30. Parvizi J, Sullivan TA, Trousdale RT et al.: 30-day mortality after TKA. JBJS 83A(8): 1157–1161, 2001
31. Pavone V, Boettner F, Fickert S et al.: Total condylar knee arthroplasty: a long-term follow-up. Clin Orthop 388: 18–25, 2001
32. Peersman G, Raskin R, Davis J et al.: Infection in TKR. Clin Orthop 392: 15–23, 2001
33. Peterson CA, Lewallen DG: Periprosthetic fracture of the acetabulum after THA. JBJS 78A(8): 426–431, 1996
34. Robertsson O, Dunbar M, Pehrsson T et al.: Patient satisfaction after TKA: a report on 27,372 knees operated on between 1981 and 1995 in Sweden. Acta Orthop Scand 71(3): 262–267, 2000
35. Rodriguez JA, Bhende H, Ranawat CS: Total condylar knee replacement: a 20-year follow-up study. Clin Orthop 388: 10–17, 2001
36. Rorabeck CH, Bourne RB, Mulliken BD et al.: The Nicolas Andry award: Comparative results of cemented and cementless THA. Clin Orthop 325: 330–344, 1996
37. Schinsky MF, Nercessian OA, Arons RR et al.: Comparison of complications after transtrochanteric and posterolateral approaches for primary THA. J Arthroplasty 18(4): 430–434, 2003
38. Schwartz JT Jr, Mayer JG, Engh CA: Femoral fracture TKA's failing today? CORR 404: 7–13, 2002
40. Towheed TE, Hochberg MC: Health-related quality of life after THR. Sem Arthr Rheum 26(1): 483–491, 1996
41. Von Knoch M, Berry DJ, Harmsen WS et al.: Late dislocation after THA, JBJS 84A(11): 1949–1953, 2002

Minimally Invasive Total Joint Arthroplasty and Direct-to-Consumer Advertising

J.L. Schaffer, L. Krishnamurthi, Ying Xie

Introduction

One of the most important functions of any organization is the marketing of their products or services to the consumers of those products or services. The predominant force for both the marketer and the consumer is to increase welfare for both parties, the marketers by selling their products or services, the consumers by using those products or services to increase their quality of life. Marketing has a wide variety of roles to play starting with understanding customer needs, both articulated and latent, translating these needs into appropriate language for research and development and design specialists, assisting product management with pricing and distribution, and informing customers through advertising. Customers cannot buy a product they are not aware of, so advertising plays a critical role in creating awareness as well as in educating customers about the product or service.

The advent of minimally invasive arthroplasty, combined with the increasing population of those over the age of 55 years, has provided a unique opportunity for the manufacturers of arthroplasty implants to promote their products directly to the patients. The major goals of promotion are to provide information, stimulate demand, influence purchasing behavior and differentiate products through a variety of vehicles such as print, video, audio, electronic and billboards. Additionally, the traditional lines of communications between marketer and consumer have been blurred with information posted on the web sites of manufacturers, patient organizations (often supported by the manufacturers) and supposedly third-party web sites with no apparent connection to any manufacturer. In health care, the users of a product or service could be defined as either the physi-

cian or patient, depending on the vantage point being examined.

Health care is a unique industry in that the traditional definitions of users and buyers of a product or service are not always clear. Arthroplasty components are prescribed and inserted by the surgeon, initially purchased by the hospital facility, ultimately paid for by the patient's insurer and used in perpetuity by the patient. The surgeon does have a vested interest in the short- and long-term performance of the implant in the patient. As with pharmaceuticals, orthopedic arthroplasty implants offer their manufacturers the opportunity to promote their products to the penultimate user, the patient. In turn, the patients, often with limited knowledge about these products and services, turn to their physicians to fill this knowledge gap while simultaneously creating increased demand for the specific service and the company's products. This discussion will focus on DTC advertisements in the context of the regulations in the United States.

Definitions

Direct-to-consumer (DTC) advertising refers to any advertisements that are directed to the final consumer of the product (◘ Fig. 33.1). Recent experience has shown that DTC advertising has increased dramatically in the past 5 years with consumers being bombarded by advertising from hospitals, insurers, providers, pharmaceutical manufacturers especially for over the counter drugs, advocacy groups and fitness centers. The Food and Drug Administration (FDA) regulations divide DTC advertising into three categories: promotion of a specific product, providing information on specific dis-

33

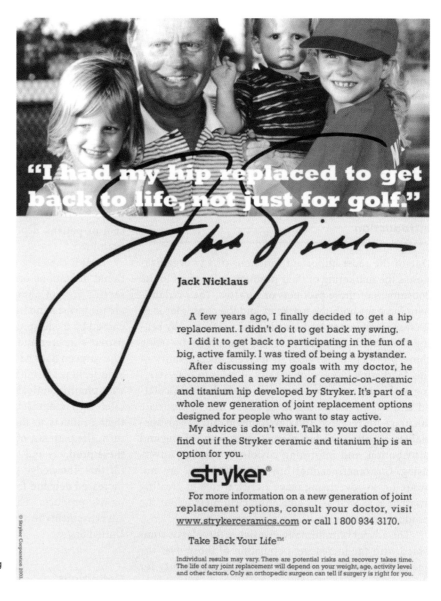

Fig. 33.1. Example of DTC advertising for arthroplasty implants

eases and reminder advertisements [1]. The FDA has very specific regulations for these different types of drug ads. The advertising regulations further distinguish between print and broadcast advertisements. Print advertisements must include the brief summary of information "relating to side effects, contraindications, and effectiveness", while advertisements broadcast through mass media such as television, radio, or telephone communication systems must disclose the product's major risk in either the audio or audio and

visual parts of the presentation [2]. The regulation also requires the sponsors of broadcast advertisements to make "adequate provision" for dissemination of the product's approved labeling.

Help-seeking ads that provide information on specific diseases aim to alert consumers about an illness and its symptoms and let them know the treatment is available. These types of ads are not brand-specific. The FDA specifically regulates that a drug's brand name cannot be used in this type of ads, although the company sponsoring the ad is identified. Help-seeking ads are used to motivate people to see their doctors to discuss the advertised condition. Advertisements for arthroplasty implants typically fall into this category. By providing assistance to patients with specific symptoms or diagnoses, the companies paying for these ads hope to provide directed information that will drive patients to surgeons using the companies' products.

Reminder ads are advertisements that "call attention to the name of the drug product but do not include indications or dosage recommendations for use of the product, or any other representation" [3]. These ads give the proprietary name of the prescriptive drug or device and the established name of each active ingredient. They may also contain additional limited information, such as the name of the sponsoring company, price or dosage form, but can not specify the dosage recommendation. However, these reminder ads do not mention any disease or condition to be treated. They are designed to build brand recognition and prompt people to ask their doctors about the advertised drug.

Product-claim ads mention both a drug's brand name and its intended use. They aim explicitly to prompt people with a specific disease or condition to go to the doctor to inquire about the drug. These ads contain general information about the category, as well as brand differentiating information about a specific drug. According to FDA rules, help-seeking and reminder ads do not have to contain detailed information on a drug's effectiveness or potential side effects. However, product-claim ads must present a "fair balance" of benefit and risk information, and must contain prominent mention of a drug's side effects and important contraindications.

Tactics of DTC Advertising

The target audience for DTC advertising is the potential user of the drug or device. This could include a diverse audience ranging from individuals with limited access to technologically sophisticated outlets such as Internet, as well as those who may not be comfortable in actively requesting or searching for product information. In order to provide reasonably convenient access to the advertised product's approved labeling to fulfill the "adequate provision" requirement, a broadcast-advertisement sponsor is required to provide four additional

sources from which the consumer could obtain the labeling information in the advertisement:

- a toll-free telephone number;
- a currently running print advertisement that contained the labeling information;
- referral to a health-care provider;
- an Internet web page address (URL) [4].

An increasing number of the pharmaceutical advertisements offer a monetary incentive, either a rebate and/or a free sample with a filled prescription, and make available additional information in printed or audio/video form [5]. In an analysis of magazine advertisements for prescription drugs, it was found that about two-thirds were for drugs to ameliorate symptoms, a quarter for drugs to treat disease, and the remainder to prevent illness. Emotional appeals were the most common type of promotion, followed by advice to consumers to understand their medical condition. The benefits were largely described in qualitative terms, while the side-effects were typically described with data. The cost of therapy was not mentioned in any of the ads [6]. A large number of DTC advertisements are targeted to women, even when the drug in question is non-gender-specific like arthritis. This is because research shows that women pay more attention to health than men, are more likely to visit the doctor, and are more open in discussing health problems with their doctors. Bhattacharyya et al. have demonstrated that half of the claims in advertisements directed to orthopedic surgeons were not supported by data that could be used in the clinical decision-making process [7]. Advertisements directed towards consumers for identical products have been too few to provide a similar examination but provides sufficient warning that the advertisements may be misconstrued by consumers.

Participants in DTC Communication

The stakeholders in the DTC marketing efforts for orthopedic implants include patients, physicians, manufacturers and media. Obviously the two most important agents involved in the decision process are the patient and the physician. They are responsible for two sequential decisions in the prescription process: the treatment-incidence decision and the prescription-choice decision. For any prescription to be written for a

33

pharmaceutical or an implant prescribed for the patient, the patient has to initiate the treatment process, i.e., the patient has to decide whether he or she needs to visit the doctor's office and discuss his or her illness. Conditional on the patient's visit, it is the physician's decision to prescribe a specific course of action that may include a prescription for a drug or implant. Here, the physician acts as an informed agent to maximize the patient's utility with the patient's health needs and, in some cases, financial constraints in mind. For the orthopedic industry, increasing the number of patients who seek treatment is the primary focus of the DTC efforts as the local representatives will have greater influence on the surgeon's choice of implants. However, the surgeon's choices could be affected by a multitude of patients who discuss the DTC ads they saw or request the operation using a specific implant.

To summarize, we show in ◻ Fig. 33.2 a graphical illustration of the sequential decision process of the prescription-decision process and how the different components in the companies' promotion mix can affect this process. The top panel of the graph shows the

patient's treatment-incidence decision where the patient decides whether or not to visit the doctor and discuss his or her condition. The total DTC advertising effort in the therapeutic class can provide information to increase the likelihood of a potential patient's visit to the doctor. Once in the physician's office, it is the physician's decision as to which drug or device to prescribe. The physician, however, acts as the patient's agent to maximize the patient's health outcome with patients' pros and cons in mind. Therefore, it is not only physician promotions, but also price, and brand level DTC advertising, which play a role at this stage to drive physician-prescription choice.

Historical Context

The majority of DTC ads have been focused on prescription medications. Wilkes et al. note that medications were directly advertised to the public through newspaper ads from the early 1700s to the 1930s [8]. For example, 90% of the marketing expenditures for drugs

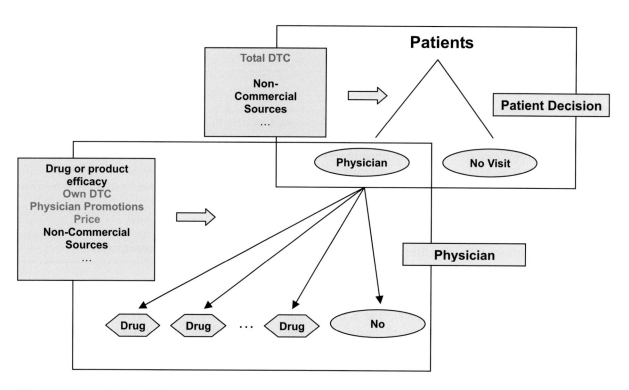

◻ **Fig. 33.2.** Prescription drug-decision process

in 1930 were for advertising in newspapers and popular magazines and only 5% was spent on detailing, samples, and technical journal advertising [9]. The Food, Drug, and Cosmetic Act (FDCA) of 1938 gave authority to the FDA over the labeling of pharmaceutical drugs, both over the counter (OTC) and prescription, but the intent of FDCA was not to be overly restrictive. Oversight of drug advertising still remained with the Federal Trade Commission (FTC). Lyles and Wilkes et al. provide a background on the changes in the laws that have taken place since the 1930s [4, 8]. Until 1951, the pharmaceutical companies made the determination of which drugs were to be available by prescription. Although the FDA could disagree with those decisions, it was not until the Durham-Humphrey amendment of 1951 that the distinction between over-the-counter (OTC) and prescription drugs was clarified [4, 8]. In 1962, the Kefauver-Harris drug amendment strengthened the laws protecting consumers, made the drug approval process more stringent, and transferred authority for prescription drug advertising to the FDA. Specific regulations were written to govern dissemination of drug information.

By 1972, there was a complete turnaround in the allocation of marketing expenditures with 75% of the spending on detailing, sampling, and technical journal advertising [9]. The requirements of fair balance and brief summary of drug performance essentially ruled out the use of broadcast media, such as radio and television. Even print advertising was not considered a positive media because of the regulations which required a statement of all the side effects and contra-indication warnings. Starting in the 1980s, drug manufacturers began to press the FDA on relaxing the rules governing direct communication with consumers. U.S. society was changing from being paternalistic to individual consumer empowerment. Still, the FDA kept the rules in force until 1997. Following a public hearing and debate, the FDA relaxed the rules for broadcast media. For the first time manufacturers could provide the drug name, the medical condition and the important risks, but not have to mention all of the product's risks, although they had to mention sources where such information can be found. Since 1997, spending on DTC advertising has skyrocketed.

Only recently in 2003 have the orthopedic implant manufacturers run ads for knee arthritis and regaining youthful function [10]. Many of the ads refer to a condition-specific web site that contains a physician locator where a limited number of surgeons are listed, presumably all of whom use the company's implants. The efficacy of this type of campaign is not yet known. However, these campaigns have already increased tensions between manufacturers and hospitals. As the hospitals attempt to contain spending on supplies and implants through aggressive negotiations and standardization, patients demanding or at least having knowledge about a specific implant may influence the physician's implant choice, and consequently adversely affect the hospitals' cost-containment efforts.

Economics of DTC Advertising [11]

DTC ads can affect the demand for prescriptive drugs and devices in a number of different ways. First, the industry's total DTC advertising effort in the category can increase patient awareness about a particular illness and the corresponding medical treatment, so as to encourage visits to the doctors' office to discuss their condition. For the people who are affected but not aware of their medical problems, DTC advertising serves as a major information source to facilitate the point of entry into the category. In this sense, total DTC advertising in the category drives the primary demand for the entire therapeutic class by converting non-users into users. This effect might be most pronounced in the categories with chronic conditions such as arthritis that may require arthroplasty, for which a large population is affected by but may not be adequately treated.

Among the three types of DTC drug ads that we discussed in the previous section, both help-seeking ads and product-claim ads contain information about the disease or condition, and therefore have an effect in encouraging the affected people to seek treatment. One would expect that these ads might be beneficial to the firm's competitors as well, because of the primary demand-stimulating effect on the entire category.

Secondly, once in the physicians' office, the patients can ask their doctors about the drug or product they saw in the DTC ads, and even request a specific brand to be prescribed. The doctors, targeted by the professional detailing programs, choose a specific drug or product to treat their patients, with the patients' therapeutic needs and financial constraints in mind. After receiving the prescription for a pharmaceutical agent, it is the patient who is responsible for having the prescription filled at the pharmacy and taking the drug as suggested. At this point, DTC ads remind them to take their medication regularly and refill it at proper intervals. These together determine the secondary demand for a specific brand in a therapeutic class. For patients who require an implant, the scenario is different. The pre-operative detailing of the surgeon who will make the implant choice combined with the promotion and information provided to patients through DTC advertisements will be the primary determinants of implant choice. Once the surgery is completed, there is little benefit in manufacturer–patient promotion, but this represents a fertile area for establishing a referral pool of interested parties.

The brand specific drug ads, i.e., reminder ads and product claim ads, might be most effective in driving the secondary demand, although the non-brand specific help seeking ads might also have some effects in differentiating the brands by associating the ads with the sponsoring company. For orthopedic patients, this may influence their decision to undergo an operative procedure, but in this case the patient–physician relationship will probably be of greater importance in influencing the implant choice. The brand-specific ad category of DTC ads may be of more importance and have a greater influence on investors than on patients or surgeons.

Synergies Between DTC Advertising and Physician-Directed Promotions

One of the key factors that determine the impact of DTC advertising on the demand for pharmaceutical products is the extent to which patients can influence the choice of drugs prescribed for them – something that largely depends on how amenable physicians are likely to be to their requests. This likelihood can be greatly enhanced if physicians are well informed by the pharmaceutical company about the drug via a professional detailing program. Otherwise, a DTC campaign can backfire, when consumers are encouraged to visit their doctor but are prescribed a rival product. Bristol-Myers Squibb's failed DTC campaign for its cholesterol reduction drug, Pravachol, is a good example. Bristol-Myers Squibb launched an extensive DTC ad campaign for Pravachol, but did not follow through with significant detailing effort targeted to physicians. The campaign increased the primary demand for cholesterol reduction drugs by prompting patients to ask doctors for prescription drugs

to lower their cholesterol. However, Pravachol did not get its share of this market growth, because physicians largely prescribed Lipitor, which was marketed to them exclusively via detailing by Pfizer. In order to prevent such unintended help for competitors, it is essential for pharmaceutical firms to treat these two promotional efforts as an indispensable part of one integrated marketing communication strategy, rather than two separately operating promotional tools. The orthopedic manufacturers have a long history of direct promotion to orthopedic surgeons as an integral part of the support program that includes the presence of a representative in the operating-room environment to assist with inventory and in-service training sessions. However, making the surgeons acutely aware of the DTC campaign is critical to the success of the marketing campaign and can be extended by a simultaneous campaign from the surgeon to prospective patients within their market.

Current DTC-Spending Trends

Since the FDA relaxed guidelines in 1997 for disseminating information about prescriptive agents through broadcast media, such as television and radio, spending on DTC advertising has sky-rocketed. To date, the vast majority of this spending has been on pharmaceutical agents and only recently have the implant manufacturers started DTC advertising. The total promotional spending by pharmaceutical firms for prescription drugs grew at an annual rate of 16% from 1996 to 2001 (◘ Fig. 33.3), while the average annual growth rate in DTC drug-ads spending was 28% between 1996 and 2001 [12]. In 2000, the promotional expenditure in the pharmaceutical industry had reached $ 15.7 billion, among which 25.5% was spent on doctor's office detailing, and 15.9% on DTC advertising (◘ Fig. 33.4). In the same year, Merck spent $ 160 million in DTC advertising to promote its anti-arthritic drug, Vioxx, in contrast to Pepsi's $ 125 million ad budget for its core brand – Pepsi Cola, and Anheuser-Busch's $ 146 million ad spending on Budweiser beer [13].

The spending for DTC drug advertising tends to be concentrated in a relatively small number of products. The top ten brands accounted for 36% of total DTC advertising spending in 2001. Six of these top ten drugs with DTC spending were also among the top ten drugs promoted to physicians by detailing and journal adver-

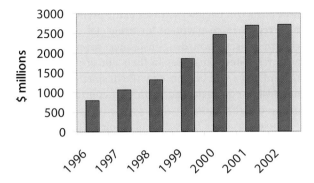

◻ Fig. 33.3. DTC drug ads spending trend (1996–2002)

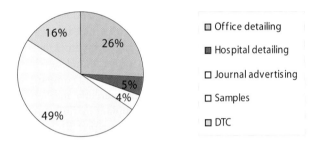

◻ Fig. 33.4. Promotional spending on prescription drugs, year 2000

tising. The drugs most heavily promoted to consumers as well as physicians are typically drugs that treat chronic conditions. They tend to be newer, and more expensive than the drugs they are intended to replace [12]. With the arrival of MIS arthroplasty, manufacturers have found a unique opportunity to approach consumers directly through DTC advertising using primarily television and the web. The use of sports stars in these advertisements is not unusual, especially given the improved performance desired with orthopedic operations and implants. Moreover, associating a sports star and improved function with an arthroplasty implant provides the consumer with positive images of their potential outcome.

Increased Awareness

A study reported in the *Journal of General Internal Medicine* found that 43% of respondents in a telephone survey thought that only "completely safe" drugs could

be advertised [14]. The same data also noted that respondents would be disappointed if their physician did not fill the drug requested on the basis of DTC advertising, that some would consider obtaining the prescription elsewhere, and would be dissatisfied with their physician [15]. This issue has not been studied in DTC arthroplasty implant advertising. Another study found that clinicians presented with a stylized scenario in which patients requested information based on exposure to DTC advertising were annoyed with the patient request, less likely to provide information, or provide samples of the requested drug [16]. However, clinicians might respond very differently in real situations when there are patients in their offices asking for a specific advertised drug. This issue is addressed in the following study which gathered information from patients prior to seeing the physician and information from the physicians after the patient visit. The study found that 7.2% of patients requested an advertised drug that the physician prescribed the requested drug in 78% of the cases, that patients who requested the advertised drug received more drug prescriptions than those who did not, and that physicians were somewhat ambivalent about prescribing the requested drug [17]. The evidence is clear that consumers are becoming aware of more new drugs through DTC advertising. In a survey of 1200 consumers conducted by *Prevention* magazine and the American Pharmaceutical Association, 39% said they had talked with their doctor about a drug they had seen advertised, 28% of these individuals requested one of the advertised drugs, and the drug was prescribed by the doctor in 84% of the cases. The difference in prescribing rates may be due to the drugs being advertised, the geographic variations or the type of physician. A positive outcome was that a third of those who had seen an advertisement for the medication they were taking said they were reminded to fill their prescription [18]. Similar results were reported in a 1999 telephone survey conducted by the FDA [19]. Another report indicated that awareness of a heavily promoted drug did not necessarily translate to knowledge of the medical condition for which the drug was suited. Of ten heavily promoted drugs, only Claritin had awareness and knowledge levels above 70%; Lipitor's was 40%, and the others were below 32% or less [20]. The promotion and information blend of DTC advertising represents an opportunity to increase awareness and knowledge for consumers.

33

Ethical and Regulatory Issues

The debate is still growing on whether DTC advertising in healthcare has positive or negative effects. This is a complex issue because there are multiple stakeholders from patients to doctors to managed care to insurers to the government and to society as a whole. A positive argument is patient empowerment; that educating patients is beneficial and those patients who have a better understanding of their medical conditions can interact more intelligently and more effectively with their doctors. A second argument is that DTC advertising raises public awareness of medical conditions that are age-, gender- or race-related, which in turn results in these target populations visiting doctors' offices to be screened for the condition. The counter argument is that the basic objective of advertising is to sell more products, that DTC advertising is not different and that patients are not well served by the information available through broadcast DTC advertising.

The impact of DTC advertising on doctors is mixed. One might believe that doctors would like to interact with patients who are engaged and informed. At the same time, doctors would not like to be pressured by their patients in prescribing drugs when the knowledge base of the patients is television advertising. Many surgeons are bombarded with patients presenting a stack of information from web sites that do not present entirely accurate information. A survey of 2000 physicians in 1998 found that more than a third felt that DTC advertisements confused patients, about 40% were ambivalent, and about 16% thought that DTC ads did more harm than good. The majority of the doctors surveyed (64%) would like to see DTC advertising decreased or discontinued [21]. An AMA member pulse poll found that 72% of the respondents felt that DTC advertising had a negative impact on their practice.

Expenditure on drugs and implants that require a prescription for dispensing to patients is increasing faster than hospital-spending or physician services for managed care organizations and insurers. Pharmacy-spending has risen from the mid-single digits to double digits for most insurance plans. A big factor in the increased expenditures is the high prices of new drugs. A second factor that is being blamed is DTC advertising [22]. With the introduction of ceramic technology and MIS procedures, orthopedic surgery is also experiencing significant growth in implant costs. The increases in these costs will trigger increases in the premiums as well as increases in co-payment for drugs. Of course, those without prescription drug-insurance coverage will be faced with steep increases in their out-of-pocket costs. Implant costs will be borne by the hospital unless their purchasing contracts and insurance contracts account for these higher costs.

Society at large faces difficult choices. The products depicted in DTC advertising represent a small part of overall health expenditures but are rising at a fast rate and are a very visible component. In 1997, pharmaceuticals represented 7.2% of total national health expenditures and are expected to account for 11.2% in 2008. Similar data is not available for arthroplasty implants but are the active focus of our research. Needless to say, if a positive interaction between DTC advertising and new products is observed by manufacturers, the increase will be further exacerbated. Although drug companies spend more money on marketing than research and development, similar data is not available for implant companies. Will opportunities to spend money directly marketing products to consumers make the implant manufacturers appear more like a merchandising company?

References

1. Direct-to-consumer promotion; public hearing. 16th August, 60 Federal Register 158: 42581–42584, 1995
2. U.S. Department of Health and Human Services, FDA, CDER, CBER and CVM: Guidance for Industry: Consumer-Directed Broadcast Advertisement. August 1999
3. Food and Drug Administration, U.S. Department of Health and Human Services, CFR 202. 1(e): Prescription Drug Advertising
4. Lyles A: Direct marketing of pharmaceuticals to consumers. Ann Rev Pub Health 2002, 23: 73–91
5. Bell RA, Kravitz RL, Wilkes MS: Direct-to-consumer prescription drug advertising, 1989–1998: A content analysis of conditions, targets, inducements, and appeals. J Family Pract 2000, 49; 329–335
6. Woloshin S, Schwartz LM, Tremmel J, Welch HG: Direct-to-consumer advertisements for prescription drugs: what are Americans being sold? Lancet 2001, 358: 1141–1146
7. Bhattacharyya T, Tornetta P, Healy W, Einhorn TA: The validity of claims made in orthopaedic print advertisements. J Bone Joint Surg 2003, 85A: 1224–1228
8. Wilkes MS, Bell RA, Kravitz R: Direct-to-consumer prescription drug advertising: trends, impact and implications. Health Affairs 1999, 19: 110–128
9. Temin P: Taking your medicine: drug regulation in the United States. Cambridge, MA; Harvard University Press, 1980
10. Becker C: Skipping the hospital. Implant campaign goes straight to the patient. Modern Healthcare 2003, 33: 16

11. Ying Xie: Essays on promotion mix management: an application to the prescription pharmaceutical industry. Dissertation, Northwestern University, Evanston, Il, 2003

12. Kaiser Family Foundation: Impact of direct-to-consumer advertising on prescription drug spending, 2003

13. IMS Health Inc., Integrated Promotion Service, and Competitive Media Reporting 1996–2002

14. Bell RA, Kravitz RL, Wilkes MS: Direct-to-consumer prescription drug advertising and the public. J General Int Med 1999, 14: 651–657

15. Bell RA, Wilkes MS, Kravitz RL: Advertisement-induced prescription drug requests: patients' anticipated reactions to a physician who refuses, J Family Pract 1999; 48: 446–452

16. Zachary WM, Dalen JE, Jackson TR: Clinicians' responses to direct-to-consumer advertising of prescription medications. Arch Intern Med 2003, 163: 1808–1812

17. Mintzes B, Barer ML, Kravitz RL et al.: How does direct-to-consumer advertising (DTCA) affect prescribing? A survey in primary care environments with and without legal DTCA. Can Med Assoc J 2003, 169: 405–412

18. National Survey of consumer reactions to direct-to-consumer advertising. Prevention Magazine, July 1999

19. Attitudes and behaviors associated with direct-to-consumer promotion of prescription drugs. Center for Drug Evaluation and Research, FDA, Spring 1999

20. Lyles A: Direct marketing of pharmaceuticals to consumers. Ann Rev Public Health 2002, 23: 73–91

21. Findlay S: Direct-to-consumer promotion of prescription drugs: economic implications for patients, payers and providers. Pharmacoeconomics 2001, 19(2): 109–119

22. Hunt MI: Factors contributing to rising pharmacy costs. Available on Blue Cross Blue Shield Association Web Site, 2000

Ethics and Minimal Incision Total Joint Arthroplasty

J.R. Lieberman

Introduction

The fact that this whole text is devoted to minimal incision total joint arthroplasty clearly demonstrates that this technique has captured the attention of orthopedic surgeons and the public. In general, orthopedic surgeons embrace new surgical procedures and new technology because there is a belief that new methods will enhance patient outcomes. However, when using a new surgical technique, patient safety is a critical issue. Careful assessments of patients that receive new treatments are necessary to determine that the technology is actually cost-effective. There are a number of important issues that require clarification within the orthopedic community in order to enhance the development of minimal incision total joint arthroplasty and other new surgical procedures but also to protect patient safety. These issues include the following:

- establishing guidelines for the use of the regulatory ethics paradigm particularly related to the implementation of new surgical procedures that do not require FDA approval;
- recognition of the importance of providing patients with true informed consent about both the potential benefits and the complications associated with a new surgical technique;
- the potential pitfalls associated with collaborative relationships with industry and their impact on patient safety [2, 5].

When Is Innovation Really Experimentation?

The development of new surgical techniques is clearly necessary if patient care is going to be improved over time. According to the regulatory ethics paradigm (REP), any drug or innovative surgical technique would need to be placed into an institutional review-board-approved protocol in order to protect patient welfare [1]. Clearly, this has been well accepted with new drugs because they require rigorous pre-clinical studies, clinical trials and FDA approval. However, the question is: how does the regulatory ethics paradigm apply to the use of new surgical procedures that typically do not require FDA approval? The proponents of the regulatory ethics paradigm argue that the development of new surgical techniques is really human experimentation and therefore must be evaluated in IRB-approved protocols. If there is no IRB-approved protocol then the implementation of the new surgical intervention would not meet appropriate ethical standards [8]. This standard has been set in order to protect patient welfare.

In a provocative essay, Agich stated that the regulatory ethics paradigm may not be necessary for the development of certain surgical procedures [1]. In clinical situations where present treatments are not optimal or even ineffective, the REP may not be applicable. However, an IRB-approved n=1 trial could be implemented in such cases [4]. In addition, IRB approval is not possible in emergency situations and surgical innovations can be used as long as informed consent is obtained. Using an IRB protocol may be difficult during the developmental phase because the development of a surgical technique requires frequent adjustments. Major or minor modifications of the surgical approach, the design of new surgical instruments and identifying the appropriate patient population are usually necessary [5, 8]. However, the development of an institutional review-board-approved protocol to assess a new surgical procedure should not be avoided because it is inconvenient [2, 5].

There is also confusion about the necessity of an IRB-approval protocol when a surgeon innovator modifies an established procedure. Historically, IRB approval has not been obtained. It may be argued that the application of a minimal incision total hip arthroplasty where the same approach is used but the incision is shorter does not require an IRB-approved protocol. However, the use of two-incision technique may require IRB approval because it is a more radical change from established techniques. Again, the goal is to maintain patient safety. The potential problem with eliminating IRB-approved protocols during the initial implementation of surgical procedures is that the new procedure may not be studied in a rigorous fashion in order to determine its true efficacy and cost effectiveness. This is what has already happened with minimal incision total joint replacement. Surgeons have embraced this technique but there is little data regarding efficacy or complication rates. Patients must understand that a smaller incision does not equate with fewer complications or that a smaller incision will insure better long-term outcomes. The optimal way to truly determine the efficacy of minimal incision hip or knee arthroplasty is to perform a randomized trial comparing mini-incision and standard-incision total joint arthroplasty. A randomized trial also needs to be performed comparing a two-incision total hip arthroplasty with a single-incision mini-total hip arthroplasty to compare the efficacy and safety of these techniques. Finally, the term minimally invasive surgery should be eliminated. This term suggests that in some way the total joint arthroplasty performed with this technique is less invasive. This is actually misleading and may suggest to the patient that a minimally invasive hip is in some way safer for them.

Surgeon innovators must also be aware that there is potential conflict of interest with their patient because a surgical technique may not be better than the standard procedure [5, 7]. Patients often assume that new techniques are better than the old ones. McKneally has proposed that the term non-validated be used instead of innovative when describing a new surgical procedure. In western society, innovation implies added value and this by definition suggests that any new procedure will lead to enhanced outcomes. Patients may also not be aware of the potential for increased risks [6]. For

example, patients may not realize that at the present time the prostheses used are the same whether a standard or a minimal incision total hip arthroplasty is performed.

Another important question is when should a new technique be made available to the general orthopedic community? In general, the widespread use of the new technique or new technology should be delayed until the indications, pitfalls and potential complications have been identified. This has been a common problem in orthopedic surgery for many years. There are surgical techniques and technologies that have been employed for the past few decades and their outcomes have not been established in clinical trials nor has a prospective analysis of a specific patient population ever been performed. For example, the microfracture technique and autologous chondrocyte transplantation to treat cartilage defects and the use of non-vascularized or vascularized bone grafts to treat osteonecrosis of the hip have not been assessed in rigorous randomized multi-center clinical trials [2, 5]. The success of these techniques is still questioned by many in the orthopedic community. The recent focus on minimal incision surgery suggests that the efficacy of these techniques may not be determined in randomized trials either. It is doubtful that decreasing an incision from 6 inches to 4 inches with a posterolateral or lateral approach will have a significant benefit with respect to long-term outcomes. However, the use of a two-incision technique could have an impact on the outcomes and on peri-operative complication rates either positively or negatively but this can only be truly determined by a randomized trial. However, once a surgical procedure spreads to the orthopedic community, a randomized trial becomes difficult to perform. Patients want the new procedure because they believe anything that is new is better.

Clearly, there is no consensus regarding the precise line between innovation and experimentation. One argument for performing a clinical trial in such cases is that when the patient is a research subject they are more likely to understand that there is a lack of evidence regarding the efficacy of the new procedure and long-term outcomes. Therefore, under all circumstances it is imperative that the surgeon have a candid discussion with the patient about the potential benefits and the risks and complications of using a new procedure and the lack of evidence-based information [5].

Informed Consent and New Surgical Techniques

Over the next two decades, the advent of computerized technology will lead to adaptations in a variety of surgical procedures. A major issue that needs to be resolved is what are the best ways for surgeons to learn these new procedures? What training is necessary to learn how to use a new surgical technique? The answer to these questions will obviously be influenced by the type of procedure that is being performed, techniques that are being learned and the surgeon's prior surgical experience. There is pressure on surgeons to use new techniques even if their efficacy has not been established in order to maintain market share in their community and be recognized as a cutting-edge physician. This type of pressure can obviously lead to problems in patient care and patient outcomes [2, 5].

Although firm guidelines may not need to be established, it is imperative that surgeons receive adequate training before using a new procedure in their practice. Surgeons must also fully comprehend the indications and contra-indications for the new technique. It is also quite important that the surgeons have a frank discussion with their patients about the potential benefits and risks of any new procedure and the surgeon's experience with that procedure [2, 5]. As stated previously, patients usually assume that a new procedure should have a better outcome than an old procedure. In addition, patients may assume that new procedures particularly those using minimal incision techniques or computerized technology may have lower risks and complication rates. Patients may not understand that although minimal incision surgery has a small skin incision the decreased exposure may lead to complication rates that are equal to or even greater than those associated with the standard procedure [2, 5]. Surgeons need to thoroughly discuss the advantages, disadvantages, outcomes and complication rates associated with any surgical procedure. If there is no evidence-based data or long-term outcomes information available, then patients should receive this information, too. Finally, surgeons must candidly discuss their experience with a new surgical technique. Recently, the first information regarding the learning curve associated with the two-incision total hip arthroplasty was reported. The initial results of 423 total hip arthroplasties performed by 89 surgeons revealed an operative fracture rate of 6.7% and an early revision rate of 0.9%. Although operative time decreased between a surgeon's first case and tenth case, critical complications such as femoral fracture, nerve injury and dislocation did not decrease [9]. The question is: will surgeons share this information with their patients and compare their own results to this group? Would this information dampen patients' enthusiasm for this type of procedure?

Surgeon and Their Industrial Partner

The current economics of healthcare and limited resources available to most surgeons make it extremely difficult to develop new technology without an industrial partner [3, 5]. Industry has the infrastructure to develop new technology and the resources to make the new technology available to a wider audience. Numerous advances in orthopedic surgery have occurred as a result of successful collaborations between orthopedic surgeons and their industrial partners [3, 6]. However, the surgeon that is involved in one of these relationships must remember that the ultimate goal is to maintain patient safety. Surgeons must realize the conflicts of interests inherent in the surgeon-industry relationship and its potential impact on patient care. For example, a company has a significant financial interest in the development of a new technology and may be under pressure to obtain a return on an investment [2, 5]. Therefore, the use of a new technology may be brought to the market place before it has been adequately assessed. In the particular case of minimal incision surgery, for the first time manufacturers have become actively involved in promoting a surgical technique. In this instance, manufacturers may not be interested in supporting clinical trials in order to save resources especially if the benefits are uncertain or a randomized trial is not required by the Food and Drug Administration.

Manufacturers are now marketing directly to consumers to move the marketplace in a specific direction. These advertisements seem to urge patients to seek physicians that prescribe specific drugs, use new devices and use new surgical procedures, even though better outcomes may not have not have been established. Paradoxically, this may lead to a conflict of interest between the surgeon and the patient. Surgeons may feel pressure to use a device that is not ideal for a particular patient because of concerns that the patient may seek treatment elsewhere. In a recent report regarding the two-incision technique, a 93-year-old patient received a total hip arthroplasty using this non-validated technique [9].

In conclusion, minimal incision total joint replacement has the potential to enhance the care of orthopedic patients. It is appropriate for surgeons to embrace this new technique in order to enhance outcomes and practice efficiencies. However, the orthopedic community must temper its enthusiasm for new surgical techniques by remembering our responsibility to protect the safety of our patients. It is imperative that surgeons determine the appropriate indications for the use of this technique and to demonstrate its benefits and limitations. In addition, surgeons must take the appropriate steps necessary to become facile with these procedures so that patient care is not jeopardized [5]. The doctor–patient relationship continues to evolve as a result of the internet, direct marketing to consumers and the expansion of managed care. However, it is essential that patients continue to believe that physicians are acting on their behalf or we will lose the public's trust.

References

1. Agich GJ. Ethics and innovation in medicine. J Med Ethics 2001; 27: 295–296
2. Berry DJ, Berger RA, Callaghan JJ, Dorr LD, Duwelius PJ, Hartzband MA, Lieberman JR, Mears DC. Symposium: Minimally invasive total hip arthroplasty. Development, early results, and critical analysis. J Bone Joint Surg 2000; 85-A: 2003
3. Boyd EA, Bero LA. Assessing faculty financial relationships with industry: A case study. JAMA 2000; 284: 2209–2214
4. Larson EB, Ellsworth AJ, Oas J. Randomized clinical trials in single patients during a 2-year period. JAMA 1993; 270: 2708–2712
5. Lieberman JR, Wenger N. New technology and the orthopaedic surgeon. Are you protecting your patients? Clin Orthop (submitted)
6. McKneally MF, Daar AS. Introducing new technologies: protecting subjects of surgical innovation and research. World J Surg 2003; 27: 930–934
7. Miller FG, Rosenstein DL, DeRenzo EG. Professional integrity in clinical research. JAMA 1998; 280: 1449–1454
8. Wheeler R. One person's innovation is another's experiment. BMJ 2000; 320: 1548
9. White RG, Archibeck MJ. Learning curve for the two incision, minimally invasive total hip replacement. Presented at the annual open meeting of the Hip Society. American Academy of Orthopaedic Surgeons, San Francisco, CA, March 13, 2004

Is MIS a Faulty Paradigm?

J.J. Callaghan

Those of us in the medical profession have pledged to provide the best care of our patients with medical problems. Both hip and knee replacement have been shown to safely and effectively relieve pain, restore motion, and improve function. Over the past three to four decades the procedures have been refined so as to be performed efficiently and predictably with excellent long-term durability. If the procedures could be performed with less tissue trauma but not at the expense of safety, efficacy, durability and overall patient satisfaction, it would be desirable to both the patient and the surgeon. During this long experience with hip and knee arthroplasty, investigators and surgeons have documented some of the complications and shortcomings of the procedure as well as some of the potential innovations which through the test of time were considered "steps backwards." The potential benefits of the mini-invasive approach have been outlined in this book and early reports [1–3] (i.e. cosmesis, quicker functional return, short length of stay, fewer transfusions).

The surgeon should remember that these are only short-term goals. If these goals can be accomplished while still addressing the major issues which confront the orthopedic surgeon performing total hip and knee replacement today, there may be a place for this enthusiasm. However, as will be argued in this chapter, there are several reasons for skepticism as well as concerns for the approaches that have been implemented to encourage the widespread use of the minimally invasive approach.

What is the major problem with total hip and knee arthroplasty today? More data concerning this topic is available in the hip literature than the knee literature; however, the trends are similar. From both an economic perspective, as well as from the perspective of the patient requiring a total hip or knee arthroplasty, the need for further surgery following the index procedure is of paramount concern. The hip-replacement revision burden in the United States is 18–20% and unfortunately it is twice that of some other countries such as Sweden where that burden is 8% [4]. More data is arising to suggest that the volume of surgery performed at an institution as well as the volume of surgery performed by individual surgeons is a major factor in contributing to the revision burden [5]. However, the practical reality is that more, not less, total hip and knee replacements will be indicated in the aging and active population as data suggest people will be living longer (hence have an increase risk for developing disabling hip and knee arthritis) and the "baby boomer" generation is reaching the peak onset age for developing disabling hip arthritis. These replacements cannot all be done at centers doing over 500 to 1000 hip and knee replacements a year. There will still be a huge need for surgeons doing less than 50 hip and knee arthroplasties a year and they need to be performed with the least complications and with the least possible need for revision as both are costly to the patient and society. In addition, the rise in obesity may prohibit more and more patients with disabling hip and knee arthritis from being optimal candidates for the mini-invasive procedure. Proponents of the procedure recommend a body mass index of less than 30 for performing the mini-invasive procedures. All of the initial procedures and data collection are being performed on the younger, healthier, physically fit patients. They are not being performed on hips and knees with complex deformity (i.e. severe hip dysplasia). These results cannot be generalized to many hip- and knee-replacement practices.

What are the major complications following total hip replacement that require revision? Failure of fixation, instability and infection have been documented as the major causes of re-operation following total hip replacement. To minimize failure of fixation, implant bone interfaces must be optimally prepared. To minimize dislocation, components need to be properly positioned and hip stability needs to be assessed. To minimize infection, tissue trauma needs to be minimized, as does the time of operation. Small incisions do not address these problems and they could potentially increase each of these problems, especially in the hands of the less skilled surgeon or the surgeon who is doing fewer procedures. Some enthusiasts of the minimally invasive procedure assert that combining the minimally invasive procedure with computer-assistive surgery will compensate for the lack of visualization allowed by the small incision and the approach. This presents a tremendous risk for very little if any proven benefit. If the surgeon needs accurate positioning of markers which need to be secured throughout the case, how can he or she be sure they correctly positioned the marker and that the data collected is accurate? Have these systems been validated for all the variances of anatomy?

Is the comparison of minimally invasive hip- and knee-replacement surgery to the conversion from knee arthrotomy to knee arthroscopy accurate? There are reasons why this argument may not hold. The short- and long-term results of knee arthrotomy unlike total hip and knee replacement were not optimal. In addition, it has been documented that visualization is actually better with arthroscopy. This claim has not and cannot be made for minimally invasive hip and knee surgery. Minimally invasive hip and knee surgery may turn out to be more akin to endoscopic carpal-tunnel surgery or minimally invasive direct coronary artery bypass surgery than to the knee-arthroscopy explosion. Endoscopic carpal tunnel was touted for its ability to provide a smaller scar and early return to work. The peer-review publications demonstrated no long-term benefit. Today, questions arise as to whether the potential early return to work after the procedure was more perceptual (the surgeons enthusiasm for the procedure and the patients' desire to please the surgeon) than reality. The major complications, including nerve laceration and tendon injury, still occurred after experience was gained with the procedure. For these reasons, endo-scopic carpal tunnel, which initially gained enthusiasm and popularity, has been abandoned by the vast majority of hand surgeons. With minimally invasive coronary artery bypass surgery only 25% of cardiac surgeons use the technique and some use it selectively. Wound infection, myocardial infarction, atrial fibrillation, stroke, and mortality continue to be problems. Properly performed prospective studies are lacking. This skeptic questions whether a joint-replacement surgeon, who selects out the most motivated and fittest patients, preloads those patients for early discharge, and performs the standard incision with optimal pre-operative, intra-operative and post-operative anesthesia, pain management and rehabilitation, would not match the early and long-term results of the surgeon using the minimally invasive approach.

Is there medically legal liability issues associated with implementing the mini-invasive hip-replacement approach? The argument has been stated that since the patient has come to the surgeon desiring the technique that he or she must understand there is a learning curve including increased potential for nerve palsy and component mal-position. Legally, the surgeon should recognize he or she will be judged by the same standards as the surgeon using conventional incisions. It will be hard to defend a new "norm" which allows for a higher complication rate. It will be difficult to define competence, proficiency and qualifications for performing a new and potentially risky procedure. In addition, complications may not be as well understood by patients with extremely high expectations of the surgery.

Has the mini-invasive hip-surgery movement been appropriately implemented? The Internet and advertising have allowed patients to seek new treatments before traditional peer review can be completed [6]. This creates potential problems for both the surgeon and the patient. There are many examples of self-aggrandizing promotions of unique treatments outside the peer-reviewed system that have not held up to the scientific review process or have not withstood the test of time. Our medical profession has been designed for us to self-regulate. We have an obligation to educate the public and help them interpret non-scientific premises and promotions. Developers of groundbreaking treatments for patient care are obligated to promote their ideas through the scientific peer review of their data, which can substantiate their enthusiasm. In this era, evidence-based studies should be mandatory. In the case of the mini-invasive approach to hip surgery, the promoters have rarely recognized the work of Keggi, as reported by Light in 1980 [7], of a similar mini-invasive approach for performing total hip replacement which never became popular. One surgeon has sought and obtained a methodology patent on performing hip surgery through two small incisions and inserting the components through the different incisions (acetabular component anteriorly and femoral component posteriorly). If a treatment does prove to be an improvement, it should not be limited to a selected group of surgeons. These premises are the basis for the respect the public holds for the medical profession today.

It is the job of a skeptic to ask tough questions. This skeptic hopes that the mini-invasive hip surgery enthusiasm proves him wrong for this skeptical stance.

References

1. Wenz JF, Gurkan I, Jibodh SR. Mini-incision total hip arthroplasty: a comparative assessment of perioperative outcomes. Orthopedics 2002; 25: 1031–1043
2. Waldman BJ. Minimally invasive total hip replacement and perioperative management: early experience. J Southern Orthop Assoc 2002; 11: 213–217
3. DiGioia AM III, Plakseychuk AY, Levison TJ, Jaramaz B. Mini-incision technique for total hip arthroplasty with navigation. J Arthroplasty 2003; 18: 123–128
4. Maloney WJ. National joint replacement registries: has the time come? J Bone Joint Surg 2001; 83A: 1582–1585
5. Mahomed NN, Barrett JA, Katz JN et al. Rates and outcomes of primary and revision total hip replacement in the united states medicare population. J Bone Joint Surg 2003; 85A: 27–32
6. Hozack WJ, Ranawat C, Roth RH. Editorial: How to deliver the word? J Arthroplasty 2002; 17: 389
7. Light TR, Keggi KJ. Anterior approach to hip arthroplasty. Clin Orthop Rel Res 1980; 152: 255–260

Perspective on MIS and CAOS: What Can the Engineer Do for These Concepts?

J.L. Moctezuma de la Barrera

Introduction

Computer-assisted surgery has enabled the clinician to quantify findings less subjectively by providing measurement tools adequately tailored for different assessment activities. Tools range from image analysis for 3D exploration of diagnostic information to surgical navigation where the geometrical relationships of instruments and implants are displayed relative to anatomical structures. These capabilities have led to a re-thinking process on how anatomical structures and their relationships should be adequately described. Also, through a less subjectivity-prone relationship description–methodology, an effort to more accurately understand the consequences of a certain therapy action involving geometrical re-alignment of anatomical structures is underway. Studies involve short-, mid- and long-term follow-ups.

Minimal invasive surgical techniques reduce direct visualization of the anatomical structures of relevance sometimes dramatically reducing the surgeon's ability to properly assess the biomechanical arrangement during therapy. This in turn presents a challenge for the engineer in providing adequate technology to overcome this deficit. This article gives an overview on how technology can assist in providing the orthopedic surgeon with reliable methods to assess geometrical and biomechanical relationships under limited or without direct visualization of the surgical field.

Understanding Biomechanical Relationships

In total hip and knee arthroplasty the description of the biomechanical relationships of the implants has been traditionally limited to the frontal plane, where the interaction of forces with weight-bearing surfaces and interfaces are analyzed for the static upright-standing loading scenario. Other relationships are often derived from morphological analysis which leads to an averaged anatomical description that maybe sometimes biased by the chosen ethnic group for the analysis and from time to time fails to accurately fit the patient-specific situation. In hip arthroplasty, for example, while orientation of the cup can be assessed in a standing X-ray film, the true relationship between pelvis flexion and its influence to anteversion and inclination is not known.

In knee arthroplasty, alignment in the coronal plane, facilitated also by the ability to capture the projected mechanical axis on standing X-rays, has always played an important role in determining the degree of varus/valgus mal-alignment and provide means for planning of the corrective measure. In contrast, alignment of the other degrees of freedom of the prosthesis components is achieved intra-operatively, following more or less prominent anatomical landmarks. Especially flexion has not been addressed satisfactorily by conventional surgical instrumentation. Surgical navigation provides methods not only to intra-operatively define the mechanical axis but also the other necessary degrees of freedom to establish an orthogonal reference system where rotational orientation of the surgical components can be described. Flexion can then be described relative to the mechanical axis in the sagittal plane instead of the arbitrary description based on the inserted intramedullary rod which approximates the distal anatomical femoral axis as a secant of the arched femur. Depending on the anterior height of the opening of the femoral canal, the degree of curvature of the femur in the coronal and sagittal planes as well as the inner diaphyseal diameter a different flexion is achieved.

Surgical navigation with its ability to intra-operatively analyze and establish patient-specific anatomical and biomechanical relationships will doubtlessly play a key role together with modular implant systems that will allow the surgeon to accommodate for patient-specific arthroplastic requirements and demands.

Integrated Instrumentation

State of the art navigation is generally achieved by retrofitting tracking technology onto existing instrumentation. One major inconvenience is that existing instrumentation obviously was not designed in the first place to accommodate for such adaptation, thus making a calibration necessary. This step is in turn needed to establish the relationship between the instrument's effectuating tip and the tracking unit. Another inconvenience is the often awkward arrangement which results from the need to securely attach the tracking unit via a coupling mechanism onto an available mating surface or feature of the instrument. A further downside of ad-hoc adaptation of tracking technology is the fact that the mechanical coupling relies on friction and is therefore susceptible to impaction. If loads barely exceed the coupling's threshold, a shift of the relative position of the tracking unit may occur, leading to inaccurate readings of the position of the tracked instrument. Especially slight alterations of the calibrated situation may be difficult to perceive with the naked eye. ◘ Figure 36.1 shows a comparison of ad-hoc adapted instrumentation and integrated instrumentation.

In summary, the biggest downsides of adapted instrumentation are:

- calibration required,
- decreased ergonomics,
- impaction susceptible.

Integrated instrumentation not only overcomes these problems but also opens up new opportunities for further optimization and simplification of the procedure. Seamless integration of tracking technology makes instrumentation ergonomic and ready to use without delays and constraints. Nevertheless, tracking technology only covers one aspect of modern instrumentation. A classification of orthopedic instrumentation functionality can be shown in ◘ Fig. 36.2.

Conventional instrumentation implements the diversity of the required functionality throughout the procedures by providing a specific mechanical solution for each of step. The result is a complex and vast array of

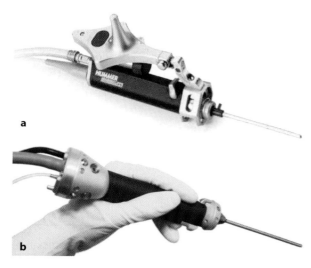

◘ Fig. 36.1. **a** Ad-hoc adaptation, **b** integrated solution

instruments which ultimately make the procedure lengthier and costlier.

◘ Figure 36.3 demonstrates the potential for integration of not only tracking technology for alignment purposes but further technology to implement required complimentary operations in order to reduce procedural complexity. An example borrowed from the knee arthroplasty is a dedicated cutting jig that combines computer-assisted alignment with suspension and motion constraining capabilities (◘ Fig. 36.4).

Also, consequent utilization of navigation capabilities together with geometric and kinematic information of the used implants can lead to further obviation of manual steps as gauging and sizing, which in such case would result as a by-product of anatomical and biomechanical initialization. For this purpose a readily accessible database can be made available where information is directly stored as an integral part of implants and instrumentation or it is downloaded through the network from a central data warehouse or a combination of both.

◘ Table 36.1 gives a comparison of the potential for OR-time reduction in relation to the degree of instrumentation integration.

Flexibility of Surgical Protocol

Analysis of the workflow of a surgical procedure is essential for the design of a computer application aimed to assist the surgeon. Nevertheless, concentrating too much on a specific flavor of a surgical protocol or other preferences leads often to rigid applications that do not accommodate easily for eventualities departing from the implemented application's workflow. However, technical solutions with too much flexibility tend to be hard to manage and are abandoned after the hype has settled. In this case, the added value to improve the outcome is certainly diminished by the increased time that the surgeon has to spend interacting with the assisting application.

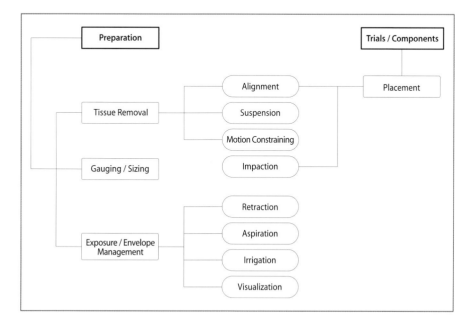

Fig. 36.2. Orthopedic instrumentation functionality

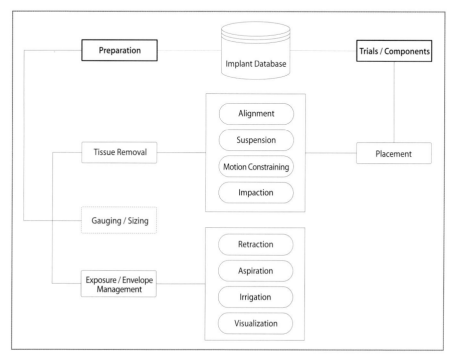

Fig. 36.3. Potential for functionality integration

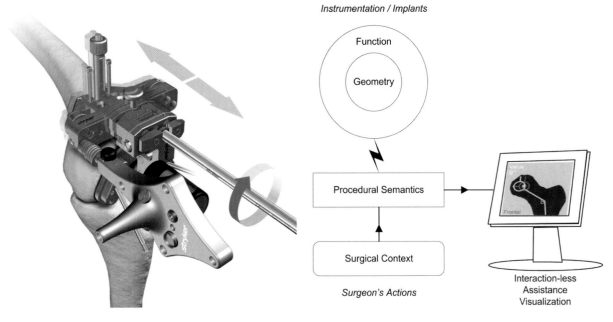

Fig. 36.4. Integration example

Fig. 36.5. "Reactive Workflow" concept

Table 36.1. Comparison of the potential for OR time reduction in relation to the degree of instrumentation integration

Instrumentation Type	Potential for OR Time Reduction
Ad-hoc adaptation	–
Seamless tracking technology integration	0
Smart instrumentation	++

Instead of targeting a happy medium with conscious trade-offs for an application, technology can help here again to free up the surgeon from performing tasks that do not relate immediately to the surgical procedure as e.g. pushing buttons on a screen to be able to visualize alignment of the instrumentation.

Reactive Workflow Through Linked Smart Instrumentation

Embedding information in instrumentation can be efficiently achieved by e.g. placing a silicon chip directly onto the body of the instrument. Wireless communication technologies make it possible to retrieve and store data from an application. Bringing the gathered information from the smart instrumentation together with the procedural semantics and the surgical context enables the assisting application to react to surgeons' actions and deliver automatically adequate procedural information and support, completely obviating the need for the surgeon to interact with the system-user interface and thus sparing time, but more important letting him dedicate undivided attention to his surgical actions and performance (■ Fig. 36.5).

Summary

Close integration of technologies into modern dedicated instrumentation will contribute to the reduction of procedural complexity. Technologically enhanced and streamlined-navigated instrumentation together with computer assistance will contribute to improve the efficiency and reproducibility of minimal invasive surgical techniques overcoming the downsides of poor visualization. Theses will in turn continue to advance tissue-sparing techniques and with it the entire patient-related benefits.

How Should We teach MIS?

A.G. Rosenberg

There are few studies that have effectively evaluated real-time surgical performance characteristics in a meaningful way. More fundamentally, there is, unfortunately, little research in the realm of surgical education to determine the performance requirements of surgical procedures in general and those of less invasive procedures in particular. However, it is ethically incumbent upon those surgeons promoting new techniques to evaluate not only their effectiveness but the most appropriate methods of teaching these techniques [1].

The old adage that it takes one year to teach someone how to operate, 5 years when to operate and a lifetime when not to operate seems to make the point that surgical skills (particularly psychomotor skills) are the easiest and most readily taught of the surgeon's repertoire. The implication is that psychomotor skills are substantively different from cognitive skills. But to the surgeon who gives this only a little thought it is clear that surgical performance is based on a continuous feedback loop of psychomotor performance and cognitive function. It is the continuous and ongoing decision-making (albeit almost always at a subconscious level) in the midst of physical performance that influences the quality of the physical intervention. Where the acquisition and execution of psychomotor skills is critical, it is still pre-requisite and symbiotic with the cognitive skill set applied during real-time performance This is the case for all high-performance occupations whether it is the airline pilot, combat soldier, or surgeon.

To what extent the development of these cognitive and motor skills (and their interaction) governs the eventual outcome is a complex problem that has not yet been fully investigated and remains poorly understood. Indeed, to paraphrase Bob Booth, "many more surgeons have done a video analysis of their golf swing than have evaluated their operative performance."

The question implied in the title of this chapter can only be answered by understanding both the current methods of surgical training and their relationship to the practice requirements of contemporary and more specifically minimally invasive surgery. Further implied is the question: are the specific surgical requirements of the MIS procedure such that they require an alteration in the manner in which we train surgeons? An additional implied assumption in the evaluation of these issues is the perception, which appears to be correct but as yet not rigorously established, that the performance of minimally invasive procedures in the training environment substantially alters the educational experience for the learning surgeon [2].

There is a host of subsidiary questions thereby raised and which require answer:

- What are the performance requirements for MIS surgery?
- Do they differ substantially from that of routine non-MIS surgery?
- What are the relationships between surgical training methods and patient outcomes and do we understand these relationships sufficiently well to proceed to alter them in a meaningful fashion?
- Does the routine adoption of MIS surgical procedures alter the current teaching environment in a way that is deleterious to the learning surgeon?
- To what extent do the answers to the proceeding questions demand the development of new methods for surgical teaching as regards the MIS procedures?
- What form might these take?

The simple answer to the first question regarding performance skills is that the requirements of MIS surgery are simply those that are found in standard surgical procedures but taken to a higher level. This arises from two specific conditions inherent in MIS surgery: first that the ability to protect structures in the standard fashion are eliminated or altered in specific ways unique to the surgical procedure, and second that this results in a concomitant and directly proportional decrease in the margin of error for various intra-operative maneuvers. Small errors during the course of the operation are less easily recognized and adjusted for as the procedure progresses and the implications of these small errors are thereby potentially magnified. In addition, the specific anatomic features that may increase the degree of difficulty for the "open procedure" are magnified when the procedure is performed in a minimally invasive fashion. Finally, and perhaps most importantly, the development of minimally invasive techniques frequently involves the removal or diminution of traditional feedback signals or clues that the surgeon normally uses and have come to rely upon (sometimes unconsciously) to make continuous adjustments to his performance. Thus, skills that are little needed, infrequently utilized, or have not been previously recognized become of greater consequence. Indeed, the loss of these cues may need to be compensated for in technique-specific ways. Training surgeons to perform these techniques would therefore seem to require the development of both traditional surgical skills as well as new ones in ways that guarantees a higher performance level than has traditionally been required [3].

The need for new training methods implies two separate factors that may be driving this concern. First: are the training methods as currently employed adequate to the task as currently envisioned? And secondly: does the conversion in the training environment from open to MIS procedures degrade the actual training experience in general? As the latter is more readily answered than the former, we will begin there.

The performance of MIS procedures does alter the current training environment [2]. Visibility of the surgical field is reduced, compromising visual feedback not only to the performing surgeon but also to the learning surgeon dependent upon observation and demonstration. Are the traditional residency education and CME surgical training methods capable of meeting this standard? Unfortunately, the answer to this question is a rather harsh indictment of the current state of surgical training in general. This system is derived (with little improvement and perhaps even some newer flaws) from

the traditional systems of apprenticeship that began in the Italian city states following the Dark Ages. As initially adapted by the German schools of Kocher and Billroth, and modified in the United States by Halsted with the influence of Osler and others, the training methodology we use to teach surgical skills remains primitive and has enjoyed little improvements in either theory or practice over the decades, while the specific technical requirements of the surgical procedure itself seem to increase steadily. The combined requirements of service and education seem to serve the best interest of neither. The current training methods are in general applied unevenly and randomly to the resident participants. The common cliché – see one, do one, teach one – seems to summarize the cavalier approach to procedural teaching that has been the mainstay of surgical pedagogy. It is clear that future medical manipulative technologies whether they be traditional surgical or otherwise procedurally interventional will require more rather than less highly structured training and assessment methods [4]. The current crisis in resident education will be exacerbated by the reduction in effectiveness of the training environment and with the current trends in continuing education of moving to a rigorous demonstration of competency model, it is clearly not too soon to be seriously concerned with how surgery is being taught (and learned).

The performance of surgery is dependent on several factors. Historically many of these factors have only been available to the surgeon during the performance of actual surgical procedures and therefore presented the surgeon with no real opportunity to "practice" either the cognitive or psychomotor skills required in the performance of surgery [5]. In addition, there is little in the way of immediate information available to the surgeon during the course of the operation that would allow him to make the type of adjustments that are based on cause–effects/feedback loops.

With modern technology, many of the factors that contribute to surgical performance can be simulated and repeatedly experienced with immediate feedback on the correctness of decisions and behaviors [4]. Development and utilization of this technology would be expected to result in any given surgeons moving more rapidly along the learning curve, allowing the surgeon to perform at a higher level during the actual surgical encounter [6]. Despite the obstacles present to the current employment of actual psychomotor skills simulation, these devices will eventually be part of the surgical training environment.

The characteristics that make up surgical performance include pre-operative, intra-operative and post-operative factors. While the focus on surgical training must be on all three arenas, it is mainly in the intra-operative phase, where actual physical skills are required, that is seen by most trainees as being the area where there is the least opportunity to develop experience. Ideally experience is gained in an environment where feedback is immediate and mistakes are tolerated as part of the learning experience [1]. One of those things that have prevented surgeons from acquiring greater levels of skill prior to entering practice or even during practice is the lack of such a practice environment.

However, even in the performance of physical skills, there are multiple cognitive processes which must function correctly and efficiently to maximize surgical performance. In the coming era of virtual reality environments and surgical training simulators, there is good reason to believe that coupling of these technologies to assist the surgeon in acquiring both motor and cognitive skills will result in improved surgical performance as well as improved patient outcomes as a result of the clinical encounter [6, 7].

A current potential model for improving surgical responsiveness and judgment can be obtained by using the interactive video game as a model. The choices of this paradigm are the several features of the modern interactive video game that make it so compelling and popular. One primary attractive feature is the need for continuous involvement by the participant. Lapses of attention cause failure (or loss to an opponent). This need for continuous vigilance by the participant is structured into the gaming environment. This forcing function of involvement leads to a "flow" experience which has been described as exhilarating and involving, compelling attention and participation. Appropriately structured, the same environment can be used to improve both cognitive responses as well as judgments and response times as has been demonstrated in flight simulators. The application of structured learning experiences in this type of environment might be expected to achieve remarkable improvements in information transmission, a primary goal of the educational experience

Of additional import is the current status of computer guided and assisted procedures to the surgeon's armamentarium. As these technologies become more widely available, the surgeon will need opportunities to practice in the new environment created by the addition of a computerized guidance interface during surgical performance. Familiarity with the structure and content of guidance information as well as integration of this information with the traditional inputs acquired during surgery will be needed to improve the real time intra-operative judgments and physical performance measures needed to perform surgery. This familiarity can best be accomplished in a highly integrated simulation environment [4].

Enhancements can be introduced to this environment that will further improve surgical performance. Appropriately structured to approximate the real life decisions and judgments that the surgeon will be called upon to make, the addition of creative elements such as complication/disaster management, head-to-head- or machine-based competition, continuous probing for knowledge deficits, and reinforcing functions used to transmit important supplementary and supporting content, will produce a robust learning environment that will make the educational experience engaging, stimulating, challenging and fun.

In order to structure an environment that would provide for progressive advances in cognitive skills acquisition, several requirements must be met. First, we must create a knowledge base that will be utilized as the cognitive foundation for the simulation technology. This so-called "content knowledge" currently exists in the mind of the surgeons who currently provide education to trainees. Second, we must structure the knowledge base so that it can be represented in an algorithmic format with eventual conversion of these algorithms into the type of appropriate branching-chain pathways environment, which can be made accessible and modifiable at the computer interface. Third, multiple supplemental elements must be developed to provide for a more challenging and robust learning environment. Fourth, an assessment module with accompanying grading mechanism must be developed to couple the quality and intensity of the learning experience to the performance level and other individual educational needs of the learner.

Work on cognitive skills development, as well as visual skills acquisition, can be accomplished with little other than content knowledge coupled to appropriate software and computers. It should be the initial focus of development efforts for several reasons. First, our investment need not be particularly large for the development of the cognitive skills applications of this technology. Much of the appropriate software currently exists and is utilized in the video-gaming industry to structure and create complex inter-active environments where multiple elements combine to provide an ever changing and stimulating participatory environment. Second, the necessary knowledge capture process will facilitate a careful, but rigorous, review and assessment of the knowledge, skills, and competencies required for high performance surgery.

If surgical education is going to be approached from a performance perspective much work will need to be done to develop detailed task inventories and decision-making algorithms. Competency models can then be developed that can be integrated into both the simulated training environment and the traditional training environment.

To eventually arrive at a complete re-design of surgical education, both short and long-term goals need to be set. Foremost, opportunities to improve the current training/learning environment must be exploited. Cameras and other multimedia technology can be installed in ORs to improve visual access to the surgical field. OR team training programs can be implemented and scenario-based modules can be developed for surgeons to practice the cognitive skills required for MIS surgery. Lastly, the long-term development of new practice environments must begin in order to ensure the effective education of future generations of surgeon practitioners.

Acknowledgements. I would like to thank Dana Kolflat, who was most helpful in augmenting and providing feedback and criticism of many of the ideas presented here.

References

1. Rogers DA. Ethical and educational considerations in minimally invasive surgery training for practicing surgeons. Semin Laparosc Surg 2002; 9(4): 206–211
2. McCormick PH, Tanner WA, Keane FB, Tierney S. Minimally invasive techniques in common surgical procedures: implications for training. Ir J Med Sci 2003;172(1): 27–29
3. Gallagher AG, Smith CD, Bowers SP, Seymour NE, Pearson A, McNatt S, Hananel D, Satava RM. Psychomotor skills assessment in practicing surgeons experienced in performing advanced laparoscopic procedures. J Am Coll Surg 2003; 197(3): 479–488
4. Kneebone R. Simulation in surgical training: educational issues and practical implications. Med Educ 2003; 37(3): 267–277
5. Dincler S, Koller MT, Steurer J, Bachmann LM, Christen D, Buchmann P. Multidimensional analysis of learning curves in laparoscopic sigmoid resection: eight-year results. Dis Colon Rectum 2003; 46(10): 1371–1378;
6. Seymour NE, Gallagher AG, Roman SA, O'Brien MK, Bansal VK, Andersen DK, Satava RM. Virtual reality training improves operating room performance: results of a randomized, double-blinded study. Ann Surg. 2002 236(4): 458–463; discussion 463–464
7. Wilhelm DM, Ogan K, Roehrborn CG, Cadeddu JA, Pearle MS. Assessment of basic endoscopic performance using a virtual reality simulator. J Urol 2003; 170(2 Pt 1): 692

CAS as a Training Tool for MIS

B. Jaramaz

Introduction

Computer-assisted surgery (CAS) can be used in several ways as a training and performance assessment tool in orthopedic surgery, especially in less and minimally invasive applications. While the traditional teaching methods of training by observing experienced surgeons, and by practicing on cadavers are not likely to be replaced in the near future, CAS brings some valuable complementary models to the learning process. It also makes simulation, training and teaching, a continuous process that extends into daily surgical practice, and works as its integral part. With the intense development and growing popularity of less and minimally invasive surgical (MIS) procedures, the role of CAS in surgical training is becoming even more essential. As surgical exposures are becoming less open, it becomes more difficult to teach a surgical procedure solely in a traditional way. There are several levels at which CAS can help in the training for MIS, specifically: to improve planning, to teach the basic surgical skills, to provide feedback on how well the conventional MIS procedure is conducted, or to validate one CAS procedure with a more descriptive or more accurate one. CAS can also provide additional visualization in the training phase; and can offer tools for accurate post-operative measurements in order to validate the process and "close the loop".

Improved Planning

Patient-specific planning and simulation can provide a new insight into the clinical problem at hand. At the basic level, it can provide 3D visualization of the diseased joint, and a virtual environment in which the surgical plan can be simulated, and the effects of the plan on the anatomy examined. For instance, it can enable selection and virtual placement of implant components, show in 3D how the components will interact with bone, and where the osteotomy cuts will be made. Additionally, the effects of the planned procedure can be calculated, and key variables like cup medialization, or leg-length change in THR can be displayed.

At the highest level, a virtual simulation of some aspects of the post-operative outcome, such as the ROM simulation after THR, can be performed. Even when this type of computer-aided planning is not performed on a routine basis, it still presents a valuable teaching tool and helps surgeons better visualize and understand the task at hand (◘ Fig. 38.1).

Teaching Basic Surgical Skills

More complex simulations, such as relating gait measurements to surgical planning, may be too difficult or impractical on a patient-specific basis, but may still be of great value for training. They could provide a virtual environment that will enable surgeons to relate the cause and effect in surgical planning and form a mental model that will help them in making better planning decisions in their routine surgeries. Such simulators are aimed at improving surgeons' technical skills and dexterity, and typically focus on acquiring certain motoric skills, or improving surgeon's reaction under adverse and unexpected circumstances. Surgical simulators have been developed for a variety of procedures: endovascular repair, sinus surgery, gynecologic surgery, orthopedic

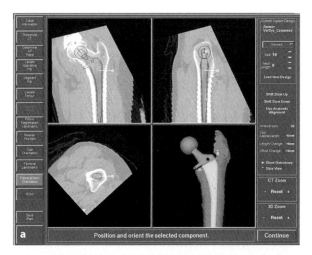

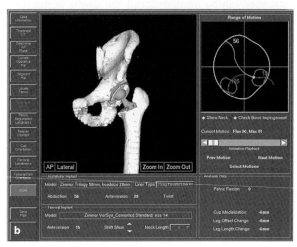

□ Fig. 38.1a,b. HipNav planning and simulation for total hip replacement. **a** Selection and placement of a modular femoral component (**b**) ROM simulation – the example shows the prosthetic impingement position in combined extension and external rotation [3]

the physical world and replicates the visual, mechanical, and behavioral aspects of the knee. Task-oriented programs monitor specific performance, such as executing a proper examination of the knee or shaving a torn meniscus. This includes moderating the haptic interface and simultaneously executing a collision-detection algorithm that prevents the instruments from moving through "solid" surfaces.

In training for actual procedures, simulators help to ease trainees' transition to actual patients, which seems inherently beneficial as a means to avoid adverse events. There is currently no evidence that simulation-based training leads to improved patient outcome. Proving this would require large cohorts of patients to be followed during and after care by clinicians in randomized trials, so the surgeon's performance on a simulator is used as a surrogate outcome instead [6]. It is likely that simulators will continue to be used and their role in training of medical personnel will grow.

There are, however, potential risks to simulation-based training. If the simulator cannot properly replicate the tasks or task environment, the clinicians might acquire inappropriate behaviors, or develop a false sense of security in their skills that could theoretically lead to harm. Although there are no data to suggest that this currently happens, such risks will have to be weighed and evaluated as simulators become more commonly used [6].

Providing Feedback on Conventional Procedure

Another mode of using CAS in the training of surgical skills is the use of surgical navigation to provide supplemental information to the surgeon about the performance of a conventional procedure. DiGioia et al. used the HipNav system for CT-based surgical navigation to understand how the pelvis moves on the operating table during surgery, and how accurate the cup alignment is with the conventional cup-insertion tool [3]. The results showed a wide variability of pelvis orientation throughout the surgery, and also pointed out a systematic error and a wide variability in cup alignment, when a conventional mechanical cup-alignment guide is used alone. When used in this fashion, the CAS system can also pinpoint the main sources of the inaccuracy and variability in conventional approaches. It can point to a systematic error introduced in the proce-

surgery, prostatic surgery, amniocentesis procedures, and oral surgery. Several training simulators have been developed for orthopedics, mostly with a focus on knee arthroscopy. Mabrey et al. [7] have developed a virtual-reality arthroscopic knee simulator that consists of a computer platform, a video display, and two force-feedback (haptic) interfaces that are linked to the instruments in the user's hands. The forces that the user would normally apply to the lower limb during arthroscopy are directed through an instrumented surrogate leg. The software provides the mathematical representation of

dure, typically by following incorrect assumption, and can also suggest a possible correction.

Noble at al. [8] described the use of navigation technology and pre-operative planning software to train surgeons in the workshop environment using cadavers. The surgeon sets the values of the parameters that define the technical outcome of the surgical procedure. During the surgical procedure on the cadaver, the surgeon receives no information regarding placement or orientation of the instruments and implants. These data are calculated after the procedure, and displayed in comparison with the original target values describing the intended position of the femoral prosthesis and the acetabular cup. This approach allows training in a non-clinical environment, and the procedure can be repeated until each technical step is mastered, with a quantitative assessment provided by the computer-based system. The authors state that at this point, it is unknown how successfully the lessons learned in the laboratory transfer over to the operating room, although experience with surgical navigation suggests that after relatively few cases, surgeons can identify systematic errors with their surgical technique and re-adjust their perception of correct component alignment and position.

Validate one CAS Procedure with a More Descriptive or more Accurate One

The concept described above can be extended to help train less expensive, but potentially less intuitive and accurate CAS procedures using the ones that are more accurate but also more expensive. For instance, an image-free navigation procedure could be performed in parallel with a CT-based procedure, to provide full visualization and strengthen the confidence in the system during the training phase. One example is the KneeNav hybrid system designed in our lab for clinical validation of the surgeon's ability to correctly identify the bone landmarks using the image-free navigation approach. The patient's CT scan is obtained and used for ground-truth definition of anatomic landmarks. Initial intraoperative steps follow the typical CT-based navigation protocol. Optical tracking is used for positional tracking of bones and tools of interest. The coordinates of points on the exposed bone surface are acquired using a tracked point probe. To map the CT-based landmarks to the surgical site, the surface-based registration is per-

formed during surgery by matching the cloud of bone surface points. After this registration step is completed, the position of bones in space is known at any time and related to the pre-operative model. The surgeon will verify the registration by placing the pointer on the bone surface. However, the landmark information from the planner will not be displayed, and the surgeon will proceed to define the landmarks according to the image-free procedure, selecting them either directly with the point probe, or the relative centers of rotation will be calculated from relative motions of the bones.

Additional Visualization in Training Phase

Providing three-dimensional models of the interaction between the anatomy and related implants and tools can help surgeons visualize their actions and complement the information obtained by direct vision. Supplemental displays, such as the ones showing the real-time updated 3D model on a monitor can help surgeon understand the link between global alignment of bones and tools and the local alignment observed through the incision or arthroscopic camera. Augmented reality displays that overlay the 3D virtual model correctly over the surgical site can further solidify the connection between the direct visual exposure and the supplemental information offered by the CAS system. Image overlay [1] shown in ◘ Fig. 38.2 is an example of such application. Image

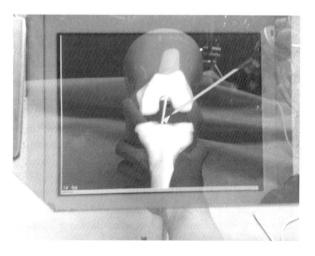

◘ **Fig. 38.2.** Image overlay. Images of 3D models of the femur and tibia are overlaid over their true position

Overlay is a computer-display technique which superimposes computer images over the user's direct view of the real world. The images are transformed in real-time so they appear to the user to be an integral part of the surrounding environment. By using image overlay with three-dimensional medical images such as CT reconstructions, a surgeon can visualize the data in vivo, exactly positioned within the patient's anatomy, and potentially enhance the surgeon's ability to perform a complex procedure.

The example shows models of the femur and tibia reflected in a semi-transparent mirror to appear overlaid over their true position inside the leg. Augmented reality displays like this will gain in importance with the increasing role of minimally invasive computer-assisted procedures and, if implemented correctly, could add a layer of safety and confidence to those procedures.

Closing the Loop

Relating the surgical variables to the outcome is crucial in improving the surgical process. In order for this concept to work, the ability to measure the surgical variables post-operatively should be at the same level of accuracy as the surgical navigation system used for precise planning and accurate placement of implants (typically in the order of 1 mm positional and 1 deg rotational accuracy). Traditional radiographic measurements, due to their 2D nature, perspective distortion, and unknown source position can produce measurements that are much less accurate. For example, the apparent version of the cup in AP radiographs after THR can be inaccurate 10–15 deg just because of the perspective projection of the cup. Furthermore, variations in patient's pose, such as pelvic flexion, between the functional and the X-ray position can be of such magnitude to obfuscate any meaningful interpretation of X-ray images. Yet, the using radiographs is the main method of post-operative evaluation, used in virtually every orthopedic practice. Although inherently two-dimensional, radiographic images are of very high resolution compared to other medical imaging modalities. Some computer-assisted tools have been developed recently to allow for highly accurate post-operative measurements from conventional X-rays (Fig. 38.3). In addition to patient-specif-

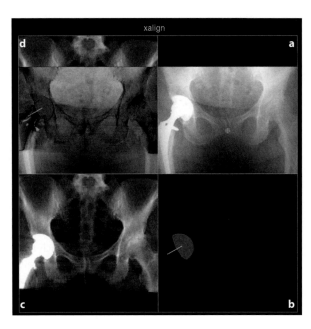

 Fig. 38.3a–d. Post-operative measurement of cup orientation using Xalign. **a** Post-operative X-ray, **b,c** virtual projection of the cup rendered from a 3D model (synthetic X-ray projection generated from CT, **d** images **a**, **b** and **c** overlaid

ic feedback, a new insight in anatomic variability and its effect on surgical referencing [5] and functional post-operative performance of implants [2, 4] is becoming available with these tools. Furthermore, by establishing a stable 3D reference system using a pre-operative CT scan, it is possible to detect gradual changes such as implant migration much earlier. Many surgeons consider the cost of a CT scan to be too high to justify its use in a routine primary TJR surgery. However, if used as a reference for post-operative evaluation, the CT scan could be re-used many times in combination with freshly acquired radiographs, and yield useful follow-up, data which in turn would have a great educational value.

All the outlined modes in which CAS can aid surgeons' training at different stages in their practice, are becoming significantly more important when considered in the context of minimally invasive surgery. The further integration between the MIS and CAS approaches will open new possibilities for more efficient training and directly and positively affect patients' outcomes in the future.

References

1. Blackwell M, Nikou C, DiGioia AM, Kanade T. An image overlay system for medical data visualization. Med Image Anal 2000; 4(1): 67–72

2. Dennis DA, Komistek RD, Mahfouz MR et al. Multicenter determination of in vivo kinematics after total knee arthroplasty. Clin Orthop 2003; 416: 37–57

3. DiGioia AM, Jaramaz B, Blackwell M et al. An image guided navigation system to intraoperatively measure acetabular implant alignment – The Otto Aufranc Award. Clin Orthop Rel Res 1998; 355: 8–22

4. Komistek RD, Dennis DA, Mahfouz M. In vivo fluoroscopic analysis of the normal human knee. Clin Orthop 2003; 410: 69–81

5. Jaramaz B, Levison TJ, DiGioia AM, Nikou C. Postoperative radiographic measurement of pelvic and implant orientation in the supine and standing positions. Abstracts from CAOS-International 2001. Comp Aided Surg 2001; 1: 62, 2001

6. Jha, AK, Duncan, BW, Bates DW. Simulator-based training and patient safety. In: Making Health Care Safer: A Critical Analysis of Patient Safety Practices. Evidence Report/Technology Assessment: Number 43. AHRQ Publication No. 01-E058, July 2001. Agency for Healthcare Research and Quality, Rockville, MD

7. Mabrey JD, Gillogly SD, Kasser JR et al. Virtual reality simulation of arthroscopy of the knee. Arthroscopy 2002; 18(6): E28

8. Noble PC, Sugano N, Johnston JD et al. Computer simulation: how can it help the surgeon optimize implant position? Clin Orthop 2003 (417): 242–252

Subject Index